Applied Nutrition

Fourth Edition

<u>Fourth Edition</u>

Applied Nutrition

(Late) *R.Rajalakshmi*
Former Professor, Biochemistry Department
M.S. University of Baroda, Baroda, India

<u>Revised by</u>:
K.K. Sakariah
Former Head,
Human Resource Development and Deputy Director
Central Food Technological Research Institute Mysore, India

Oxford & IBH Publishing Co. Pvt. Ltd.
New Delhi

Oxford & IBH Publishing Company Pvt. Ltd.
113-B Shahpur Jat, Asian Village Side
New Delhi 110 049, India
Fax: (011) 4151 7559
Email: oxford@oxford-ibh.in

Cover Illustration

Radiological status of children fed lime treated dhokla, a popular dish of Western India. Note the greater number of ossification centres in the hands of lime treated dhokla fed children on the right. (*Results of Baroda studies by the author's group*)

ISBN 978-81-204-1766-3

Printed at Chaman Enterprises, New Delhi

Foreword by *Uma M. Iyer*

The text book on Applied Nutrition was written by a professor who had exceptionally wide experience in clinical biochemistry and nutrition. The book has been aptly coined as applied nutrition as it bridges the knowledge gaps that exist between theory and practice. The book was very popular with students studying nutrition, dietetics and biochemistry in various colleges and universities of India. It was also used as a reference book in universities and research institutions abroad. Gujarat Government had translated it in Gujarati so that village workers could use it.

After the third edition publishers stopped printing it since the author fell sick and could not revise it. Now Dr. K.K. Sakariah, an excellent teacher, accomplished researcher and former Deputy Director of CFTRI, Mysore has revised it by including the recent updates and newer topics. IBH/Oxford is publishing it as its fourth edition

I am sure students studying nutrition and dietetics would use it as an additional reference text book and will be able to enrich the practical knowledge in the field of nutrition.

Prof Uma M. Iyer
Head,
Department of Foods and Nutrition
Faculty of Family and Community Sciences
The M S University of Baroda.

Foreword by *V. Prakash*

It is a great pleasure to write this Foreword for the book entitled "Applied Nutrition" by late Dr. Rajalakshmi, Former Professor of Biochemistry Department of the M.S. University of Baroda, Baroda and revised by Dr. K.K. Sakariah, Former Dy. Director of CFTRI, Mysore, India. This book has been devoted to Prof. C.V. Ramakrishnan as I understand and he was one of the great teachers and a leading Biochemist and the ambience of Baroda strongly has an aura of such a doyen in the area of Biochemistry and also in Applied Nutrition. There are several editions of this book but at the same time when I see the contents of book I feel it gives a very big canvas for the students and teachers to know the basics of nutrition.

I have gone through the book and I have seen the authors have divided the book into several Parts and under each part there are Chapters which deals with specific topics of nutrition.

I have separately treated each of the part in my Foreword and in the end I have tried to consolidate my generic comments keeping all these four parts of the book in view.

In Part I, the book addresses the various food fuels used by the body for the energy metabolism, water, minerals and vitamins, digestion, absorption and metabolism, formulation of dietary supplements and nutrition in relation to gene and I am even glad that nutrigenomic and epigenetic aspects are also addressed and covered. This is a very fundamental part of the Book and puts a firm basis for the flavour parts of the Book.

Part II looks at the use of food with a focus an specific raw materials such as cereals and millets; legumes oil seeds and nuts; fats and sugar; vegetables and fruits; foods of animal origin and miscellaneous foods and drinks. The additional Chapters in Part II also deals with the role of heat on the nutritive value and digestibility, a very important Chapter to look at. Chapter 17 in this part focuses on Food Safety indirectly through food microbiology and hygiene point of view even though a separate chapter on Food Safety and Standards is dedicated in Chapter 19 of this Part. These two forms a sandwich for Food preservation Chapter 18 in this Part and has been by design an important logistic.

Part III deals with diets such as meal planning, the need of nutrition at different ages, (the need of nutrition for the aged and geriatrics and perhaps what is relevant to India today), how does one modify diets for special diseases, the food for such problems as hypercholesterolemia, diabetic etc., This is a very important area of work that the Researchers have to focus for tomorrow and this Part addresses it adequately.

Part IV especially deals with community nutrition which is so important and is relevant to today's situation. This Part addresses in detail the diet and nutrition service, nutrition and human development improving nutritional status and community participation and more importantly how the food security is in relation to population growth.

Overall, the book has large appendices consisting of information on preservation of foods, composition of cooked food, diet survey proforma etc., The glossary and the index and the selected references and even the scientific names of foods stuffs and their Hindi versions add more weight to the scientific content of the book.

Even though there is a huge plethora of information in this very needed book on Applied Nutrition, but perhaps what is important for the students and for the teachers is being able to readily digest this book with at least the basics knowledge in Biochemistry. That will make the subject of nutrition easily digestible! This book should not be considered as to advise for an individual or a group or a group of people in a region what to eat or what not to eat but it is the scientific relevance of traditional foods , ethnic foods as well as the cultural aspect of food with a firm scientific understanding of the metabolism and catabolism that makes nutrition a very vibrant subject through this Book. It is this aspect the readers must realise. One easily realises this when one reads this book end is exposed to Applied Nutrition fundamentals. However, you can enjoy reading this Book if your level of knowledge of Biochemistry and Chemistry along with Physiology is sufficient to appreciate the treatments of each subject. I am sure the void in the literature, the void in the need for such a book of this quality for teachers and students, academia and researchers would be filled in by this Book.

I congratulate the Authors on this very important area of Applied Nutrition which today should be nurtured and I strongly feel this should be a part of a large number of Libraries both professional and personal ones and it surely can become a reference book as we move forward. But we need to remember in Applied Nutrition the bell can only ring when we wipe out malnutrition in the villages and remote areas and in urban slums by nutritional intervention not only through Government programmes but also through public awareness. I am sure this book will also fill in that void in the public domain for such needed agenda of social nutrition which is very critical.

I wish the Reader of this Book a wonderful journey in reading through.

Dated : 11 Feb. 2013

Padmashree Dr. V. Prakash
Distinguished Scientist of CSIR –INDIA
Director of Research, Innovation & Development
at JSS Institutions, Mysore, India
Former Director, CFTRI, Mysore, India
Former Coordinator, United Nations University, Mysore, India
President, International Society for Nutraceuticals and Nutritionals and Naturals
Council Member, International Union of Nutritional Sciences
Council Member, International Union of Food Science and Technology

Foreword by *K. Bhaskarachary*

Elevating levels of nutrition and the standards of living of the people of India requires a combination of key initiatives including agricultural development, strengthening of food systems, social and economic progress and nutrition, health and education programmes. This resource book will assist teachers in institutions to explain why these factors are important and how they are related to each other. This book APPLIED NUTRITION is divided into four parts and each part plays a vital role in nutrition. The need for a comprehensive source of resource materials based on Indian food systems has long been recognized. To address this need, Dr. K.K. Sakariah, Former Head, HRD, CFTRI has revised this text. The book is a rich source of practical information drawn from the scientific literature, nutrition databases and field experiences from India.

The important contribution of (late) Dr. R. Rajalakshmi, former Prof. Biochemistry Dept. M.S. University of Baroda, India, compiled the book with wealth of information, drawing from her years of teaching and research experience in India.

The introduction part gives brief description regarding the important aspects of nutrition while first part covers the importance of carbohydrates, fats, proteins used as fuels by the body and detailed mechanism of energy production in the cell. Even minerals, vitamins, digestion, absorption, metabolism, different formulation of dietary allowances, genes related to nutrition are well discussed. The second part covers use of food tables, different foods, and drinks, effects of cooking, nutritive value of foods, hygiene, food preservation, safety and standards. The third part mainly concentrates on diet and part four deals with community nutrition.

Thus this book addresses a wide range of topics with various chapters that offer original synthesis of knowledge, providing a fresh perspective in nutritional science. Thus the information on basic nutritional science, clinical nutrition and public health nutrition are each addressed very nicely which is very useful for advanced undergraduate students, dietitians, researchers, university teachers, policy makers and nutrition and health professionals. I am confident that this book will enable to create innovative training programmes which contribute to long-term improvements in the food and nutritional situation of India.

Dr. K. Bhaskarachary
Vice President, Indian Dietetic Association (IDA) and
Senior Research Officer
Food Chemistry Division
National Institute of Nutrition
Jamiaosmania
Hyderabad-500007AP, India

Preface to the Fourth Edition

I would like to start the preface of this book with the dictum that Science is only one and is all pervading. Judicious application of knowledge of the Science of Nutrition can be adapted to any given situation based on the available food resources, tradition, ethnicity and socioeconomic status of the people. Application of this principle will go a long way in alleviating nutritional problems of the country and improving the health status of the people at different stages of growth and development.

I found a reflection of this thought in me when I went through the book applied Nutrition originally written by Prof. R. Rajalakshmi in the year 1969 and subsequently revised twice the third and the last being in 1981.

There has been emergence of knowledge in the field of Nutritional Science and Food Science since its last edition. During the gap of more than three decades newer knowledge has emerged in Basic Sciences that have direct relevance and application to health and well being of mankind. Number of compounds other than the classical nutrients have been identified and the mechanisms by which they support health deserve a place in the revised edition of this book. Besides, the health attributes of ingredients that are commonly used in traditional and ethnic foods are better understood today in terms of their chemical nature and mechanism of action. Many of these components are traditionally consumed in India in the form of several recipes. The original book has given wide coverage of such recipes. The practical acumen and multidimensional approach of the author of this book is reflected through the length and breadth of the book and I felt the book needs to be revised without changing the original style but with more back up with the science content in the light of publications emerged after its last edition. When I proposed this idea to Prof.C.V.Ramakrishnan he kindly agreed and gave me permission to do so. I put on record my gratefulness to him for the support.

I am thankful to the publisers for their interest in bringing out the Fourth Edition of this book. I am thankful to Ms.Uma Devi for the secretarial service in the preparation of the manuscript of the revised edition.

January, 2013   K.K. Sakariah
                                                                                          Kottayam

Contents

Foreword by Uma M. Iyer   v
Foreword by V. Prakash   vii
Foreword by K. Bhaskarachary   xi
Preface to the Fourth Edition   xiii

PART I: Nutrition

1. Introduction   3
2. The Fuels used by the Body-Carbohydrate, Fat and Protein   7
    Fat as Fuel   10
    Protein as Fuel   11
    Carbohydrates   11
        Carbohydrates in foods   12
        Digestibility of carbohydrates   14
    Proteins   17
        Dynamic state of protein metabolism   18
        Nutritional classification of proteins   21
        Ideal essential amino acid pattern   21
    Protein Requirement   26
        Protein and amino acid requirement of   27
            infants and children
        Protein requirement during pregnancy   28
        Protein requirement during lactation   28
    Protein Gap in India   29
    Plant Sources the Ultimate Source of Proteins and Energy 30

		Fats	30
		Functions of Fat	30
		Lipid Components	31
		Sources of Fat in the Diet	32
		Endogenous Synthesis of Fat	33
		Recommendations on Dietary Fats	34
		Fat Metabolism	34
3.	Energy Metabolism		36
	Energy value of foods		37
	Basal Metabolic Rate (BMR)		38
	Factors affecting BMR		40
		Age	41
		Sex	41
		Pregnancy	41
		Thyroid function	41
		Other conditions	41
	Energy requirements of individuals		42
	Measurement energy requirement for physical work		42
		Douglas Bag	42
		Max-Plank Respirometer	42
		Determination of energy requirement	44
4.	Water and Minerals		49
	Water		49
	Sodium		52
	Potassium		54
	Calcium and Phosphorus		54
		Calcium deficiency	58
	Phosphorus		62
	Magnesium		62
	Sulphur		62
	Trace elements		63
		Iron	63
		Copper	65
		Cobalt	67
		Iodine and Fluorine	67
		Selenium	71
		Other minerals	71
5.	Vitamins		72
	Fat Soluble Vitamins		75
		Vitamin A	75

Effects of vitamin A deficiency	79
Prevalence and prevention of vitamin A deficiency	82
Hypervitaminosis A	83
Vitamin D	83
Hypervitaminosis D	86
Resistant rickets	87
Vitamin K	87
Vitamin E	87
Amount in ordinary diets	88
Water soluble Vitamins	89
Thiamine (Vitamin B1)	89
Riboflavin (Vitamin B2)	92
Nicotinic acid	94
Sources of niacin	96
Vitamin B12	97
Functions of Vitamin B12	97
Folic acid	99
Pantothenic acid	100
Biotin	101
Vitamin C	102
Vitamin C and collagen synthesis	105
Vitamin C and intestinal absorption of iron	105
Vitamin C and cardiovascular system	105
Vitamin C and immune system	106
Vitamin C and steroid biosynthesis	106
Vitamin B6	107
6. **Digestion, Absorption and Metabolism**	109
Digestion in the buccal cavity	111
Digestion in the stomach (Gastric digestion)	112
Digestion in the intestine	113
Metabolic fate of nutrients in the body	119
Metabolic fate of carbohydrates	119
Non-fuel functions of carbohydrates in the body	122
Non-essential amino acids	122
Metabolic fate of dietary fat	122
Metabolic fate of protein	124
Vitamins and minerals	124
7. **Formulation of Dietary Allowances**	128
Assessment of nutritional status	129
Body measurements	129
Prevention and cure of deficiency symptoms	130

	Balance studies	131
	Biochemical status	134
	Other criteria	134
	The epidemiological approach	135
	Requirements and recommended amounts	135
8.	Nutrition in Relation to Genes— Nutrigenomics and Epigenetics	139
	Chemical nature of genes	139
	Human genome project	140
	Single Nucleotide Polymorphism (SNP)	141
	SNP as a risk factor	142
	Apolipoprotein E (ApoE)	142
	ApoE and atherosclerosis	143
	Epigenetics	143

PART II: Foods

9.	Use of Food Tables	149
10.	Cereals and Millets	154
	Rice	156
	Cooking of rice	157
	Old rice and new rice	158
	Other rice products	160
	Fortification of rice	160
	Wheat	161
	Wheat Milling	162
	Bajra, Jowar and Maize	163
	Bajra	163
	Jowar and Maize	164
	Ragi and Kodri	165
	Use of cereals in infant feeding	166
	Sprouting and roasting	166
	Parched grains	167
	Professional methods used for parching in India	167
	Paddy and rice	167
	Other products	168
	Role of millets in food security in India	169
	Use of fermented foods in infant feeding	169
	Idli	170

	Khaman	170
	Dosa	171
	Dhokla	171
11.	**Legumes, Oilseeds and Nuts**	173
	Dals	176
	Toxic materials in pulses	178
	Aspergillus flavus	180
	Soya bean	180
	Preparation of soya milk	182
	Preparation of Tofu	182
	Oil seeds	183
	Sesame seeds	185
	Poppy seeds	185
	Nuts and other seeds	185
	Fenugreek	185
	Processed foods based on legumes	186
12.	**Fats and Sugars**	188
	Fats	188
	Sugars	195
13.	**Vegetables and Fruits**	198
	Starchy vegetables	199
	Leafy vegetables	203
	The use of vegetables and fruits	205
	Soups	205
	Juices	206
	Vegetables	208
	Fruit salad	208
	Baked dishes	208
	Chutneys	208
14.	**Foods of Animal Origin**	211
	Milk	211
	Evaporated milk	215
	Condensed milk	215
	Toned milk	215
	Dry milk	215
	Pasteurization of milk	216
	Meat	217
	Eggs	219
	Fish	219

15. Miscellaneous Foods and Drinks   221
        Beverages   221
            Coffee   221
            Tea   224
            Cocoa   225
        Miscellaneous foods and drinks   226
            Aerated drinks   226
        Spices, condiments and herbs   227
        Phytonutrients in the diet   231
            1. Antioxidants   231
            2 Phytosterols   233
            3. Natural acids   233
            4. Non-digestible carbohydrates   233
            5. Enzymes   234
            6. Papaya and Jack fruit   234
            7. Bioactive compounds in spices and herbs   234

16. Effects of Cooking on the Digestibility and Nutritive   236
     Value of Foods
        Cooking under pressure   237
        Dry methods of cooking   238
        Leavening agent   239
        Frying   239
        Repeated use of oils for frying   241

17. Food Microbiology and Hygiene   244
        Microorganisms in fermented foods   245
            Curd   245
            Bread   245
        Commercial uses of microorganisms   246
        Intestinal microflora   247
        Pathogenic microorganisms and parasites   247
        Milk   248
        Catering institutions   249
        Care of utensils   249
        Drinking water   250
        Intestinal parasites   250
        Disposal of night soil   251
        Personal hygiene   252
        Microorganisms involved in food and water   252
            borne diseases

18. Food Preservation   255
         1. Rodents and pests   255
         2. Microbial   255
         Principles of Food Preservation   256
               Water activity   256
         3. Freezing preservation of foods   259
         4. Cold sterilization using hydrogen peroxide,   261
               ethylene oxide and ionizing radiation
         5. Chemical preservation of foods   261

19. Food Safety and Standards   265
         Addition of extraneous matter   266
         Mixing inferior quality materials with superior ones   266
         The use of prohibited dyes and preservatives   266
         Extraction of valuable ingredients   266
         Fats and oils   268
         Milk   268
         Spices   270
         Coffee, tea and cocoa   271
         Eggs   272
         Meat   272
         Vegetables   273
         Other foods   273
         Pesticides   273
         Radiation   274
         Food Safety and Standards Authority of India (FSSAI)   274

PART III: Diets

20. Meal-Planning   281
         Food exchange system   283
               Cereals   283
               Leaf greens   283
               Starchy roots and tubers   283
               Other vegetables   284
               Fruit   284
               Sugar   284
               Legumes   284
               Fat   284
               Milk and milk products   284
               Flesh foods   284

21. Nutritional Care of Particular Groups   289
       Infants   290
       Birth to three months   292
       Vitamin C   295
           3-6 months   297
           6–12 months   297
           1–5 years   299
       Adolescents   299
       Expectant and nursing mothers   302

22. Diseases Caused by Malnutrition   304
       Under nutrition and malnutrition in children   305
       Kwashiorkor   306
       Marasmus   307
       Disorders of the skeleton   308
       Rickets   309
       Osteomalacia   311
       Osteoporosis   311
       Undernutrition in adults   312
       Protein deficiency in adults   314
       Obesity   314
       English formula   315
       Metric formula   315
       BMI classification   315
       Deficiency of vitamin A   320
       Scurvy   321
       Ariboflavinosis   322
       Beriberi   322
       Pellagra   323
       Nutritional anaemia   323
       Lathyrism   325
       Goitre   325
       Fluorosis   326
       Diseases of the skin   327

23. Modification of the Normal Diet in Selected Conditions   328
       Diabetes mellitus   329
       Hypercholesterolemia   330
           Aim of therapy   332
           Modifications suggested   332

Diseases of the digestive system 333
    Inflammation of the intestine 333
    Diarrhea 334
    Constipation 335
    Ulcers of the stomach and duodenum 335
    Gastritis 337
    Disease of the liver 337
    Renal disease 339
    Other conditions associated with uraemia 342
    Gout 343
    Urinary calculi 343
    Gluten-free diet 344
    High protein diets 344

PART IV: Community Nutrition

24.   Diet and Nutrition Surveys 347
    The oral survey 347
    Weighment of foods 350
    Determination of dietary intake from cooked foods 351
    Food intake of particular groups 354
    Institution diets 355
    Anthropometric measurements 356
    General appearance and clinical symptoms 358
    Other criteria 358

25.   Nutrition and Human Development 361
    Physical stature 362
    Psychological status 365
    Mortality and longevity 366
    Nutrition and human development 366
    Malnutrition and productivity 367
    Malnutrition among the rich 368

26.   Improving Nutritional Status of Community 370
    Neonatal period 370
    Pre-school children 371
    School boys 373
    Other groups 374
    Nutrition education 374
    Food fads 378

27. Food Production in Relation to Population Growth 381
and Need
Agricultural production 381
Sources of nitrogen 385
Household food security 387
Dairy farming 389
Poultry-farming 392
Fisheries 394
Vegetables and fruits 394
Our immediate problem 395
Future prospects of agricultural production 395
Conclusion 396

APPENDICES

I. Preservation of Foods 399
II. Some Foods Suitable for Young Children and Others 407
III. Proforma for use in Diet Surveys 410
IV. A. Volume-Weight Equivalents of Selected Foodstuffs 410
B. Approximate Composition of Cooked Foods 420
V. Nutrition Education—Specimen Lessons 424

Selected Reference 435
Scientific Names of Foodstuffs with their Hindi Versions 438
Glossary 450
Index 467
About the Authors 479

Part I:
Nutrition

Chapter 1

Introduction

All living things need foods. Plants require soil nutrients, water, air and sunlight in order to thrive. Every farmer knows from experience what type of plants thrive on what kind of soil and under what conditions of cultivation. The development of agriculture as a science has enabled us to identify the specific nutrients needed by different plants and the proportions in which they are needed.

The health, physical appearance and performance of farm animals and pet animals reflect the quality and adequacy of the food they eat. The poorly nourished animal has a poor coat with loss of hair, dull lustreless eyes and poor appearance. A good dairy or poultry farmer has to know about the food needed for good health and productivity, if he wants to be successful.

Multicellular organisms are made of cells and extra-cellular fluids. All living cells contain water, proteins, nucleic acids, lipids and carbohydrates and minerals such as calcium, phosphorus, magnesium, iron and many others. Most of the cell constituents are synthesized from relatively simple substances like glucose and amino acids. Substances essential for cellular synthesis and various life processes are called nutrients. The nutrients required by different classes of organisms vary with their physiology and biosynthetic capacity. While plants and certain microorganisms can synthesize cellular constituents from few nutrients, higher animals require a greater number of nutrients to be supplied in the diet **(Table 1)**.

Every culture has its own dietary patterns based on the use of varied sources of foods such as cereals, legumes, vegetables, fruits, nuts, milk, meat, fish, poultry and eggs. In some cultures, the use of animal foods may be taboo whereas in other groups such as the Eskimos and hunting tribes the diet may consist predominantly meat and fish.

Table 1. Nutrient requirements of different classes of organisms.

Organism	Nutrients required	Major constituents synthesized
Plants algae, CO_2-fixing bacteria	CO_2, water, minerals, nitrogen Source	carbohydrates, fats, amino acids and proteins, vitamins
most microorganisms[1]	performed carbon source, Water, minerals, nitrogen Source	Fats, amino acids and proteins, vitamins, carbohydrates.
animals	carbohydrate, protein or amino acids, linoleic acid, water, minerals and vitamins	body protein (from dietary proteins, amino acids) fats, vitamin C (in most species), vitamin D, carbohydrates

[1] Some microorganisms also require particular amino acids or vitamins for growth and survival.

The basic food patterns followed by our ancestors have been largely adequate as evident from the very fact that man has survived for so many thousands of years. But, as a result of modern innovations resulting from technology and urbanization, food patterns have changed which in some cases was not desirable in terms of health. Some examples of such changes are the introduction of refined flour and sugar in the diet of the Eskimos, Red Indians and others, and the introduction of highly milled rice in this country. Milled rice is nutritionally inferior to hand pounded rice which is rich in B vitamins. Even in western society which has almost eliminated nutritional deficiency diseases, food patterns have changed for the worse in some respects. The western diet of today contains a far greater proportion of sugar and fats than was the case in the past resulting in faulty nutrition. While primitive man might have instinctively formed adequate dietary habits modern man is so far removed from nature that he has acquired artificial tastes for foods that are neither essential nor conducive for health and well-being. His instinct might have been a guide for the wise selection of foods in the past but we know that it is not always the case now. Otherwise, we will not have disorders caused by consumption of polished rice and refined flour and excessive consumption of fat, sugar and alcohol.

More than one per cent of the population in this country is blind primarily because of failure to choose the right kinds of vegetables which are readily available. A large number of children in regions of the country die before the age of five years because inadequate nutrition.

Majority of world's population live in countries where food supply is not plentiful. Most of the people in these countries either do not have enough to eat or do not have the right kind of food. Foods available for young children are particularly unsuitable. In the year 2010, 7.6 million children under five died, down from 8.1 million in 2009, 8.8 million in 2008 and 12.4

million in 1990. About half of child death occurs in Africa. Malnutrition is the cause of most childhood death in these countries. Poor nutrition results in poor resistance to infection and greater incidence of diseases such as tuberculosis.

Diseases caused by a faulty diet are very common among the poor. In some of the poor sections of the population there is prevalence of kwashiorkor and marasmus in children apart from night blindness, total blindness, beriberi and pellagra. Work performance is affected by poor nutrition and it has been also reported that poorly nourished people are more likely to get into accidents.

Recently, it has been suggested that severe malnutrition in early, childhood may interfere with normal psychological development. Thus a poorly nourished child may fail to benefit from schooling. This means that as an adult, he will not be able to benefit effectively from the latest advances that take place around him.

The emergence of nutrition as a science in its own right has enabled us to identify the nutrients needed for a sound state of health, the foods in which they are present, the approximate proportions in which they are needed and the consequences of a diet lacking in them. Our ancestors knew, for instance, that milk is good for health, but we know today that the nutritive value of milk is due to the protein, calcium and vitamins present in it. This knowledge enables us to supply these nutrients from other cheaper and more readily available foodstuffs if enough milk is not available. With the knowledge available to us it is possible to eliminate nutritional deficiency diseases which affect a large proportion of the world's population. This has already been done in western countries.

This book is divided into four parts for the sake of convenience. However, mention needs to be made that each part is not dealt with in isolation and there has been interfaces among the four parts. The objective of Part 1 is to cover the Science of Nutrition from the very elementary level in form and content that is understood by a heterogeneous group who might use this book. Recent findings and information as applicable are incorporated at appropriate places. The science part of the book is only one and it is all pervasive. Judicious application of the Science of Nutrition adapting to various socio-economic and geographical conditions, available food resources, culture, traditions and habits will go a long way in alleviating malnutrition and improving health status of the population of India. The book "Applied Nutrition originally authored by (late) Dr. R. Rajalakshmi and revised by Dr. K.K. Sakariah embodies this knowledge. It is hoped that the message embodied in this book will reach the remotest regions of the country which is vital in fulfilling the objective of writing this book.

Part 2 deals with the entire gamut of food resources that is available in India and the agricultural production status in various sectors. The quality aspects of these food raw materials and the various ethnic products prepared from them in relation to chemistry and nutrition are narrated from a Food Science perspective. Part 2 culminates from Part 1 and hence the reader may find interface and repetitions to a limited extent though. The author felt it appropriate to do so and the editor has retained the original style as it offers continuity of the subject matter to the readers.

Part 3 and Part 4 are application oriented chapters. The various nutritional deficiency diseases, their causes, aetiology and prevalence and the management of these diseases with the judicious use of locally available food raw materials in a form and combination that is normally accepted by people of various regions are dealt with. Part 3 deals with a highly discussed issue, that is, Food Safety and Standards and Processed Foods. This aspect has been covered along with practical aspects of food microbiology and hygiene. Attempts have been made to highlight this topic to the attention of practicing nutritionists and housewives. Part 4 deals with methodologies and strategies that can be adopted to take the science of nutrition at grass root level and this part is applied in nature. Several practical hints, useful data, methodologies and ready reckoners are given at the end in the form of appendices.

During the revision of this book the editor has taken special care to include newer knowledge emerged after its last edition. The concept of phytonutrients and nutraceuticals was introduced at appropriate places. The editor thought it is appropriate add one chapter on nutrition in relation to genes. Nutrigenomics and epigenetics are newly acquired dimensions of Nutritional Sciences and students of advanced nutrition will benefit from this section.

This book is an attempt to communicate, to the layman as well as to students of nutrition, the nutrients needed by man, the amounts in which they are needed, and the sort of diet which can provide good nutrition and improve the health and well-being of people by correcting the common deficiencies in their diet. Special efforts have been made to formulate dietary patterns based on foods which are easily available and which are within the purchasing or productive capacity of the poor man in this country. As such the book differs from text books by western authors which do not always provide information appropriate for conditions prevailing in this country or in other developing countries. It is hoped that this book will be found useful by students of nutrition, public health workers, school teachers, extension workers, officials concerned with community development, municipal authorities, medical men and housewives, in other words, all those who have to apply a knowledge of nutrition for the welfare of those under their care.

Chapter 2

The Fuels used by the Body-Carbohydrate, Fat and Protein

Food is a prime necessity of life. The Bhagavad Gita recognises the basic dictum, "of food are beings made". Warm-blooded animals maintain a specific body temperature which is generally above the surrounding temperature and the lack of this characteristic constitutes one of the obvious differences between a living body, a dead body and non-living matter such as stone. This require a continuous supply of heat or energy, which is provided by the slow burning or oxidation of food. However, this must be regulated so that the resulting temperature is neither higher nor lower than the normal temperature of the body.

Machines require some source of energy in order to work. Mechanical energy is required in the case of machines operated manually, electrical energy in the case of flour mills and chemical energy in the case of machines using coal or diesel oil. In the ultimate analysis, the energy supplied is converted to kinetic energy needed for "work". The work we do also requires energy. The body is more efficient than the machines we generally use. Our teeth chew food more efficiently than grinders. The work done by the brain is accomplished at a very low cost of fuel as compared to electronic computers. The brain is like a very compact portable computer weighing only 1.5 kilograms. The brain function is carried out by highly specialized cells called neuronal cells. The brain function is an electrophysiological process and it requires energy.

The work of the heart in continuously pumping blood can well be imagined. The mechanical energy required for muscular work must also come from the oxidation of FOODS in the body. The oxidation of carbon compounds in our body differs from that of carbon in a furnace. The coal in a furnace burns in one step producing large amount energy instantaneously whereas the carbon compounds in the body are burned step by step in a controlled manner in such a way as to make available the energy in the right amount at the right time. In both cases carbon dioxide and water are formed as end products. The process of release of energy contained in fuels of the body namely carbohydrates, fats and proteins taking place in a living cell is called metabolism. In the living cell the energy released in the metabolism is used to synthesize a molecule called Adenosine Triphophate (ATP). The terminal phosphate bond of ATP is energy rich and this bond is formed using the energy released during the metabolism of carbohydrates fats and proteins. ATP is the readily transactable energy coinage that can be used in all energy requiring processes in the living cells.

Oxidation is a process where energy is released and reduction is a process where energy is absorbed. In photosynthesis atmospheric carbon dioxide is reduced by hydrogen of water absorbing solar energy. This is the first step in the trapping of solar energy in biological systems which take place in the plant kingdom where chlorophyll is present. Photosynthesis is a series of reduction reactions with starch the major carbohydrate in plants as the end product. The starch is a polysaccharide made up of repeating units of the monosaccharide, glucose which is accepted as a fuel in most of the living cell, be it plants, animals or microorganisms. Glucose is a highly reduced form of a substance and the chemical energy contained in it can be used as a fuel in all energy requiring biological processes. The carbon skeleton of glucose can be converted to other fuels like fats and protein in the living cells and this process energy contained in glucose is transferred to these fuels and the energy content of these fuels varies with level of reduced state of the fuels concerned. Thus fat has more energy content than carbohydrates.

Man and animals consumes carbohydrate, fat and protein in the form of food and they oxidize these fuels and derive the chemical energy contained in them and in this process the energy released is transferred to ATP. Therefore, we can trace the source of chemical energy contained in ATP molecule to solar energy.

There are some common features in the step by step process by which the energy contained in the three fuels namely carbohydrate, fat and protein is harnessed in the form of ATP. Basically they are all oxidative processes. In biology, oxidation can be either addition of oxygen or removal of hydrogen. Essentially, in photosynthesis solar energy is harnessed in the form of starch by a reductive process in which there is addition of hydrogen. And the reverse process happens when carbohydrate is utilized in the body for releasing the energy.

If we consider the step by step process of oxidation of glucose in the body we will be covering the major features of fat and protein oxidation as well. In the initial reactions of glucose metabolism, one molecule of glucose which is a 6 carbon compounds is broken down to two molecules of 3 carbon compound namely pyruvic acid. This step by step process involves removal of hydrogen from glucose and this series of enzyme catalyzed reactions is known as glycolysis. This is the anaerobic phase of glucose metabolism which does not involve oxygen. The further metabolism of pyruvate is different in different living systems including the various tissues of man. We will now consider the further metabolism of pyruvic acid completely to carbon dioxide and water. The aerobic phase of carbohydrate metabolism starts with the conversion of pyruvic acid to acetyl coenzyme A (acetyl CoA) which is a 2 carbon compound the third carbon being liberated as carbon dioxide. A few molecules of pyruvic acid undergo carbon dioxide fixation to form a 4 carbon organic acid namely oxaloacetic acid. The further metabolism of pyruvic acid completely to carbon dioxide and water is brought about by a cyclic series of reactions known as Krebs Cycle named after Hans A Krebs who has elucidated this series of reactions. The first reaction in this series of reaction is the condensation between acetyl CoA and Oxaloacetic acid to form citric acid which is a 6 carbon compound. Citric acid undergoes a series of dehydrogenation reactions in the Krebs Cycle whereby hydrogen atoms are removed from intermediate compounds. Some of the reaction of Krebs Cycle involves liberation of carbon dioxide by decarboxylation. Dehydrogenation steps are catalyzed by enzymes known as dehydrogenases.

At the end of the Krebs Cycle oxaloacetic acid is regenerated. The net result of the Krebs Cycle is the oxidation of a molecule of acetyl CoA to carbon dioxide and water. Oxaloacetic acid regenerated condenses with a second molecule of acetyl CoA to form citric acid and the Krebs Cycle is continued for a second time and the process is continued for the further metabolism of pyruvic acid formed from glucose completely to carbon dioxide and water.

The complete oxidation of glucose involves glycolysis followed by Krebs Cycle. All the six carbon atoms are converted to carbon dioxide and all the hydrogen atoms are converted to water by this process. Complete oxidation of one molecule of glucose in this manner release the energy contained in it which is sufficient to synthesize 38 molecules of ATP. An outline of this process is given in **Fig 1**. The aspect of energy transduction as to how the chemical energy in glucose is converted to chemical energy in ATP when fuels in the living cells are oxidized has been dealt with in more detail in chapter 6.

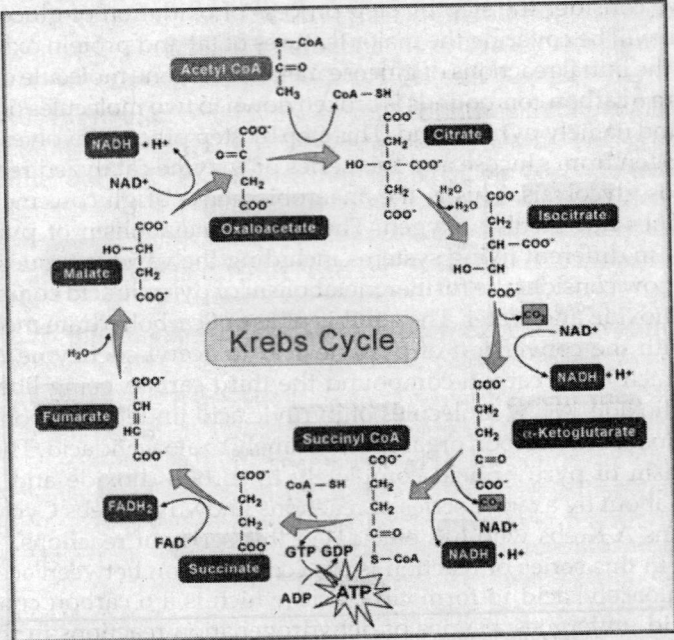

Figure 1. Schematic outline of oxidation of glucose.

Fat as Fuel

As mentioned, the process of fuel oxidation in the body described above is common for carbohydrate, fat and protein. In the case of fats, the fatty acid part undergoes a process called beta oxidation which is the initial phase of fat oxidation. As an analogy to glycolysis in the case of glucose oxidation, the fatty acid undergo a series of breakdown reactions whereby 2 carbon moieties of fatty acids are removed from the beta position to produce acetyl CoA. At the end of one cycle of beta oxidation a molecule of acetyl CoA and fatty acid shorter by 2 carbon atoms are produced. For instance, in the beta oxidation of palmitic acid which is a C16 fatty acid, at the end of one cycle of beta oxidation one molecule of acetyl CoA and a C14 fatty acid is produced. At the end of 7 cycles of beta oxidation the entire palmitic acid molecule is converted to 8 molecules of acetyl CoA. As in the case of glycolysis, hydrogen atoms are removed from fatty acid intermediates during beta oxidation. The complete oxidation of a molecule of fatty acid palmitic acid by beta oxidation followed by Krebs Cycle yield energy sufficient to synthesize 129 molecules of ATP. This is a higher energy yield when compared to the energy yield of 38 molecules of ATP when 1 molecule of glucose is oxidized in the body. On a gram to gram basis the energy yield of fat is slightly more than double that of carbohydrate.

Protein as Fuel

The major function of proteins in the food is to supply the amino acid required for the synthesis of body proteins. However, part of the amino acids derived from the dietary proteins are also oxidized for energy purpose. This happens when there is an excessive intake of proteins. Proteins act as fuel when there is severe non-availability of stored carbohydrate and fat in the body. This happens in prolonged starvation when stored form of carbohydrate like glycogen in liver and fat stored in the adipose tissues are depleted. The body metabolism then turns on to the breakdown of tissue proteins to amino acids. The amino acids are then channelled to direct oxidation and for the synthesis of glucose. The formation of glucose from amino acid is a requirement of the body for the maintenance of blood sugar level. It should be mentioned here that blood sugar is the major source of energy in vital organs like brain and inadequate supply of glucose by the blood will affect the brain function which will lead to serious complications.

The first step in the utilization of amino acids as fuel is the removal of amino group of amino acids by a process called deamination. Deamination of amino acids produces organic acids from amino acids and ammonia.

Many of the organic acid formed by deamination of amino acids are intermediates of carbohydrate metabolism. For instance, puruvic acid from alanine, oxaloacetic acid from aspartic acid, alpha ketoglutaric acid from glutamic acid and so on. The organic acids so formed from amino acid join the common pathways of carbohydrate metabolism whereby they are completely oxidized to carbon dioxide, water and ATP. The organic acids can also be converted to glucose by the reverse reactions of glucose breakdown. When proteins are oxidized for fuel purpose the nitrogen of amino acids is converted to ammonia which is eliminated from the body as urea. Part of the ATP formed on oxidation of amino acids is used for the synthesis of urea. If one takes into account of total energy produced and used up for urea synthesis it can be seen that on a gram to gram basis the number of ATP molecules formed is the same for carbohydrate and protein.

The body is composed of mainly water, protein, fat and carbohydrate and minerals mainly calcium, phosphorus, magnesium, sodium and potassium. Although carbohydrate is the major source of fuel the total amount of carbohydrate at any moment is limited and the carbohydrate required is either derived from food or formed from protein as needed. The approximate composition of the body is shown in **Table 2.**

Carbohydrates

Carbohydrates are compounds of carbon, hydrogen and oxygen conforming to the general formula $C_n H_{2n} O_n$ or $C_n H_{2n-2} O_{n-1}$. They are the most

Table 2. Composition of the adult human body[1]

	Approximate Amount	%
Total body weight	65 kg	100
Major constituents		
Water	41.0 kg	63
Protein	10.0 kg	16
Fat	9.0 kg	15
Carbohydrate	0.5 kg	0.7
Minerals	4.5 kg	7.0
Minerals		
Calcium	1200 g	1.7
Phosphorus	670 g	1.0
Potassium	245 g	0.35
Sodium	105 g	0.17
Magnesium	25 g	-
Zinc	1.2-2.3 g	-
Iron	3-4 g	-
Vitamins		
Vitamin C	5.0 g	-
Vitamin A	90–152 mg	-
Thiamine	25 mg	-
Vitamin B12	750–11900 µg	-
Total vitamin	6.0 g	-

The data given are based on the following sources:
1. Davidson, S., R. Passmore and J.F. Brock (1973*). Human Nutrition and Dietetics*, 5th Edition, the English Language Book Society and Churchill Livingston, Edinburgh.
2. Beaton, G.H.and McHenry, E.W.(1964). Nutrition, Vols.I and II. Academic Press N.Y
3. Moore, C.V (1964). Modern Nutrition in Health and Disease, Edited by Wohl, M.G. and Goodhart, R.S.3rd Edition, Lea and Febiger, Philadelphia.

widely available and economic source of energy. Although carbohydrate forms less than 1% of body weight, it is a major component of the diet and the staples used by man (Table 3). Ordinary diet based on cereals contains approximately 400g of carbohydrate as against 50g of protein and 40g of fat.

Carbohydrates in foods

Monosaccharides—Hexoses such as glucose, fructose, mannose, galactose, pentoses and deoxypentoses.

Table 3. Calorie, protein, fat and carbohydrate contents of selected foods*.

	Amount in 100 g of edible portion				% of total calories derived from		
	Calories (kcal)	Protein (g)	Fat (g)	Carbohy-drate (g)	Protein	Fat	carbohy-drate
Rice	345	6.8	0.5	78.2	6	1	91
Wheat	346	11.8	1.5	71.2	14	4	82
Maize	342	11.1	3.6	66.2	13	10	77
Bajra	361	11.6	5.0	67.5	13	12	75
Jowar	350	10.4	1.9	72.6	12	5	83
Kodri	310	8.3	1.4	65.9	11	4	85
Ragi	328	7.3	1.3	72.0	9	4	87
Bengalgram	372	20.8	5.6	59.8	23	13	64
Blackgram	347	24.0	1.4	59.6	28	4	68
Redgram	335	22.3	1.7	57.6	27	4	69
Greengram	334	24.0	1.3	56.7	29	3	68
Soyabean	432	43.2	19.5	20.9	40	40	20
Sesame	563	18.3	43.3	25.0	13	69	18
Groundnut	567	25.3	40.0	26.0	8	46	26
Milk: Human	65	1.1	3.4	7.4	7	47	46
Cow	67	3.2	4.1	4.4	19	56	25
Buffalo	117	4.3	8.8	5.0	11	68	31
mutton	194	18.5	13.3	neg**	38	62	neg**
Ckicken	109	25.9	0.6	neg**	95	5	neg**
Fish (pomfret, black)	111	20.3	2.6	1.1	73	21	6
Egg	173	13.3	13.3	Neg**	31	69	neg**
Leafy vegetables (a)	30–45	2.5	0.3-0.9	3–7	27–45	2–18	40–60
(b)	80–120	1.4	0.2	18–28	5–7	1-2	90–93
(c)	24	1.5	0.2	18–20	25	8	70–77
Fruits (d)	75–120	1.0	0.4	17–27	3–5	3–5	57–90
(e)	30–70	0.6-1.0	0.1	7–10	5–8	1–3	57–93

* In this and other tables giving food composition the values are mostly derived from:
(1) Gopalan, C., B.V Ramasastri and S.C. Balasubramaniam. 1971. Nutritive value of Indian Foods, National Inst. Nutr., I.C.M.R. Hyderabad.
(2) Watt, B.K. and A.L. Merrill. 1963. Composition of Foods, Agriculture hand book No. 8, USDA, Washington, D.C.
  (a) based on commonly consumed vegetables such as fenugreek, amaranth, spinach, etc.
  (b) based on vegetables such as potatoes, elephant yams, sweet potatoes etc
  (c) based on vegetables such as brinjals , bitter gourd etc.
  (d) based on fruits such as banana, mangoes, chikku etc.
  (e) based on fruits such as melon, grapes, oranges, papaya etc.
**neg; negligible

Disaccharides—Sucrose made up of glucose and fructose (present in sugar Cane)

Maltose made up of glucose and glucose (present in malt)

Lactose made up of glucose and galactose (present in milk)

Oligosaccharides—Made up of few monosaccharide units (Beta glucan, Galactomannan,Inulin)

Dextrin—Made up of a number of monosaccharide units (Maltodextrins made up of glucose)

Starch—Made up of large number of glucose units by alpha 1,4 glycosidic linkage(amylose and amylo-pectin).

Cellulose—made up of large number of glucose units by beta 1,4 glycosidic linkage

Pectin—made up of sugar acids such as glucuronic acid and galacturonic acid.

Distribution of carbohydrates in foods

Plant foods show wide variation in their carbohydrate composition. The major carbohydrate in cereals, pulses and tubers is starch

Fruits contain primarily, glucose, fructose, sucrose and pectin. Oligosaccharides are present in agave and elephant yam. Fructose is the major sugar in honey.

Fibre in foods

Cellulose, oligosaccharides and pectin constitutes the fibre part of the food. Cellulose is the insoluble fibre and pectin and oligosaccharides are soluble fibre.

Digestibility of carbohydrates

Among the polysaccharides starch (amylose and amylopectin) can be digested by hydrolysis by the digestive enzyme amylase present in the intestine because the monosaccharides are linked together by alpha 1,4 glycosidic linkages. Cellulose is not digested by amylase because the beta 1,4 glycosidic linkage of cellulose is resistant to amylase. Soluble fibre is also not digested by amylase.

Carbohydrate an essential part of diet

Although carbohydrate is the major fuel source of the body, the carbohydrate stores of the body are limited as can be seen from Table 2.

Can we live without dietary carbohydrate? Although protein and glycerol part of fat can be converted to carbohydrate in the body, at least a small quantity of carbohydrate is necessary in the diet. However when fatty acids are the major fuel used in certain situations they are first converted to acetyl CoA as mentioned earlier. For the further metabolism of acetyl CoA is the Krebs Cycle, oxaloacetic acid is required. Oxaloacetic acid is formed from carbohydrate and hence in the absence of carbohydrate there will be a limitation of oxaloacetic acid leading to sluggish fatty acid oxidation. The accumulated acetyl CoA in converted to acetoacetic acid and beta hydroxy butyric acid rendering the pH of the blood acidic. This condition is known as metabolic acidosis.

The person falls into a state of coma during acidosis because of the resulting disturbances in body and brain function. This can be prevented by adding a small quantity of carbohydrate to the diet.

The Eskimo who thrives on a diet almost free from carbohydrates does not suffer from acidosis. It has been suggested that this is because the fats in the diet consumed by the Eskimos are derived from fish and whale and contain large quantities of linolenic acid and the oxidation of this fatty acid does not result in the excessive formation of ketone bodies. This may also be because of adaptation to diets low in carbohydrate for a long period. Such adaptation was shown by subjects who voluntarily took a meat and fat diet for several months. In the beginning their blood showed increased levels of ketone bodies but the same diminished gradually. It is doubtful, however, whether such adaptation can occur in young children who are more prone to ketosis.

Some individuals, particularly obese persons, are able to utilize fats without abnormal accumulation of keto acids. However, women who have more fat in the body than men are more prone to ketosis. It also occurs more readily in pregnancy. The muscles and other tissues can utilize fats as fuel but the brain cannot do so normally and must have a continuous supply of glucose which is maintained even when a dietary supply of carbohydrate is absent by converting the glycerol derived from fat and some of the amino acids derived from protein into the same. Glucose is also essential for the red cells in blood. In adult man, the brain accounts for 20–25% of resting metabolism as measured by oxygen consumption so that there is an obligatory requirement of 75–100 g of glucose.

The need of the brain for glucose does not, however, mean that we have to take glucose or 'glucose biscuits' as the carbohydrates in foods are readily converted to glucose.

When a man is fasting, his carbohydrate reserve is rapidly exhausted as the body contains a reserve of less than 500 g. He has thereafter to live mostly on fats stored in the adipose tissue and on the proteins derived from tissue breakdown. In human system there is a limitation of conversion of fat into glucose. Therefore, only the glucogenic amino acids are the only source of glucose formation in acute starvation. With prolonged starvation, the brain regains some of its ability to use fatty acids as fuel, an ability that is present in the new born infant.

Although only a small quantity of carbohydrate is required in the diet, most ordinary diets, except those of groups such as hunters or Eskimos living on animal foods, contain carbohydrate as a major component. It is wasteful to the body to use protein or fat as the major fuel source as they are not completely oxidized in the body. To use an analogy, varieties of coal which burn almost completely and do not leave behind much ash, or fuels such as kerosene which burn completely, are preferable to those which leave behind a large amount of residue.

Since both starch and sugar are carbohydrates the question arises whether there is any difference between the two. Although a gram of starch and a gram of sugar have nearly the same fuel value they may not always be the same from the nutritional standpoint. An animal given a diet composed mainly of starch (80%) and including adequate quantities of other nutrients will grow at a much more satisfactory rate than one given the above diet with sugar substituted for starch.

Animals fed sugar and starch are also found to differ in many other respects. Intestinal absorption of simple sugars like glucose and sucrose is fast and this will tend to raise the blood sugar level suddenly necessitating the release of more insulin by the pancreas. This increase in insulin in the circulating blood is necessary for the further metabolism of sugar so that the blood sugar level is maintained within the normal range. In the case of starch sugar is formed gradually by digestion in the gastrointestinal tract and the product of starch digestion namely glucose is absorbed gradually and hence the tendency of sudden spurt in blood glucose level does not happen. Carbohydrates of different structures vary in their capacity to cause spurt in blood glucose level upon their digestion and absorption. This capacity is known as glycemic index. Those which cause high spurt in blood glucose level are the ones with high glycemic index and the ones which cause low spurt in blood sugar level have low glycemic index.

A high sugar diet is found to increase blood cholesterol and one including complex starches found to lower it. Dental caries is found to occur more frequently in children consuming excessive amounts of sugar, particularly in the form of sweets between meals. Further, except in the case of people living on foods such as tapioca or sago, starch is seldom consumed as such but in the form of cereals, legumes, etc. These foodstuffs contain not only starch but other valuable nutrients including water soluble vitamins which are necessary for the metabolism of carbohydrate in the body. Refined sugar and fat on the other hand, are devoid of vitamins and minerals. It is not surprising that upper class people in this country consuming excessive amounts of refined sugar and fats often show symptoms of vitamin deficiency and anemia.

Although our diet includes vitamins some of them are synthesized in the intestine. The extent of synthesis depends to some extent on the source of carbohydrate in the diet and is more with certain starches.

It would appear from the foregoing that it may not be wise to substitute a large quantity of sugar for starch in our diets. But when they are combined in reasonable proportions, as they usually are, the nutritive value of a diet is not affected. The amount of carbohydrate we need in the diet depends on the amounts of protein and fat included and our energy requirements which will be dealt with elsewhere (Chapter 3).

In ordinary diets about 10% of total calories are supplied by proteins and 20–25% by fat and the remaining 65–70% in the form of carbohydrate.

Proteins

The presence of sugar, starch and fat in foods was recognized and techniques for their extraction from various foods known from very early times. Subsequently it was found that many foods contain nitrogenous matter which is different from starch and fat and which yields ammonia when subjected to destructive distillation. Such a compound (gluten) was found in wheat after all the starch was washed off. These substances were found to be similar to nitrogenous substances of animal origin such as casein, egg albumin and collagen. As they are the primary substances in the 'cell barring water, they came to be called proteins (i.e. prime substances).

Proteins are compounds of carbon, hydrogen, nitrogen, oxygen and usually sulphur. Barring water, they are the chief substances in the cell and form about 45% of the dry matter of the body. They form an important constituent of muscle and other tissues and vital fluids such as blood. They form a major building material of the body and make good the wear and tear of tissues which is a constant feature of the process of life.

The protein content of some common foods is shown in **Table 3**. It can be seen from the same that foods such as mutton, fish, chicken, egg, dals etc. contain more protein than cereals. Roots and tubers contain even less. However, the percentage of protein is not always a reliable guide in the case of foods such as milk or leafy vegetables. Both these foods contain a lot of moisture, but in terms of dry matter, they are quite rich in protein. That is why the percentage of calories provided by protein is a better index.

Proteins are made up of various combinations of amino acids. There are about 18–20 amino acids commonly found in proteins. These amino acids are combined in various ways and proportions so as to form a practically unlimited number of proteins just as any number of ragas can be formed from a few basic notes.

Plants can synthesize all the amino acids needed for protein synthesis from nitrogenous compounds and carbohydrates. The animal body can synthesize only some of these amino acids and the rest have to be provided in the diet. The former are called 'non-essential' meaning that the body can do without them in the diet and the latter 'essential' meaning that they have to be provided in the diet. However, both essential and non-essential amino acids are necessary for protein synthesis and the many metabolic reactions carried but by the body. Both are found in most proteins. The essential amino acids are isoleucine, leucine, lysine, methionine, phenylalanine, tryptophan, threonine and valine. Arginine and histidine are not essential for the adult but essential for the young infant till the ability to synthesize them develops in the body.

Because non-essential amino acids can be synthesized in the body we should not conclude that their inclusion in the diet has no value. Some non-essential amino acids can be synthesized only from other essential amino acids. This means that, if they are not supplied in the diet, some of the essential amino acids will have to be used for their synthesis. For instance, cystine can be synthesized from methionine and tyrosine from phenylalanine, but more of methionine and phenylalanine will have to be consumed to make these conversions possible. Thus although non-essential amino acids can by synthesized in the body, they have a sparing action on essential amino acids. In the absence of non-essential amino acids, the amount of essential amino acids supplied may have to be doubled or trebled.

The proteins we eat are not assimilated as such but broken down into amino acids during the process of digestion. This was first recognized from studies on animals which were given perforated metal capsules containing meat. The meat in the capsule was found to disintegrate progressively by the action of the digestive juices, till finally, almost all the material had seeped out in a few hours. The amino acids liberated after digestion enter the blood stream from the intestine and the blood carries them to the liver and to different parts of the body where they are used for protein synthesis. Amino acids are also oxidized for energy purpose. When amino acids are oxidized ammonia is formed which is converted to urea and excreted in the urine

Dynamic state of protein metabolism

That the body proteins are being continuously broken down (catabolism) and resynthesized (anabolism) was established by Shemin and Rittenberg as early as 1946. This phenomenon is known as Dynamic State of protein metabolism .There is a certain concentration of free amino acids in every cell and this constitute what is known as the free amino acid pool. There are various ways by which amino acids contribute to the pool and ways by which amino acids are drained off from the pool. The Dynamic State of protein metabolism is depicted in **Fig. 2**. The degradation of tissue proteins to amino acids, amino acids derived from dietary proteins and de novo synthesis of amino acids constitute the ways by which amino acids are added to the pool. Synthesis of tissue proteins, oxidation of amino acids for energy and pathways of nitrogen excretion constitute ways by which amino acids are drained off from the pool. The rate at which these various ways operate depends on several factors such as (a) dietary intake (b) metabolic state of the individual and (c) stage of growth.

At the growing stage the rate of anabolism is more than catabolism. This is governed by the homeostatic mechanism built in nature as the growth requires more of tissue formation. In growing children the dietary proteins and the amino acids formed are retained as tissue protein and hence the nitrogen excretion in the urine is less than nitrogen intake in the form of dietary protein. A normally growing child is in a positive nitrogen balance. After the growing stage as in an adult the rates of anabolism and catabolism are the same and hence nitrogen intake and nitrogen excretion are the same. Such a state is called nitrogen equilibrium. A third situation is when there is more of tissue protein break down due to muscle wastage. This occurs in old age, certain pathological conditions and prolonged starvation. In this case nitrogen excretion exceeds nitrogen intake through diet and this state is known as negative nitrogen balance. During prolonged starvation there is a tendency for the blood sugar to go down the normal level. This metabolic state demands the synthesis of glucose from other substances mainly some of the amino acids known as glycogenic amino acids. The synthesis of glucose from amino acids is known as gluconeogenesis. The

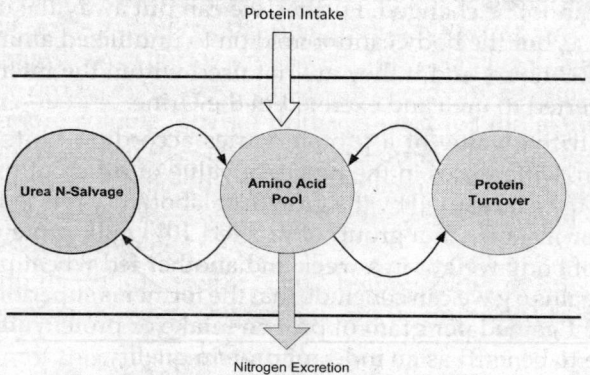

Figure 2. Dynamic State of Protein Metabolism.

glucose synthesized in this manner is used to keep the glucose level in the blood at normal range. Gluconeogenesis occurs mainly in liver and to some extent in the kidneys.

As will be discussed later, for the synthesis of proteins in the body all the essential amino acids should be there in the right proportion. When the dietary proteins are deficient in one or more essential amino acids there is insufficient utilization of amino acids for the biosynthesis of proteins in the body. The amino acids that are not utilized for synthesis of proteins are oxidized and the end products like urea is excreted in the urine. Therefore, negative nitrogen balance occurs in individuals who consume diets containing proteins that are incomplete with respect to one or more essential amino acids.

The amino acid composition of different proteins varies considerably depending on the structure and function of the tissue in which they are present. For instance, even a grain of rice or wheat contains four different kinds of proteins. The proteins in different tissues are also very different. Gelatin, a protein present in the bone contains no sulphur whereas keratin, a protein present in hair contains more sulphur amino acids than other proteins.

For the synthesis of different proteins, the body needs the amino acids of which they are composed and needs them in the right proportions. To give an example, if we knit a sweater with a particular pattern in red, white and black, needing the three colours of wool in the proportions 4:2:1, unless we, get the three colours in these proportions, we cannot use all the wool. Suppose we get them in the proportions, 1:1:1 we shall be able to use them only in the proportion 1:1/2:1/4 and 1 1/4 out of three or 42% of the wool will be unutilized. In the case of knitting, we can unwind the whole thing and change the pattern according to the proportions in which the three colours are available, but the pattern of body proteins is fixed by the genes and cannot be changed. Further, we can put away the unused wool for future use, but the body cannot hold on to unutilized amino acids fore more than 2-3 hours and if they are not used within the interval they are partly converted to urea and excreted in the Urine.

The nutritive value of a protein varies according to its amino acid composition. Differences in the nutritive value of different proteins were first sought to be measured by the growth of laboratory rats fed on different proteins. For instance, if a group of rats fed 10% milk protein in the diet gains 12 g of body weight in a week and another fed wheat protein at the same level gains 6 g we can conclude that the former is superior to the latter. Later, weight gained per gram of protein intake or protein efficiency ratio (PER) came to be used as an index of protein quality.

Nutritional classification of proteins

Nutritionally proteins are classified into three types namely complete proteins, partially complete proteins and incomplete proteins. Complete proteins contain all the essential amino acids in the right proportion. Partially complete proteins are deficient in one or more of essential amino acids. The deficient amino acids are called limiting amino acids. One or more essential amino acids are absent in incomplete proteins. Gelatin is an incomplete protein because the essential amino acid tryptophan is absent in this protein.

Protein Efficiency Ratio (PER) has been used for a long time to measure the quality of proteins. In this method a group of statistically matched weaned albino rats are fed on a standard diet containing the test protein at 10% level for a given period. The growth of the rats during the period is determined by the difference in body weight before the start of the experiment and after the experiment. Protein intake is calculated from the food consumed during the period. The ratio of weight gain and protein intake is calculated and expressed as PER. It has now been realized that animal models do not give the real picture of protein quality in the case of human subjects. Secondly, PER does not take into account the digestibility factor of proteins in foods.

Protein Digestibility-Corrected Amino Acid Score (PDCAAS) has been adopted by FAO/WHO as the preferred method of protein quality in human nutrition. The method is based on comparison of concentration of the first limiting essential amino acid in the test protein with the concentration of that amino acid in a reference (scoring) pattern. The scoring pattern is derived from essential amino acid requirement of a pre-school child. The chemical score obtained in this way is corrected for the fecal nitrogen loss of the test protein. The essential amino acid content and the PDCAAS values of proteins from commonly used foods is given in **table 4.**

Using such criteria the nutritive values of the proteins of egg, milk, wheat and corn were found to be in descending order. Subsequent studies showed that, the nutritive value of proteins such as those of corn and wheat can be improved by the addition of limiting amino acids or by the addition of other foods containing a surplus of the limiting amino acids in which the former are deficient. We can now use amino acid tables and make a reasonable guess about proteins which can be combined to form a mixture of good protein quality.

Ideal essential amino acid pattern

Milk is the food provided by nature for the growth of the young and can, therefore, be expected to contain all the essential amino acids in the right

Table 4. FAO ideal pattern and composition of common foodstuffs with regard to essential amino acids and PDCAAS values of proteins *

	Nitrogen (g per 100 g)	g/g of nitrogen										PDCAAS
		lysine	methionine + cystine	tryptophan	threonine	leucine	isoleucine	phe. alanine + tyrosine	valine	arginine	histidine	
FAO reference pattern (1984)												
Infants (milk)		0.41	0.26	0.16	0.26	0.58	0.28	0.45	0.34		0.16	
Pre-school (2–5 yrs)		0.39	0.17	0.08	0.23	0.44	0.19	0.41	0.23		0.13	
School (10–12)		0.29	0.14	0.06	0.18	0.29	0.18	0.14	0.16		0.11	
Adults		0.10	0.11	0.03	0.06	0.12	0.08	0.12	0.08		0.10	
Milk												
Human	0.18(1.13)	0.42	0.21	0.11	0.29	0.52	0.33	0.28	0.28	0.24	0.16	1.00
Cow	0.51(3.20)	0.50	0.21	0.09	0.28	0.60	0.34	0.34	0.36	0.21	0.17	1.00
Buffalo	0.69(4.30)	0.49	0.26	0.09	0.30	0.64	0.33	0.28	0.38	0.20	0.13	1.00
Egg	2.13(13.0)	0.44	0.35	0.09	0.32	0.52	0.42	0.36	0.43	0.38	0.15	1.00
Wheat	1.89(11.90)	0.17	0.23	0.07	0.18	0.41	0.22	0.28	0.28	0.29	0.14	0.40
Rice:												
Parboiled	1.02(6.50)	0.22	0.32	0.07	0.29	0.56	0.31	0.35	0.46	0.50	0.19	0.56
Milled	1.09(6.8)	0.23	0.26	0.08	0.23	0.50	0.30	0.30	0.36	0.47	0.15	0.56
Maize**	1.78(10.50)	0.20	0.22	0.04	0.28	0.72	0.24	0.31	0.26	0.17	0.17	0.43
Jowar (Sorghum)	1.66(10.4)	0.15	0.19	0.04	0.21	0.88	0.27	0.31	0.31	0.19	0.13	0.33
Bajra	1.86(11.50)	0.19	0.26	0.11	0.24	0.75	0.26	0.30	0.35	0.33	0.15	

Ragi	1.17(7.40)	0.22	0.35	0.10	0.24	0.69	0.40	0.33	0.41	0.28	0.16	0.53
Kodri	1.33(08.0)	0.15	0.29	0.05	0.20	0.65	0.36	-	-	-	-	-
Bengal gram	2.74(17.0)	0.44	0.12	0.05	0.22	0.58	0.32	0.36	0.28	0.59	0.16	0.60
Red gram (tur dal)	3.57(22.3)	0.48	0.12	0.04	0.20	0.45	0.25	0.52	0.23	0.30	0.23	-
Cow Pea (lobia)	4.00(25.0)	0.43	0.14	0.07	0.23	0.44	0.24	0.32	0.28	0.40	0.20	0.57
Lentil (mazoor)	3.87(24.2)	0.45	0.11	0.07	0.25	0.45	0.27	0.33	0.31	0.54	0.17	0.52
Green Peas	3.60(22.5)	0.47	0.13	0.07	0.25	0.43	0.27	0.29	0.29	0.59	0.14	0.50
Green gram	3.84(24.0)	0.46	0.14	0.06	0.20	0.51	0.35	0.31	0.26	0.35	0.18	-
Soya bean	6.90(43.0)	0.40	0.18	0.08	0.24	0.48	0.32	0.31	0.30	0.45	0.16	0.94
Ground nut	4.10(25.0)	0.23	0.14	0.06	0.17	0.40	0.24	0.31	0.26	0.69	0.15	0.69
Fish	2.80(17.5)	0.56	0.26	0.07	0.24	0.47	0.36	0.25	0.38	0.35	0.22	1.00
Chicken	4.41(26.0)	0.49	0.26	0.09	0.31	0.34	0.36	0.25	0.32	0.35	0.16	1.00
Mutton	2.96(18.7)	0.51	0.27	0.07	0.29	0.48	0.31	0.25	0.31	0.43	0.17	1.00

* Some of the values for amino acid content are derived from Amino acid Content of Foods and Biological data on protein. FAO Report No. 24, 1970, Third print 1981.

** values are approximate as maize varieties have varying protein content. values of nitrogen are converted to protein and given in paranthesis.

proportions. The amino acid composition of human milk has, therefore, been used as a standard for evaluating the quality of different proteins. The proteins of whole egg and egg albumin have also been used as 'reference proteins' because they are completely utilized. Studies have been carried out on children and adults using diets providing synthetic amino acids and either no protein or minimal amounts of a protein such as casein or egg albumin. One amino acid at a time is omitted from the diet and then increased gradually till it is enough to restore adequate nitrogen retention. On the basis of such studies, the Food and Agriculture Organization (FAO) proposed an ideal pattern in 1957 for the proportions in which amino acids should be present in the diet. This pattern has been termed the FAO reference protein or pattern.

This pattern has now been revised by the FAO to take into account differences in the amino acid requirements of children and adults. The latter require protein mainly for the renewal of tissues whereas the former require it for the formation of new tissues as well so that their need for essential amino acids can be expected to be greater. The amino acid composition of proteins in a food can be compared with that of a standard protein or pattern and any deficiencies in the former recognized. These can be made up by combining them with foods which have an excess of these amino acids. Proteins which can be combined so that the protein value of the resulting mixture is greater than that of any of them alone are called 'complementary' proteins.

There are examples of complementary foods in terms of mutual supplementation of amino acids in Indian diets. Rice with sambhar and chapati with dal are familiar examples of cereal pulse combination. Other examples in Western diets are white cheese with whole wheat pasta, Spinach salad with sesame seed and yogurt with sesame and flax seeds.

The important point to be noted is that vegetarians should include proteins from various sources in their diet to meet the essential amino acid requirement.

The amino acid composition of certain foods is compared in Table 4 with that of standard protein and FAO reference pattern. It can be seen from the table that cereals, millets, ground nut and sesame are deficient in lysine but pulses, soya bean and animal food are rich in the same. Pulses in general are rich in lysine but deficient in methionine where as cereals in general are rich in methionine but deficient in lysine. Therefore, a combination of cereals and pulses makes good quality proteins. This point is important for people who live on vegetarian diet who depend on plant protein for their protein requirement. Even though individual foods may be lacking in a particular amino acid they can be combined with others which are rich in that amino acid.

The amino acid which is most deficient in a protein is called the first limiting amino acid. The one next in the degree of deficiency is called the second limiting amino acid and so on. For instance, lysine is the first limiting amino acid and threonine the second in most cereals. It is easy to see that increasing the amount of the second limiting amino acid without increasing that of the first limiting one will be of no value. Sometimes such addition is only found to decrease nutritive value.

The nutritive value of protein in foods may also be affected because of excess amino acids. An amino acid present in excess may interfere with the absorption of other amino acids by competing with them at the site of absorption. For instance, both jowar and maize have excess leucine which is found to interfere with the absorption of isoleucine and valine. The effects of excess leucine can be prevented by adding more isoleucine. Also excess amino acids which are not utilized for protein synthesis have to be converted to other suitable compounds mainly urea and excreted. It has generally been found in animal experiments that when a liberal amount of a single essential amino acid such as phenylalanine, leucine or isoleucine is added to a basal diet the nutritive value of the diet is decreased. The effects are more observable if the protein content of the basal diet is low. Such excesses are seldom found in natural diets but there may be an imbalance caused by the relative excess of one amino acid over another. The effects of an excess of one amino acid can be reversed by another amino acid. Some examples are threonine and tyrosine, methionine and glycine, histidine and methionine and leucine and isoleucine/valine. As mentioned earlier, protein is necessary for the building up of body tissues. This does not mean that no protein is required after growth is completed. Even in the adult, the body proteins are being broken down continuously and new proteins formed. Besides, protein is also necessary for the synthesis of enzymes, hormones and other body substances.

Some of the amino acids have synthetic functions in the sense that other biologically important compounds can be biosynthesized from these amino acids. The essential amino tryptophan is one such amino acid from which the vitamin nicotinic acid, the vasodilator serotonin and the non-essential amino acid tyrosine can be synthesized in the body. Phenylalanine is the precursor of dihydroxy phenylalanine (DOPA), and melanin pigments present in the skin.

Ordinary diets providing enough calories are likely to provide enough protein if the diets are composed of a variety of foodstuffs. But diets based predominantly on tapioca, sago and bananas are not adequate in protein. When children are fed diets based on these they develop a disease syndrome known as kwashiorkor. Diets based primarily on cereals have less protein value than those including pulses, leafy vegetables, milk, eggs, meat, fish and liver. This is particularly the case when grains such as maize and jowar are used as the staple.

Protein Requirement

The recommended Daily Allowance (RDA) of proteins for various sections of population has been calculated on the basis of protein requirement for maintenance of nitrogen balance. Since the protein in the tissues is continually broken down and products of protein metabolism lost in urine, feces and sweat as nitrogenous substances, enough protein must be available in the diet (a) to make good these losses referred to as endogenous losses (b) for growth—during growth, protein is needed for the formation of new tissue (c) development of fetus during pregnancy (d) milk production in the case of nursing mother and (e) to cover the unutilized dietary protein. We have also to allow for the fact that dietary proteins may not be completely utilized and utilization may vary from 50–70% depending on the composition of the diet.

Several studies suggest that the endogenous losses of protein are related to basal metabolism and that in order to replace these losses, we need about 10 g of protein for every 1000 Calories expended for basal metabolism. If incomplete digestion and absorption and additional losses through sweat, hair, nails etc. are taken into account, the figure could be higher. The requirement for growth can be calculated on the basis of the amount of weight (tissue) gain per day. In practice it is found that diets providing 8–10% Calories in the, form of protein are found to be quite adequate.

Habitual diets of different ethnic and geographical regions are important factors to be considered in arriving at RDA for proteins in applied nutrition. The essential amino acid content in habitual dietary protein and digestibility need are to be considered while determining the RDA of proteins. Egg protein has been used as reference protein to assess the quality of other proteins. It has been already brought out that cereals and legumes the two major proteins in India are lacking in two essential amino acids namely lysine and methionine. In spite of mutual supplementation their combination have a quality lower than that of egg protein.

The protein and essential amino acid requirement have been subjected to revisions by expert groups of FAO, WHO and UNU. The report of expert group of the Indian Council of Medical Research has come out with a comprehensive review of the recommendation made by the above international organization on the protein requirement adults. The figures arrived at are given in **Table 5.**

Mention needs to be made here that the total protein requirement of 0.66 g/kg body weight/day given in the table 5 has been computed on the

Table 5. Protein and Essential Amino Acid Requirements.
(FAO/WHO/UNU,1985, FAO/WHO/UNU 2007): Adults

Amino acids	FAO/WHO/UNU 2007		FAO/WHO/UNU 1985	
	mg/Kg/day	mg/g protein	mg/Kg/day	mg/g protein
Histidine	10	15	8–12	15
Isoleucine	20	30	10	15
Leucine	39	59	14	21
Lysine	30	45	12	18
Methionine	10	16	-	-
Cysteine	4	6	-	-
Methionine+Cysteine	15	22	13	20
Threonine	15	23	7	11
Phenylalanine+Tyrosine	25	38	14	21
Tryptophan	4	6	3.5	5.0
Valine	26	39	10	15
Total EAA	184	277	93.5	141
Total Protein*	0.66g/Kg/day		0.60g/Kg/day	
Safe level of protein	0.83g/Kg/day		0.75g/Kg/day	

* High quality protein like egg, milk etc.

basis of essential amino acid content of a high quality protein like egg protein the utilization of which is 100%. But in practical situation in a country like India, the average diet consists of cereals and legumes and the utilization of proteins in a diet of cereal-legume combination is 70–80% of that of egg protein. This factor is taken into consideration for deciding on a safe intake level of 0.83 g/kg body weight.

Nutritionist are also of the view that it is desirable to provide children diets containing 8–10% of total calories as protein calories, provided the proteins are derived from different sources such as cereals, pulses, leafy vegetables and milk and adequate in terms of total calories.

Protein and amino acid requirement of infants and children

The protein requirement for infants and children are computed on the basis of maintenance requirement and requirement for growth. It has been estimated that for maintenance the child requires 0.68 g of protein per kg body weight per day which is similar to adults. Data are now available for protein deposited in the body during growth at various ages for males and females. The protein requirement for children is based on a) maintenance of nitrogen balance and b) growth. There have been several studies of determination of nitrogen balance and protein deposition of tissues at various ages of a child's growth. Based on these data the protein requirement at various stages of growth of a child has been recommended. The recommended safe level of protein intake for a child of l month is 1.77 g/kg body weight/day. This requirement decreases to 1.14 g at the age of 1 year. There is further gradual decrease in protein requirement to 0.92 g/kg body weight/day till the age of 10 years. This pattern is same for boys and girls. After the age of 10 years boys and girls have different growth patterns but their protein deposition rates show only a small difference. There is a gradual decrease in protein requirement from 0.91 to 0.85 for boys from the age of 11 to 18 and from 0.90 to 0.80 for girls in similar age group.

Protein requirement during pregnancy

There is an additional requirement of protein during pregnancy for fetal growth and expansion of maternal tissue. There is an additional requirement of protein during pregnancy for fetal growth and expansion of maternal tissue. Requirement (additional) of a high quality protein for 10 Kg gestational weight gain are 1,7 and 23 g/day in 1st, 2nd and 3rd trimesters respectively.

Protein requirement during lactation

During lactation additional protein is required for the synthesis of milk proteins. The recommended additional safe requirement of proteins in the case of lactating women is 19 g during 1–6 months and 13 g during 6–12 months.

Because of the severe deficiency symptoms brought about by a lack of protein it used to be a practice to recommend extravagant amounts of animal protein in the diet. But we now know that this is an impossible goal. Animals subsist on plant foods whereas plants manufacture their own proteins. In order to get one kg of animal protein we have to feed the animal with about 5–10 kg of plant proteins. Similarly Production of animal proteins requires more water. Production of one pound of meat requires 25 times as much water as that of one pound of vegetables. It is, therefore, simpler and more economical to take plant proteins as such in suitable combinations as the production of animal protein to meet the needs of all the people in this world will require much more land and water than are available now.

The consumption of excessive amounts of animal protein is not necessarily beneficial. When we habitually take much more protein than is necessary, the amino acids derived from the excess protein are metabolized and the end products are excreted through the urine as the capacity of the body to store excess protein is limited. Thus a very high protein is not necessarily beneficial, and, according to some nutritionists, may, in fact impose an extra burden on the kidney. Scientists including Chittenden and his associates in U.S.A. showed many years ago that increasing the protein content of the diet beyond a certain desirable level does not have any beneficial effect. On the other hand, people who take large quantities of animal protein which are rich in methionine are found to have increased levels of cholesterol in blood.

Present day nutritionists are therefore concerned with making the quantity and quality of plant proteins adequate for human nutrition. Attempts have been made to utilize proteins from novel sources such as yeast, green leaves and algae, and to improve the quality of cereal-proteins by 'fortifying' them with lysine. However, such attempts now seem to be only of academic importance.

Protein Gap in India

The place of pulses and oilseeds in meeting the protein requirement and essential amino acid requirement in India have been discussed in the foregoing discussion. However, between per capita availability and production of pulses there has been a gap as can be seen below:

Year	Per capita availability
1958-59	27.3 kg/year
1989-90	16.0 kg/year
2006-07	12.7 kg/year
2007-08	13.9 kg/year

Production of pulses in India grew at less than 1.3% during the last 30 years while the population grew at 1.8% during this period. This disparity is the reason for the gap in the pulses requirement. This requirement has to be filled by import which is being done. The demand for pulses is projected to be over 40 million by the year 2020 by Government of India and FAO. This means an additional annual production of 25 million tons in the next 9 years. This calls for at least doubling the area of pulses cultivation or doubling the yield per hector. Both the options are not practical at present though attempts are being on developing newer varieties of the crops by the application of modern science. India will have to look at other vegetable sources to be able to bridge the gap. Soya bean which is known for high content of high quality protein is one of the alternatives suggested.

Plant Sources the Ultimate Source of Proteins and Energy

As mentioned in chapter 2, the ultimate source of energy for human physical activity and the energy required for protein synthesis is solar energy and it is the plants which have the photosynthetic machinery to harness the solar energy. Animals feed on the plants and grow and the flesh acquires part of the energy content in the form of animal protein. As the mammalian gene is akin to the human gene, protein of the flesh of the animal is akin to the body protein in terms of amino acid composition. However, it is well known that the efficiency of conversion of feed into flesh protein, that is meat, is rather low and hence in developing countries the accessibility of animal protein is rather low on account of economic factors as well as socio-religious factors. Therefore, it is expected that the future generation depending on agriculture crops that contain protein tailor made for human consumption by modification of plant genome by application of genetic engineering is a hope. Biocassava a new variety of cassava envisaged in the Bill Gates and Melinda project is one of the examples of international scientific cooperation towards filling the protein gap in developing countries of Africa and Asia. The safety of such crops is being studied by expert groups and the regulatory agencies of governments of countries are seized of this issue.

Fats

Fats are not, strictly speaking, essential, except as sources of essential fatty acids but they are very useful components of the diet. They enhance the taste, flavour and acceptability of the diet, give satiety value and are concentrated sources of calories. They form a convenient cooking medium for deep and shallow frying. They stay longer in the stomach and thereby inhibit gastric secretion and are useful in allaying the discomfort of hyperacidity. Some recent studies claim that they protect to some extent against the effects of undernutrition.

Functions of Fat

a) Provides insulation to the body tissues.

b) Source of energy. Each gram of fat when oxidized in the body gives 9 kcal.

c) Helps in the absorption of fat soluble vitamins such as vitamin A, D, E, K.

d) Acetyl CoA formed as an intermediate in the oxidation of fatty acids is the starting compound for the biosynthesis of biologically important compounds such as cholesterol, steroid hormones and prostaglandins.

Phospholipids and glycolipids formed from fatty acids are constituents of brain. Fatty acids are essential for the formation of cell membrane.

Fat is readily stored in the body as it does not have to be stored with a large amount of water as is the case with protein. This means that much less storage space is required for fat than for protein which is why even when proteins are available in excess they are converted to fat and stored in the adipose tissue. For instance, 10 kg of fat can be stored in less than 13 kg of adipose tissue but if the same amount of energy had to be stored in the form of protein, the corresponding weight of fat-free tissue would be about 112 kg.

The fat stored in the body can be readily mobilized for the production of energy, particularly when adequate amounts of the same are not available from food. As in the case of protein, there is a constant turnover of fat in the body.

Lipid Components

Dietary fat consists of mainly triglycerides which are esters of glycerol and fatty acids. Phospholipids, glycolipids, sterols such as cholesterol and other sterols are also constituents of fats and together they are called lipids. The fatty acid part of fats have various chain lengths. Based on the chain length fatty acids are classified into three types namely short chain (<10), medium chain (12 and 14) and long chain (16–24) fatty acids. Based on the number of double bonds in the fatty acids the fats are divided into three types namely, saturated fats, mono unsaturated fats and polyunsaturated fats (PUFA). The double bonds in the unsaturated fatty acids may have cis or trans configuration (trans fats). Nutritionally significant fats have double bonds in the cis configuration.

Nutritionally fatty acids are classified into 2 types, namely essential fatty acids and non-essential fatty acids. Essential fatty acids cannot be synthesized in the body and they have to be supplied by the food. The non-essential fatty acids can be synthesized in the body. The body tissues especially liver has the biosynthetic machinery to convert carbohydrates into fats.

PUFA, namely Linoleic acid (LA 18:2n-3) and alpha Linolenic acid (ALA 18:3n-3) are the essential amino acids. Both LA and ALA have 18 carbon atoms. The former has 2 double bonds and the latter has 3 double bonds. LA and ALA can be converted in the body by adding carbon atoms and more double bonds to produce Arachidonic acid (20:4n-6). Arachidonic acid has 20 carbon atoms and 4 double bonds starting at the 6th carbon atom from the omega end of the chain. The other two long chain polyunsaturated fatty acids are eicosapentenoic acid (EPA) and docosahexenoic acid (DHA). Both EPA and DHA are constituents of cell membrane structure.

Human milk is unique in the presence of DHA apart from other fatty acids. DHA has special role in the development of brain and retina in human development and hence the significance of breast feeding of babies.

The fatty acid composition of diet is one of the factors which control the cholesterol fractions in the blood namely Very Low Density Lipoprotein (VLDL), Low Density Lipoprotein (LDL) and High Density Lipoprotein (HDL). These cholesterol fractions are implicated in atherosclerosis and Coronary Heart Diseases. The ratio of the cholesterol fractions in the right proportion is now shown to be one of the factors that prevents plaque formation and constriction of blood vessels and more so the arteries that supply blood to the heart. It is now well known that fats rich in saturated fats such as hydrogenated fats and animal fat increase the risk of coronary heart disease when compared to unsaturated fats. Recent studies have shown that intake of LA, ALA, EPA and DHA lower the risk of heart disease.

Sources of Fat in the Diet

The fat content of foods varies from negligible amounts in fruits to more than 40% in nuts (Table 3). The sources of fat can be the fat that is intrinsically present in the food or the fat that is added during cooking as a cooking medium. Components of the foods such as cereals, legumes and millets contain varying amounts of fat and these fats are called invisible fat while the fat that is added during cooking is called visible fat. The invisible fat in the plant foods though a small quantity (1.5-3%) they are healthy fat in terms of fatty acid composition. The added fat present in the diet are from the various vegetable oils, hydrogenated fat and dairy fat.

The fat that is intrinsically present in animal foods such as meat fish and eggs are high when compared to the invisible fat in the plant foods. Cholesterol is present only in foods of animal origin. Cholesterol is absent in plant foods. However, cholesterol can be synthesized in the body from acetyl CoA formed as an intermediate the oxidation fatty acids. **Table 6** gives the fat and cholesterol content of selected foods. Animal fats are rich in saturated fat and vegetable fats are rich in unsaturated fats. Some of the commonly used vegetable oils rich in essential fatty acids linoleic acid are corn oil, soybean oil, sunflower oil, safflower oil, sesame oil, rice bran oil and cotton seed oil. Soybean oil is also rich in alpha linolenic acid.

Fish oil is also rich in linolenic acid.

Table 6. Fat and Cholesterol content in selected foods*.

Dairy Products	Portion	Cholesterol (mg)	Total Fat (g)	Saturated Fat (mg)
Whole milk	1 cup	33	8	5
Yogurt	1 cup	29	7	5
Cheddar cheese	1 oz	30	9	6
Fats				
Butter	1 tsp	11	4	3
Margarine	1 tsp	0	4	1
Vegetable oil	1 tsp	0	5	1-2
Egg	1	212	5	2
Salmon	3.5 oz	63	12	2
Lobster	3.5 oz	71	1	0
Tuna	3.5 oz	30	1	0
Beef	3.5 oz	80	15–40	10–20
Liver	3.5 oz	380	5	2
Chicken (no skin)	3.5 oz	85	5	1

* Cholesterol is present only in foods of animal origin.

Endogenous Synthesis of Fat

The dietary fats are digested into fatty acids and glycerol as described in chapter 6. Part of the dietary fat that is absorbed by the blood and transported to the body tissues are oxidized for energy purpose and the rest is stored in the adipose tissue as stored form of energy. Apart from dietary fat the body fat also has certain amount of fat synthesized in the body. Tissues such as adipose tissue of the body and liver have the biosynthetic capacity to convert carbohydrate into fat.

Because of high content of saturated fatty acids in coconut oil this oil was thought to be unhealthy. The controversy surrounding coconut oil is now disappearing and the oil is becoming popular in view of newer findings. The major fatty acid in coconut oil is medium chain fatty acid Lauric acid. Medium chain fatty acids are absorbed more efficiently than long chain fatty acids. Medium chain fatty acids are transported in the portal blood directly to the liver unlike long chain fatty acids which are incorporated into chylomicrones and transported through the lymph. Animal studies have shown that medium chain fatty acids are preferentially used for energy production as against long chain fatty acids and their deposition as body fat is much lesser. The sources of cholesterol in the blood are foods rich in cholesterol and endogenous synthesis. Cholesterol is synthesized in the liver from acetyl CoA formed from oxidation of fats and carbohydrates. Hypercholesterolemia can occur even in people who are perfect vegetarians who do not consume foods of animal though the prevalence of such cases are comparatively less. The rate limiting enzyme that controls the biosynthetic pathway of cholesterol synthesis in the body is Hydroxymethyl glutaryl CoA reductase (HMG CoA reductase) which converts HMGCoA to Mevalonic acid in the biosynthetic pathway of cholesterol. Most of the drugs used to reduce cholesterol level in the blood such as statins of various types inhibit this enzyme thereby reducing the cholesterol synthesis in the body.

Recommendations on Dietary Fats

The recommended daily requirement of fat is dependent on the total energy requirement of the individual which is based on the physical activities.

The recommended dietary allowance of fat is 15–30% of total energy requirement. The diets of the poor in India provide less than 10–15 g of fats and oils per day whereas upper class diets contain 40–60 g. Some tribal people such as the Bhils of Gujarat State hardly use any fat for cooking. About 20–50 g would appear to be a reasonable allowance.

As discussed, essential fatty acids are needed for the synthesis of cell membranes and for several other functions. In experimental animals, a deficiency of essential fatty acids causes loss of fur, loss of blood in the urine, necrosis of the tail and death. Generally, deficiency is not found in human beings. It is considered sufficient if the diet provides about 1% of total calories in the form of linoleic acid and this amount (2-3g) is supplied by most foodstuffs and ordinary diets. But children brought up on poor rice diets practically devoid of essential fatty acids may develop infantile eczema which is cured by the administration of essential fatty acids. However, infantile eczema may arise from other causes as well.

Fat Metabolism

Fatty acids are first converted to acetyl CoA which is a common metabolite of oxidation of fat and carbohydrate. The further metabolism of acetyl CoA requires oxaloacetic acid which is formed from carbohydrate. Therefore, when there is a severe restriction of carbohydrates in the diet oxaloacetate supply will be limiting factor in the further metabolism of acetyl CoA by the Krebs Cycle where the major amount of energy in the form of ATP is generated. Therefore, when there is a severe restriction of food as in starvation the stored fat in the body is the only source of energy and the mobilization of fat from the adipose tissue and the oxidation of fatty acid by different tissue will take place to meet the energy requirement. When there is an insufficient supply of oxaloacetate in starvation the further metabolism of acetyl CoA in the Krebs Cycle will be sluggish and the excess acetyl CoA that being formed from fatty acids will be channelled to other pathways. Two molecules of acetyl CoA combine to form acetoacetic acid and then to beta hydroxybutyric acid. The latter two compounds are called ketone bodies. Excessive amounts of these two compounds in the blood results in conditions of ketosis and acidosis. . However, adaptation to a diet practically devoid of carbohydrate has also been shown by adult male volunteers given meat diets which are rich in saturated fatty acids.

Fats are derived from wholesome foods such as nuts, oilseeds and milk which contain not only fat but also protein, minerals and vitamins. But generally we tend to separate the fats from these and take them as pure fats containing nothing besides, except for vitamins A and D in the case of butter and ghee. When excessive amounts of such pure fats or pure sugar are consumed, they reduce the intake of other wholesome foods and the diets are likely to become deficient in minerals and vitamins. Thus fats and sugars form sources of 'empty' calories i.e., they are foods which have fuel value but do not have the nutrients necessary for their metabolism. The same applies to alcohol an excessive consumption of which results in reduced intakes of other wholesome foods and the consequent nutritional deficiencies apart from the harmful effects of alcohol itself.

Chapter 3

Energy Metabolism

As pointed out earlier, the body requires energy for the maintenance of body temperature and for carrying out its normal functions. Whether we are at rest or at work, the internal organs of the body are constantly at work. For example, the lung has to suck in and press out air the heart to pump blood, the stomach to contract and expand so as to churn food and so on.

Heat is the chief end product of the foods we eat. The carbohydrate consumed is converted to glucose which is oxidized to carbon dioxide and water with the production of heat. Fatty acids are oxidized to give the same end products. A major part of the amino acids absorbed is used for tissue synthesis or repair. The remainders as well as the amino acids resulting from tissue breakdown are converted first to organic acids which may be either used for glucose and fat synthesis or oxidized to give carbon dioxide and water as end products. Hence whether we consume food in the form of proteins, carbohydrates or fats, we derive heat as a chief end product of their metabolism. The calorie value of the foods we eat can be determined by burning a sample in a bomb calorimeter, so called because the sample is ignited by a fuse wire as in a bomb. The bomb calorimeter is immersed in water at known temperature and the rise in the temperature of the water caused by the burning of food is used as a measure of the heat produced. The unit of heat used in nutrition is a large Calorie consisting of 1000 calories and defined as the amount of heat required for increasing the temperature of a kilogram of water from 15°C to 16°C. It is called a kilocalorie or a Calorie. It may be recalled that a calorie is the amount of heat required to increase similarly the temperature of one gram of water. Attempts are now being made to replace this unit by the Joule which is defined as the work done when the point of application of a force of one Newton is displaced through a distance of one meter in the direction of the force. This change is advocated on the ground that it is based on the fundamental units used to physics of mass, length and time, and does not, like the calorie, involve temperature (1 calorie =4.186 Joules).

Energy value of foods

The fuel values of a gram each of carbohydrate,fat and protein have been found to be respectively about 4.0, 5.65 and 9.3 kilocalories. However, the fuel value of protein and fat when oxidized in the body are only about 4 and 9 kilocalories respectively because of incomplete utilization. In the case of fat, absorption is incomplete. In the case of protein some amount of energy is used to convert ammonia formed when proteins are burned to urea which is excreted in the urine. The fuel value of foods when burned in a bomb calorimeter is referred to as physical fuel value and when utilized in the body as physiological fuel value. The physiological fuel value has been arrived at by making correction for the metabolic loss that occurs when carbohydrates, fats and proteins are oxidized in the body. The physiological energy value of carbohydrate, fat and protein are 4,9 and 4 kcal per gram respectively. The factors 4:9:4 are called Atwater-Bryant Factors.

The fuel value of the foods we eat can be imagined if we consider that the heat derived from one banana will be sufficient to increase the temperature of a litre of water from room temperature to boiling point.

In the body, part of the energy produced is trapped by the formation of phosphate compounds which can store up energy. The most important of these is adenosine triphosphate or ATP. When adenosine diphosphate or ADP acquires one more phosphate bond to become ATP, 8 kilocalories are trapped for each molecule of ATP formed. This energy is released when ATP is converted back to ADP. ATP is needed for the metabolic reactions involved in vital phenomena including neural transmission, muscle contraction and intestinal transport which is why the energy needed by the body has to be supplied in the form of food the oxidation of which can result in the formation of ATP and cannot be replaced by heat from outside. This explains why we need food even in a hot environment climate. The energy not used for ATP synthesis is dissipated as heat but it serves to maintain the temperature of the body above the environmental temperature which is usually lower. The energy trapped as ATP is also ultimately dissipated as heat generated in the body.

Although the body derives the energy needed for its many functions from compounds such as ATP, the synthesis of ATP depends on the amount of energy released during the oxidation of food in the form of carbohydrates, fatty acids, proteins and glycerol and that is why we are concerned with the fuel value of the foods we eat.

The energy value of the diet is a convenient index of its nutritive value. In mixed diets composed of a variety of foodstuffs, a diet adequate in energy is likely to be adequate in other respects. The major problems in the world today are under nutrition or an inadequate energy intake among the poor,particularly in developing countries, and over nutrition or energy intake in excess of requirements among the wealthier sections of the population.

When the energy value of the diet is more than the energy needed, the excess energy is stored as fat in the adipose tissue. This happens whether the calories are derived from fat, protein or carbohydrate.

When the calories in the diet are less than the calories needed, body tissue is broken down and the products of tissue breakdown are utilized for oxidation and heat production. Generally the fat in the adipose tissue is utilized. The calorie value of the tissue differs according to the composition of the tissue. One kg of ordinary tissue as gained by growing children represents a store of 2000–3000 kcalories. One kg of adipose tissue in an obese individual which contains more than 70% of fat represents a store of 6000–7000 Calories. When the weight gain is primarily due to water retention, it does not represent calorie stores.

Basal Metabolic Rate (BMR)

The total energy required by the body when at rest is referred to as basal metabolism and is generally calculated on a 24 hour basis. This requirement is measured in terms of the heat produced under resting conditions either by placing the subject in an insulated chamber and measuring the change in the temperature of the surrounding air or by making the subject breathe from an oxygen cylinder and measuring the amount of oxygen consumed by the subject in a specified period. The heat produced is calculated by multiplying with a factor 4.7 as when 1 litre of oxygen is used in the body 4.7 kcals of heat is generated. Both methods give comparable results and the latter method has largely replaced the former as it is more convenient and less expensive. An equipment known as Benedict-Roth apparatus is used in this method. Essentially this equipment measures the oxygen consumed by the subject for a period of time say 5 minutes. The measurement of the basal rate of energy consumption is generally done in the morning when the subject is relaxed and resting and has not had food for a period of 10–12 hrs.

A major part of the heat produced is lost by convection, and some amount, by radiation from the skin. It is not surprising that the basal metabolic requirement of an individual is proportional to the area of his body surface. This has been measured in large numbers of individuals and found to be related to height and weight. Of two persons weighing the same, the taller person will need more energy than the shorter one as his body surface will be greater even though he is of the same weight. Equations have been worked out for the calculation of surface area from both height and weight or from only weight by Aub-Dubois. Ready-made tables giving surface area for known height and weight are available (**Table 7**).

Basal heat production is also related to the mass of actively metabolizing tissues and is, therefore, less in individuals with more body fat as adipose tissue is metabolically much less active than, for instance, muscle.

Basal metabolic requirements are expressed in terms of either whole body requirements for 24 hours or for square meter of body surface or per kilogram of body weight per hour. The basal heat production per hour ranges from 55-60 kcalories per square meter at the age of one year to about

Table 7. Surface area in relation to height and weight (after Aub-Dubois).

Height in centimeters	Weight in Kilograms												
	25	30	35	40	45	50	55	60	65	70	75	80	85
	Surface area in square meters												
200							1.84	1.91	1.97	2.03	2.09	2.15	2.21
195						1.73	1.80	1.87	1.93	1.99	2.05	2.11	2.17
190				1.56	1.63	1.70	1.77	1.84	1.9	1.96	2.02	2.08	2.13
185				1.53	1.6	1.67	1.74	1.80	1.86	1.92	1.98	2.04	2.09
180				1.49	1.57	1.64	1.71	1.77	1.83	1.89	1.95	2.00	2.05
175	1.19	1.28	1.36	1.46	1.53		1.67	1.73	1.79	1.85	1.91	1.96	2.01
170	1.17	1.26	1.34	1.43	1.5	1.57	1.63	1.69	1.75	1.81	1.86	1.91	1.96
165	1.14	1.23	1.31	1.40	1.47	1.54	1.60	1.66	1.72	1.78	1.83	1.88	1.93
160	1.12	1.21	1.29	1.37	1.44	1.50	1.56	1.62	1.68	1.73	1.78	1.83	1.88
155	1.09	1.18	1.26	1.33	1.4	1.46	1.52	1.58	1.64	1.69	1.74	1.79	1.84
150	1.06	1.15	1.23	1.30	1.36	1.42	1.48	1.54	1.6	1.65	1.7	1.75	1.80
145	1.03	1.12	1.2	1.27	1.33	1.39	1.45	1.51	1.56	1.61	1.66	1.71	
140	1.0	1.09	1.17	1.24	1.3	1.36	1.42	1.47	1.52	1.57			
135	0.97	1.06	1.14	1.20	1.26	1.32	1.38	1.43	1.48				
130	0.95	1.04	1.11	1.17	1.23	1.29	1.35	1.40					
125	0.93	1.01	1.08	1.14	1.2	1.26	1.31	1.36					
120	0.91	0.98	1.04	1.10	1.16	1.22	1.27						

40–42 kcalories per square meter in the young adult male (**Table 8**). The standards for different ages have been worked out by Aub-Dubois and Fleisch and others. A normal young adult male of average size is found to require 1 kcalorie per kilogram per hour. For adults weighing about 60 kilos, the requirement per day will, therefore, be approximately 1500 kcalories.

Table 8. Basal metabolic rate in relation to age and sex*.

Age (yr)	Male	Female
	kcalories per square meter per hour	
Birth	31	31
1	58	58
2	57	57
3	56	56
4	55	55
5	54	54
6	53	51
7	52	50
8	51	48
9	50	47
10	49	45
12	48	43
14	46	41
16	45	39
18	43	37
19-20	42	37
20–25	41	37
25–30	40	37
30–35	40	36
35–40	39	36
40–45	38	35
45–50	38	35
50–55	37	34
55–60	36	34
60–65	36	34
65–70	35	33

* Benedict F.G,(1938), Vital energetics, a study in comparative metabolism, Publication 503, Carnegie Institute, Washington.

Factors affecting BMR

Basal metabolic requirements are likely to be similar for individuals of the same age, sex and weight and comparable build and state of health. However, they vary with factors such as age, sex and other variables.

Age

New born children have a relatively low BMR (30 kcal/sq. m/h) which rises to its peak value around the age of 1-2 years.

Young children are found to have higher basal metabolic rates than adults when considered in terms of Calories per square meter of surface area or kg of body weight. However, their total requirement for basal metabolism is less than that of adults. The reverse appears to be the case with advancing age after middle age when the basal metabolic rate shows a slow decline.

Sex

No differences in basal energy expenditure are found between male and female children of the same age. However, adolescent girls and women are found to have a lower metabolic rate than adolescent boys and men. This difference is partly due to the greater amount of body fat in the former.

Pregnancy

The extra energy required for the growth of the fetus, the placenta and associated maternal tissues as well as that required for carrying the extra load around imposes an increase in energy expenditure to the extent of 15–20% above normal towards the latter half of pregnancy.

Thyroid function

Hypothyroidism resulting from inadequate secretion of thyroxin by the thyroid gland is found to decrease the BMR. In hyperthyroidism BMR is found to be elevated.

Other conditions

Muscle tension, hormonal secretions and pathological conditions such as fever also influence BMR. A rise in body temperature of one degree (Fahrenheit) is found to increase BMR by about 7%. During sleep, BMR is decreased by about 10%.

In women BMR also varies during different phases of the menstrual cycle. It tends to rise at the time of ovulation and fall at the onset of menstruation. These changes are often associated with slight changes in body temperature.

It has been found that BMR is considerably decreased in individuals subjected to prolonged or chronic undernutrition.

Psychological tension caused by worry or mental tension increases the BMR. It is found to increase in students appearing for examination and people who are anxiety ridden.

BMR is more in people living in cold countries than people living in tropical countries where atmosphere is generally warm. This is because in cold weather body has to produce more heat to keep the body temperature in the normal range.

Energy requirements of individuals

The basal metabolic rate gives only the energy expenditure of the body at rest.

Over and above the BMR the energy requirement increases when the individual performs work. The increase in energy requirement over the BMR is called the activity increment which depends on the nature of work. For instance, sitting up requires greater energy than lying down and activities such as standing, walking and running require increasing amounts of energy.

Measurement energy requirement for physical work

The activity increment for physical activities of various kinds is determined using two equipments namely Douglas Bag and Max-Plank respirometer.

Douglas Bag

In this method the subject breaths into a 100 liter capacity bag while performing the work for a period of 5–10 minutes. The volume of the expired air and its composition of oxygen and carbon dioxide measured. The ratio of carbon dioxide output to oxygen consumed gives the respiratory quotient (R.Q). From the value for oxygen consumption and R.Q the energy expenditure can be calculated. This method is applicable for short duration physical work.

Max-Plank Respirometer

The basic principle is the same as that of Douglas Bag. The method is applicable for physical work involving longer duration.

The energy cost of activities varies not only with the nature of the activity but also with the speed and efficiency with which they are carried out. Walking fast requires more energy than cycling at 10–15 mph. Also, a person with more efficient muscular coordination is likely to require less energy than one whose coordination is poor. The energy cost of singing will be lesser in the case of of one who moves only the vocal cord and lips than in the case of one who also shakes his head and body and makes gestures with hands. This is also true of practiced activities as compared to new ones. We know from experience that walking along a familiar route is less tiring than walking the same distance in an unknown route.

In the case of walking or running the energy cost is related to body weight. Obviously, it cost more energy for a heavy individual to carry out these activities. On the other hand the energy cost talking may not be related to the body weight to the same extent as other physical work

In adult man the brain accounts for about 20–25% of basal metabolism although its weight is only 2.5% of body weight. In other words, the metabolic requirement of brain tissue is more than that of other tissues when considered on the basis of weight. But no appreciable increase in energy expenditure seems to be involved in mental work. This may be because the brain is always highly active whether we are consciously doing mental work or not.

From the available data we can conclude that mild activities such as sitting and talking require about 0.5 Calories per kg per hour whereas heavy work such as sawing wood may require more than 5 kcalories per kg per hour. A simple classification is made in Table 9. A sedentary individual or one who does not indulge in vigorous muscular exercise may require only 10–15 kcalories per kg per day for activity whereas a manual labourer may require 20–25 kcalories or more.

In estimating the energy requirements of an individual we have to take into account the requirements of basal metabolism as well as those of physical activity. In the case of the growing child or adolescent we have to also consider the requirement for growth. Other factors to be discussed below will also have to be considered.

Not all the potential energy present in foods is available to the body. About 5–10% of the energy value of the diet is lost through substances excreted in the feces and about 3% through urine. An allowance will have to be made for these losses while calculating the energy requirements of an individual. However, these losses are taken into account when energy value of food is calculated as physiological energy value. Another factor that needs to be considered is the Specific Dynamic Action of Foods (SDA). SDA is defined as the increase in the production of heat when foods are ingested. Among nutrients proteins have the highest SDA of about 30%. Rubner's theory is that the increase in the heat production represent the reactions in which part of the ingested protein is converted to glucose, the remaining protein that is not converted to glucose is burned with N carrying moiety. The heat produced in these reactions is not utilizable and hence appears as heat. SDA of carbohydrate is about 10% and fat has the lowest SDA of 2-3%. Taking the above factors into consideration the energy cost of selected activities have been determined and the same is given in **Table 9.**

Table 9. Energy Cost of Selected Activities.

Additional energy required per Kg body weight per hour (kcal)	Activities
Negligible Less than or above	Lying awake, mental work
0.5	Sitting, reading aloud, standing, personal care, eating, machine sewing, writing.
1.0	Hand-sewing, knitting, tailoring, singing dish-washing, ironing, most laboratory work (standing), household activities, type-writing.
1.5	sweeping the floor, light exercise, playing the piano.
2.0	Walking at moderate speed (about 3 mph), climbing down the stairs.
2.5	Carpentry, metal work, white-washing, cycling at moderate speed.
3.0	Walking fast, vigorous exercise.
3.5	Stone-cutting, climbing up the stairs.
4.0	Severe exercise, running, swimming, sawing wood.

An adult who is able to carry on his normal work without losing or gaining weight must be presumed to be in energy balance. That is, the energy expended by him is equal to the energy consumed. Similarly the energy intake of a child can be expected to be adequate when the child shows a normal growth rate and is reasonably active and playful.

Both activity levels and energy intakes are somewhat reduced with age in the adult. If food intake is not appropriately reduced, body weight increases which is the reason why so many people put on weight after age of 30 or 40 years.

Determination of energy requirement

To calculate the energy requirements of either an individual or a group, we need an estimate of energy needed for both basal metabolism and activity. The former can be estimated from getting information on height, weight, age and sex and making an estimate according to the information given in **Tables 8.** For instance, for a boy of age 8 years, height 120 cm. and weight 25 kg, the surface area will be 0.91 sq. m. **(Table 7...).** His BMR (kcalories per sq per hour) is 52 **(table 8...).** Total energy needed for basal metabolism will be equal to 52 x 24 x 0.91 or 1135 kcalories.

A rough estimate of the energy requirements of different groups can be made by making estimates of the approximate calories needed for basal metabolism and adding a percentage increment over the same for activity. The difference between total energy intake and basal energy needs in healthy well-nourished individuals should give us an idea of the activity increment in different groups.

Individuals who hardly indulge in activities requiring more than 1.5 kcalories per kg except perhaps for a minimum amount of walking can be considered as sedentary Those who engage for at least an hour or two in activities such as walking, running, swimming, athletics, manual work, playing tennis, etc. can be considered as moderately active. Those who perform at least four to six hours of heavy manual work or athletics can be considered as "active".

During growth, the energy requirement for tissue growth has also to be considered, but this is negligible as compared to total requirements as the tissue gained per day is not more than 10–15 g(except during early infancy) representing a gain of about 20–30 kcalories.

The above approach is useful for estimating the average energy requirements of different groups and this has been done in **Table 9A**.

The energy requirements of an individual can be calculated with greater precision by calculating energy needed for basal metabolism as mentioned above and making appropriate allowances not only for activity but also for factors such as sleep, specific dynamic action of food, environmental temperature, fecal and urine losses. For practical purposes, however, it will suffice to make a careful estimate of the energy cost of 'activities' and add this to the BMR calories.

The value arrived at by this method does not differ appreciably from that derived by detailed calculations as can be seen from **Table 9B**.

In using body weight as a standard, it is better to take desirable body weight rather than actual weight. Suppose a child weighs only 8 kg when his normal weight should be 12kg it is better to calculate the energy requirement on the basis of latter weight rather than the former actual weights. Otherwise, we can only expect the child to continue to be undernourished. On the other hand, for an obese woman who weighs 70 kg when her weight according to height should be 55 kg, it is better to calculate energy requirement on the latter basis.

Further, although BMR varies with weight during the period of growth it does not do so to the same extent after the growth has ceased. For instance, if the expected weight of a woman for her height is 55kg and she weighs 70kg her actual weight is 27% more than the expected value. But her BMR will be only 11% more than that for normal weight, as can be verified by calculation based on the Tables 7 and 8.

Table 9A. Energy requirements of individuals at different age levels.

Age (Years)		Height[1] (cm)	Weight[1] (kg)	Surface area[2] Sq. meters	Calories for			Calories[5] (per Kg)	Total calories[6] recommended by ICMR
					Basal[3] metabolim	Activity[4]	Total[5]		
1		74	9–11	0.43	600	300–600	900–1200	90–110	1200
2–4		93	13–14	0.58	800	400–800	1200–1600	90–110	1200
5–6		109	17–19	0.73	900	500–900	1400–1800	80–95	1500
7–10		123	23–25	0.92	1100	600–1100	1700–2200	70–90	1800
11–12		138	28–32	1.09	1200	600–1200	1800–2400	60–75	2100
13–15	M	150	38–42	1.30	1400	700–1400	2100–2800	55–70	2500
	F	152	39–43	1.34	1350	700–1350	2000–2700	50–65	2200
16–19	M	163	45–50	1.50	1500	700–1500	2200–3000	50–60	3000
	F	155–158	43–47	1.42	1300	700–1300	2000–2600	45–55	2200
Adults	M	165–170	55–60	1.67	1550	800–1550	2300–3100	40–50	2400–3900
	F*	155–158	45–50	1.46	1250	700–1250	1900–2500	40–50	1900–3000

* An additional allowance of about 15–300 calories and 500 calories are needed during pregnancy and lactation.
1 On the basis of data obtained on upper class subjects in Baroda.
2 Calculated from body weight for the first three groups and on the basis of Aub–Dubis standard for the other groups.
3 On the basis of 110% of Fleisch standard for the first two groups and Aub–Dubois standards for the remaining groups. The addition to the former was because of their somewhat smaller values as compared to the latter.
4 Taken as 5–100% of BMR for all age groups.
5 Rounded figures. The actual intakes in the upper class are found to be close to or less than the lower limit of the range.
6 Gopalan, C. and B.S. Narasingarao. 1971. Dietary allowances for Indians. Nutrition Research Laboratories. ICMR, Hyderabad, India.

Table 9 B. Energy requirement of selected subject.

Age, 24 years: Sex, Male	Height,	165 cm,	Weight;	55kg;
Surface area; 1.6 square				
Metres				
BMR per square				
Meter per hour according to age and sex	....	....	41	k calories
BM per day: 41 x 24 x 1.6 or	....	....	1574	k calories
BM per kg of body weight	....	....	28.5	k calories
Reduction for 8 hrs of sleep	......	....	47	k calories
Net Calories for BM	......	....	1527	k calories
Daily routine				

Activity	Duration	k cals. per kg per hr	Total k calories
Laboratory Work	4 hours	1.0	220
Attendance at work	3 hours	0.5	82.5
Study at Desk	3 hours	0.5	82.5
Relaxation	1 hour	0.5	28
Personal care	1 ½ hours	0.5	41
Meal time	1 ½ hours	0.5	41
Walking	1 hour	2.5	137
Cycling	1 hour	2.5	137
Total energy cost of Activities			770 k calories
Energy requirements for BMR + activity	......	....	2997 k calories
Allowance for loss due to specific dynamic action (6%)			
And fecal losses * (6% + 5%)	......	....	173 k calories
Total	......	....	2470 k calories
Allowance for warm environmental			
Temperature (-10%)	......	....	155 k calories
Total dietary requirement	......	....	2315 k calories
Simplified calculations			
BM per kg of body weight	......	....	28.5 k calories
BM per day	......		1570 k calories
Allowance for activity	......	....	770 k calories
Total requirements	......	....	2340 k calories

BM: Basal Metabolism.

* To be ignored if energy requirements are calculated in terms of physiological fuel value.

Calculations of energy requirements are of importance in assessing the adequacy of the diet in the case of undernourished individuals and requirement in the case of obese individuals whose body weight exceeds desirable limits. An estimate of energy requirement of population per capita is compared with energy available from food supplies in order to assess the adequacy of food supplies in a community.

Chapter 4

Water and Minerals

Proteins fats and carbohydrates are all complex carbon compounds that are referred to as organic compounds. The body also requires inorganic nutrients such as water, sodium, potassium, calcium, phosphorus, iron, iodine, etc in suitable forms. There are many other elements required in comparatively small quantities and these are called trace elements.

Water

About 60% of the weight of the body is accounted for by water. Man cannot survive for long without water although he can survive without food for quite a few days.

The functions of the body are inconceivable without water. In fact, the principle used in the preservation of foods by dehydration is that moulds and bacteria cannot survive in its absence.

Water gives form and structure to the cells and the body. It cushions the body and protects it against environmental stress. It also helps the body to maintain stable temperature because of its high specific heat. Processes such as chewing and swallowing are facilitated by the lubricating effect of water. Tasting and swallowing of foods is impossible when the throat is dry.

The metabolic reactions of the body take place in an aqueous medium. The enzymes that catalyze metabolic reactions require water for ionization of their active sites. Water ionizes substances such as sodium chloride. That is the sodium and chlorine in sodium chloride are dissociated and held as ions or electrically charged particles. Sodium ions are positively charged whereas chlorine ions are negatively charged. The ions of calcium, magnesium, potassium, and sodium are important for the 'irritability' of cell-membranes or their contraction and expansion so as to permit the flow of substances across them.

Water also enters directly into certain metabolic reactions in which a molecule of water is either added to or removed from certain substances. For instance, both reactions take place at different stages in the formation of bone from calcium phosphate.

The evaporation of water requires heat and, therefore, produces cooling. The evaporation of sweat from the body surface helps to keep the body at a temperature of about 98°F even when the surrounding temperature is high or when excess heat is produced in the body because of severe muscular exercise.

Water is necessary for the flushing out of waste products of metabolism. Urea which is the chief end product of nitrogen metabolism in mammals can be excreted through the kidneys only if there is enough water. In this connection, in mammals which drink plenty of water, the faces are moist and urea is excreted along with water in the form of urine. In birds and insects which drink less water, the faces are almost dry and uric acid is the chief end product of nitrogen metabolism and is excreted in an almost dry form. As birds have to fly, they cannot afford to carry excess luggage in the form of water. The low water requirement of insects partly accounts for their ability to survive under varying conditions.

Water is also necessary for the flushing out of toxic substances formed in the body in various metabolic processes and administration of drugs for treating various diseases.

Water is consumed as such or in the form of beverages. Most of the foods we eat contain some water. It is also formed in the metabolic reactions. The oxidation of a gram each of starch, protein and fat results in the formation respectively of 0.60, 0.41 and 1.07 g of water.

Water is lost from the body through feces, urine, sweat and expired air. These losses must be replaced by water in food and drink or that formed from metabolism. During growth, water is also required for the formation of new tissue. The normal adult is usually in a state of balance with regard to water. In other words, the water consumed by him and that produced in metabolism equal to the total amount lost through sweat, urine, lungs and faces. When the latter is more than the former, the body contains less than normal amount of water and this condition is called dehydration. In the reverse case the body contains more than a normal amount of water resulting in oedema.

In severe dehydration of the type found in extremely under nourished Children the skin is shrunk dry and wrinkled. Conditions such as vomiting and diarrhea or those such as fever or drug treatment also result in dehydration if enough water or liquids are not consumed. When the body retains more than a normal amount of water, the condition is referred to as oedema. The skin is glossy and extremities of limbs appear swollen. If the skin is pressed at the site of oedema it does not bounce back to original position almost immediately as it should, but forms a dent This condition is found in kwashiorkor the protein deficiency disease and sometimes in adults suffering from severe degree of starvation or diseases of the kidney.

Many people subject themselves to mild dehydration and consequent fatigue during working hours if drinking water is not readily available at the site of work. In warm environment it helps if water is habitually consumed between meals. Usually our intake of water is guided by feeling of thirst. This feeling is associated with dryness of throat and mouth and is believed to be regulated by the level of sodium in the blood.

This explains why sometimes salty food increase our feeling of thirst. When there is water depletion the concentration of sodium in blood is increased and this gives rise to, the feeling of thirst. However, when sodium is also lost through sweat along with water, there is depletion of both sodium and water so that the resulting concentration of sodium in blood is not altered. In this case no feeling may be experienced and, therefore, no water may be consumed and hence dehydration is the result. This happens in people such as miners, glass factory workers etc., working in a very hot environment. If a feeling of thirst is experienced under such condition, water is generally consumed resulting in a low concentration of sodium and a disturbance of electrolyte balance in the body.

The water present in cells is referred to, as intracellular water whereas that present in the space between the cells is referred to as extracellular water.

The amount of water in the body can be estimated by measuring the density of the body. The person is seated in a chair which is slowly lowered into water at known temperature and he is weighed with whole body under Water. The difference between the normal weight and weight under water gives an idea of the weight and volume of the water displaced. The density of the body can, therefore be calculated. The same is known to vary with the amounts of fat and water in the body. The body of normal individual who does not have excessive adipose tissue has a density of 1.06 and a fat content of about 14%. If the density is less than this, the fat content will be more. By measuring body density we can estimate the amount of fat in the body. Water forms about 70% of the body weight minus the weight of fat. We can therefore guess the amount of water present in the body by measuring the density of the body.

The amount of water can also be estimated by injecting into the blood a radioactive substance such as labeled potassium or substances which diffuse freely in the body such sodium thiocyanate. From the resulting concentration of this substance in blood, we can estimate the amount of water present in the body. To give an example, suppose we put a known amount of some substance, say salt, in an unknown amount of water, the concentration of salt in water will depend on the amount of water present. If 10g of salt result in a solution which contains lg of salt per 100 ml, we can infer that the volume of water used is 1 litre. The estimation of body water by injection of radioactive substances is based on similar reasoning.

Sodium

Sodium is present in many foods in the form of sodium chloride; It is also added to foods in the form of common salt. However, there are primitive people, especially those living in areas far away from rock salt or the sea, who do not add salt to their diet. Many of them ash certain plants and consume the ash, which contain sodium. They seem to have the capacity to adapt to at low salt diet and their kidneys excrete less salt in the urine. Once they learn the use of salt, it becomes a precious commodity in these areas.

The sodium and potassium contents of selected foods are given in **Table 10.** Plant foods are generally lacking in sodium and diets based predominantly on sodium require added salt. However, the amount of salt consumed by civilized man is usually in excess of requirements (5–10 g) and most of this is excreted in urine.

Diets rich in spices and condiments are prepared with more salt than bland diets. In normal healthy individuals, the excessive consumption of salt is not attended with ill effects, but this involves an unnecessary load on the kidney and is undesirable for people with kidney disorders. Restriction of salt intake is also necessary with elevated blood pressure. It is also suspected that children given too much of salty foods at a very young age (3–6 months) are more prone to develop blood pressure as adults.

The traditional practice of giving up salt on certain days may be desirable for individuals getting on in age as blood increases gradually with age.

As stated earlier sodium and potassium are present in blood and tissues. The former is present primarily in the extracellular fluid and the latter in the intracellular fluid. The traffic of these ions across cell membrane is important for many cellular functions and transport of other substances. It is therefore, important for the body to maintain normal concentration of both. As already stated,in the case of miners and others who have to work in excessively hot environment the excessive loss of sodium through sweat may result in symptoms such as fatigue, muscular weakness and vomiting. It is advisable for such people to take water to which a small quantity of salt has been added. Drinking buttermilk or lemon juice to which a small quantity of water has been added will help to prevent salt depletion during the summer. Losses of sodium and water which occur with vomiting and

Table 10. The mineral composition of common foodstuffs

foodstuff	% Ash	Sodium	Potassium	Calcium mg per 100 g	Phosphorus	Magnesium	Iron
Rice	0.6	8.0	70	10	160	48	3.1
wheat	1.7	17.1	284	41	306	138	4.9
Maize	1.5	15.9	286	10	348	144	2.0
Bajra	2.3	10.9	307	42	296	125	5.0
Jowar	1.6	7.3	131	25	222	140	5.8
Kodari varagu)	2.6	4.6	144	27	188	112	5.2
Bengalgram	3.0	37.3	808	202	312	168	10.2
Blackgram (dal)	2.7	39.8	800	154	385	185	9.1
Redgram (dal)	3.5	28.5	1104	73	304	133	5.8
Greengram	3.5	28.0	843	124	326	171	7.3
Soyabean	4.7	5	1677	240	690	265	11.5
Sesame	5.3	60	725	1450	570	181	10.5
Ground nut	2.3	5	674	90	350	206	2.8
Milk:							
Human	0.2	16	51	28	11	NA	NA
Cow	0.7	16	140	120	90	NA	0.2
Buffalo	0.8	19	90	210	130	NA	0.2
Amaranth	2.6	230	341	393	83	247	25.5
Fenugreek	1.5	76.1	31	395	51	67	16.5
Spinach	1.5	58.5	206	73	21	84	10.9
Potato	0.9	11.0	247	10	40	20	0.7
Brinjal	0.3	3.0	200	18	47	16	0.9
Mutton	1.3	32	130	15	150	65	2.5
Chicken	1.0	50	320	25	245	60	-
Fish (pomfret)	1.5	NA	NA	286	306	70	2.3
egg	1.0	122	129	60	220	125	2.1

NA- Values not available

diarrhea in infants may prove fatal because of this and can be treated by giving frequently boiled water containing sugar or jaggery and salt as well as buttermilk prepared from boiled and cooled water and salt.

Potassium

As already stated, potassium is an important constituent of intracellular fluid. A diet that is adequate in other respects is likely to be adequate with regard to potassium. Most plant foods contain several times as much potassium as sodium (**Table 10**). Potassium deficiency may be found in conditions Such as kwashiorkor and diabetic coma. It is associated with symptoms such as muscular weakness and mental apathy. As these symptoms are found in many other conditions it is difficult to identify the deficiency. Potassium and sodium are required by the body in balanced proportions and an excess of potassium intake in the face of deficiency of sodium intake is not desirable. People living on salt-free diets should take fruit juices which are rich in potassium, after dilution. It is also not generally advisable to use excessive amounts of potassium salts which have a salty taste in place of common salt in salt restricted diets.

Calcium and Phosphorus

Calcium phosphate, a salt of calcium and phosphorus, forms a major component of the skeleton which accounts for 16% of adult body weight. The newborn infant has a store of about 28 g of calcium. The body of adult man contains about 1200g of calcium, and of adult woman, a little less than this amount. The amounts of phosphorus in the body are somewhat less being about 20 g in the infant at birth and about 670 g in adult man.

The amount of different foods that can provide 100 mg of calcium are indicated in **Table 11**. It can be seen from the same that milk is by far the best source. Leafy vegetables contain liberal amounts, but the oxalate present in many leafy vegetables is believed to prevent the efficient utilization of calcium. Ragi among millets and sesame seeds among legumes also contain liberal amount of calcium but the same is believed to be poorly utilized because of the presence in the former of phytate and in the latter of oxalate.

The calcium in foods is usually present in the form of complex compounds. During digestion, the calcium is freed from these compounds so that it can be absorbed into the blood stream. The absorption of calcium depends on a number of factors.

As mentioned earlier, many plant foods contain high amounts of oxalic acid and phosphorus compounds called phytates. Calcium combines or 'chelates' with the former to form oxalates, and with the latter to form phytates. These are not soluble and cannot, therefore, be absorbed from the intestine. When the diet is rich in phytate or oxalate, we may expect the calcium in the diet to be less efficiently utilized. However, there is an enzyme phytase in the intestine which can break down phytate. This break down

Table 11. Different foods as sources of calcium.

Food stuff	Approximate amount (g) Providing 100 mg of calcium
Rice and maize	1000
Wheat, jowar and bajra	250–400
Dals(dehusked legumes)	150
Whole legumes including soyabean	50
Groundnut	200
Leafy vegetables	40
Root vegetables	500
Other vegetables	250
Cow milk	85
Buffalo milk	40–50
Skim milk powder	10
Egg	200
Fish	750–1000
Meat	1000
Selected sources:	
Ragi	30
sesame seed	10
agathi leaves	10
elephant yam	200
sitaphal (custard apple)	25
wood apple	75

of phytate by the phytase enzyme helps calcium absorption. Procedures such as sprouting and fermentation of cereals, legumes and millets reduce the phytate content of these foods significantly. Malted ragi is now a well known ingredient as a source of calcium for children. The interference of oxalate in calcium absorption may not be a serious problem as ordinary diets do not contain much of oxalate.

Vitamin D, lysine, lactose and citric acid have been found to promote the absorption of calcium. Milk calcium is very well absorbed and this may be partly due to the liberal amounts of some of these substances in milk. The mechanism of action of Vitamin D in the intestinal absorption of calcium and calcium deposition on bone are discussed in the section of Vitamin D.

The absorption and utilization of calcium are also affected by the protein content and quality of the diet. The bones of animals fed a diet poor in protein content or quality contain less calcium. They are also not as strong as bones of animals fed normal protein. Their bone resembles that of a younger animal with immature bone suggesting delayed skeletal maturation. The most crucial factor regulating absorption, however, is the need of the body. Vitamin D is necessary for this regulation . For instance, adults consuming a great quantity of milk often get more than 1500–2000 mg of calcium in the diet. Let us suppose the adult body needs about 250 mg to replace losses. In this case only about 12–17% of the calcium present in the diet will have to be absorbed. On the other hand, absorption may be as high as 70% if the diet contains something like only 350 mg.

The absorption of calcium also depends on the proportions in which calcium and phosphorus are present in the diet. The bone contains calcium and phosphorus roughly in the ratio 2:1. In addition, some phosphorus (about 10–15% of the total) is present in the soft tissues, which have a higher rate of metabolism than the bone so that the body requires calcium and phosphorus in approximately equal proportions. It is obvious that as the formation of bone requires calcium as well as phosphate neither can be utilized fully if the other is not supplied in adequate amounts. It would, therefore seem desirable to have the two approximately in reasonable proportions, (1:1 or 1.5:1). Most cereal diets are high in phosphorus and low in calcium. However, so long as both are present in the diet in adequate amounts they seem to be utilized satisfactorily even if their proportions are not ideal. This may be because vitamin D helps in their efficient utilization even when the ratio of the two is unfavorable. However, young children require relatively more phosphorus in relation to calcium than adults and by giving them a supplement of only calcium, we may disturb the Ca:P ratio which may result in the poor absorption of both. Vitamin D helps in the better utilization of phosphorus by decreasing urine losses of the same.

Bone has half the tensile strength of steel. Otherwise we should be breaking our bones so much often or bending them out of shape. How is this strength achieved? The calcium absorbed combines with phosphate and water to form hydroxyapatite crystals of calcium phosphate. First, a fibrous network made of collagen and other nitrogenous substances is formed. The bone minerals are deposited on this network as crystals. These crystals are re-dissolved and re-crystallized so as to form bone tissue. During the re-crystallization some of the water is lost and the structure of the crystals is also changed.

We may compare the change in the texture of bone material with those of a different kind achieved while making ice-cream. Milk or cream is frozen first, thawed and beaten and then refrozen in order to get a smooth creamy texture. The material obtained after the first freezing is very different in texture and quality from that obtained after the thawing and freezing. Phosphate is necessary for the formation of calcium phosphate at the bone site. The enzyme alkaline phosphatase, present at the bone site liberates phosphate from complex compounds of the same and makes it available at the bone site. The activity of this enzyme depends on many factors including vitamin D and the activity of the parathyroid gland.

Since the bone is a hard and strong structure, we may suppose that once the bone develops to its full size there is no need to worry about further supplies of calcium. This is not the case as bone matter is continually dissolved and reformed. This ensures that the structure retains its tensile strength.

A small portion of the calcium in the body is present in blood and other tissues, but this portion is most important for body functions. The calcium content in the blood is 8–10 mg per 100ml. The maintenance of calcium level in the blood is controlled by the thyrocalcitonin the the hormone secreted by the parathyroid gland. Low calcium level in the blood triggers the secretion of this hormone by the parathyroid into the blood which in turn helps the desorption of calcium from the bone into the blood. The reverse process occurs when the calcium level in the blood tends to go up, that is, more calcium is deposited to the bone. The calcium in the blood is necessary for the blood to clot. It also regulates the permeability of cell membrane, conduction in the nervous system and the beating of the heart. Calcium is a cofactor of one the enzymes involved in the coagulation of blood. Calcium in the blood is present in both ionized and bound forms. Because of the many important functions of calcium in blood it is exceedingly important for the concentration of the same, particularly ionized calcium to be maintained within narrow limits. When the calcium levels fall below critical levels, the irritability of cell-membranes and excitability of muscles are increased and convulsions may result. When it exceeds certain limits, muscular excitability is decreased. Difficulty in walking, poor gait and poor muscle tone may result.

The readiness, with which calcium can be added to or removed from the bone or in other words, its mobility, makes it possible to supply rapidly the extra calcium needed for the healing of bone injuries. Calcium is deposited in the bone in early pregnancy and utilized for fetal growth in late pregnancy and for milk production after delivery. As mentioned earlier, children require relatively more phosphorus.

How much calcium do we need? Young children obviously require more calcium in proportion to body weight in order to meet the requirements of the growing skeleton. The adult also requires calcium in the diet in order to replace the losses of calcium from the body. Some calcium is lost daily through the digestive juices which are secreted into the alimentary canal as these juices contain large amounts of calcium. A portion of the same may be reabsorbed but a substantial portion is lost through the feces.

Some calcium is lost through urine and probably a small amount through sweat. The diet must provide enough calcium so that the amount absorbed is Sufficient to replace these losses in adults and to meet the demand of the growing skeleton as well in young children. In expectant and nursing mothers it must also be enough to provide for the needs of fetal growth and milk production.

The metabolic requirements for calcium vary from 60 to 250 mg in different age groups. As all the calcium in the diet is not absorbed the diets have to provide much more than this and the amounts recommended by different authorities take this into account. The amounts recommended by the FAO are shown in **Table 12.**

Table 12. Calcium intakes as compared to recommended Allowances.

Age (yrs)	Amount (mg) of calcium Consumed[1]		Recommended[2]
	lower class	upper class[3]	
Less than one	200–300	1600	500–600
1–9	250–300	1400	400–500
10–15	300–350	1200	600–700
16–19	350–400	1200	400–600
20–40 Men	350–400	1200	400–500
Women	250–400	1100	400–500
Pregnancy and Lactation	250–400	1100	1000–1200

[1] Based on results of diet surveys carried out in different projects by the author and her colleagues in urban Baroda.
[2] FAO/WHO (1962). Calcium requirements. Report of a joint FAO/WHO Expert Group, Who Technical Report Series No. 30. World Health Organization, Geneva.
[3] Mostly derived from buffalo milk which contains 200 mg % calcium.

Calcium deficiency

Milk is by far the best source of calcium as can be seen from Table 11. Since the diets consumed by the poor do not contain enough milk they are deficient in calcium as compared to recommended amounts (Table 12). We may therefore expect high prevalence of calcium deficiency diseases, but the actual prevalence is not as much as may be expected. This may be partly because of the generous supply of sunshine to which the children are exposed and vitamin D formed helps in the more efficient utilization of the calcium available in the diet. Further, utilization is more efficient in people adapted to low intakes over a long period. However, poor bone development is found in a substantial proportion of young children on the basis of radiological examination. Normally, children show some characteristic change in the size, Shape, thickness and density of bone with growth. New centres of ossification (newly calcified areas) are also found. The rate of these changes is delayed when the child is not adequately nourished Some of these differences can be seen from the X-ray pictures of the hand of a poor child receiving the ordinary home made diet and another child of the same age given an improved meal at the balwadi **(Fig. 3).** The two differ with regard to the appearance of the long bone of the hand (1), the number and size of ossification centres (2) and the appearance of long bone in the fingers (3). Further the thickness of the outer edge of the bones (for instance 3) is also affected by nutritional status.

The delayed development of bone in young children is not only due mainly to deficiencies of calcium and vitamin D but also those of calories, protein and vitamin A. Even in upper class children receiving adequate calcium, vitamin D deficiency may be prevalent as the mothers do not permit young children to play in the sun.

The common calcium deficiency diseases are rickets and retarded bone development in children and osteomalacia in adults, particularly in women during the reproductive period. Osteoporosis occurring in the elderly may

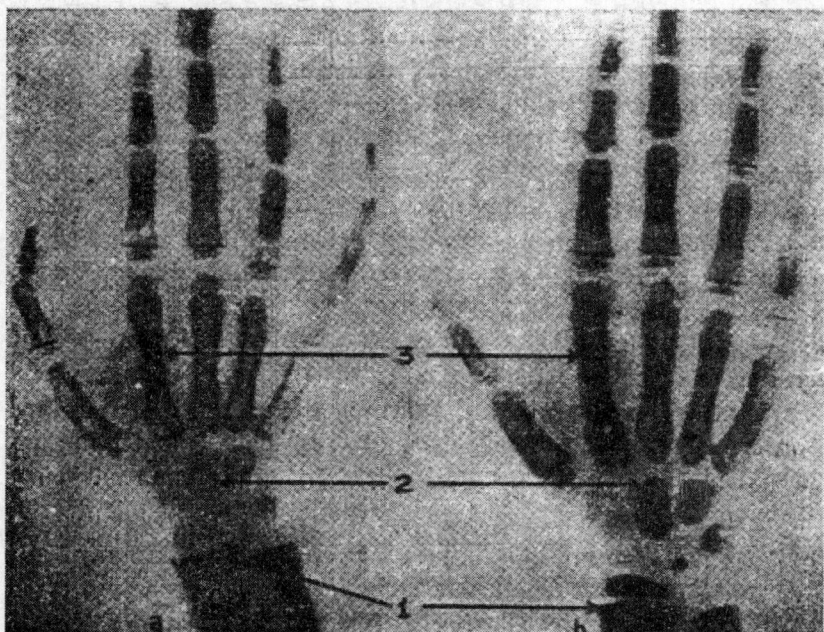

Figure 3. Radiological status of fed and control children (The fed children received a balanced lunch including lime treated dhokla. Note the greater number of ossification centres in the hand of the fed child):

a—control child; b—fed child.

1. long bone of the hand; 2. ossification centres; 3. long bone of the finger.

Table 13. Increase in calcium content of foods by lime incorporation.

Foodstuff	Ingredients		Procedure	Amount (mg) of lime powder added[1]	pH[2]	Approximate increase (mg) in calcium content
1. Dhokla	Coarsely ground wheat Bengal gram dal salt	50g 50g 5g	Batter prepared from ingredients, fermented, lime-treated, steamed, cooled, sliced and seasoned.	0 500	5.0 6.3	0 200
2. Idli	Rice(coarsely ground) Blackgram dal (finely ground) salt	77g 33g 5g	Batter prepared from the ingredients, fermented, lime –treated and steamed	0 450	4.7 6.0	0 180
3. Khaman	Bengalgram dal	100g	As for dhokla	0 350	5.2 6.5	0 140
4. Sambar (broth) used with rice	Redgram dal Vegetables Tamarind	12g 12g 3g	Vegetables added to partially cooked dal and the cooking continued. When the mixture is almost cooked, lime treated tamarind juice, salt and seasoning added and the cooking completed.	0 150	5.0 6.0	0 60
5. Sour buttermilk	Sour curd Water	20g 80g	The two churned together and treated with lime.	0 280	4.1 6.5	0 112

[1] Values are per 100g of dry ingredients in the case of items 1, 2 and 3 and on wet weight basis in the case of items 4 and 5.

[2] pH is a measure of acid-base balance. Values below 7 indicate acidity and those above 7 alkalinity.

not necessarily be due to calcium deficiency. This aspect will be discussed elsewhere.

While plant foods can be combined suitably so as to provide adequate proteins and other nutrients in the diet,it is difficult to get enough calcium from these foods for groups such as young children or nursing mothers whose calcium requirement is relatively high as compared to calorie requirement.

Studies in Baroda have shown that the calcium content of foods can be increased by adding lime or slaked lime to sour foods such as butter milk, fermented batters of idli, khaman, dhokla and sambhar. Lime is alkaline and its addition to foods results in the loss of more than 50% of thiamine and riboflavin which are destroyed in the presence of alkali. By adding lime to acid foods in such a way that the resulting foods still remain sour or at least do not become alkaline, the calcium content of foods can be increased without incurring vitamin losses as shown in **Table 13**. In studies carried out in Baroda, animals fed lime treated dhokla were found to have 50% more of calcium in their bones than those fed ordinary dhokla. Pre-school children given a daily supplement of lime treated dhokla for 8 months were found to show good skeletal development as compared to those given ordinary dhokla as judged by X ray examination (**Fig. 3**). As lime powder costs practically nothing this is a simple way to increase the calcium content of diets based primarily on plant foods especially for groups requiring more calcium and not getting enough milk.

Excess calcium and vitamin D in the diet may also cause severe disorders of calcium metabolism. In the United Kingdom the widespread prevalence of rickets and the recognition that deficiency of calcium and vitamin D are responsible led to public health measures designed to improve the intake of both. Because of the over anxiety of parents and others to protect children against these deficiencies, many children were getting much more of these nutrients than is good for them. Baby foods, breakfast cereals etc. were fortified with both calcium and vitamin D and anxious parents gave liberal doses of cod liver oil as well. This results in high intakes of both calcium and vitamin D. The consumption of the latter was often 10 times desirable amounts. Many children showed symptoms of excessive absorption of calcium with abnormally high levels of calcium in blood, a condition called hypercalcemia. This condition is characterized by loss of appetite, vomiting, weight loss, growth arrest, mental retardation and kidney damage.

Hypercalcemia is treated by diets low in calcium and vitamin D. Fortunately, such high amounts of calcium and vitamin D are not likely to be present in natural diets unless the foods are specially fortified. Normally, the regulation of calcium absorption by the body ensures that no more than what is necessary is absorbed with ordinary diets.

Phosphorus

The role of phosphorus in bone calcification has already been described. Phosphorus is also present in blood and tissues in the form of phosphate and other organophosphates that have vital functions in the body. Phosphate is required in mitochondrial oxidative phosphorylation where ATP is formed when fuels carbohydrates, fats and proteins are oxidized. Another major function of phosphate is in the formation of phospholipids of membranes and brain tissues. Cereals are high in phosphorus content and although much of it is present in the form of phytate it does not usually form the limiting nutrient in cereal diets or in diets based on natural foods. Phosphate deficiency may occur in young children because of deficiency or impaired utilization of vitamin D and this may be aggravated if they are given generous supplements of only calcium.

Magnesium

Next to calcium and phosphorus, magnesium is the major inorganic constituent in the body which contains about 25 g of this mineral. Ordinary diets contain about 300 mg and this seems to be sufficient. Rice contains less magnesium than other grains and signs of magnesium deficiency have been found occasionally in rice consuming regions like Burma. Some magnesium is derived from drinking water so that magnesium deficiency is not likely in areas where the drinking water is hard.

Like calcium, magnesium plays an important role in cell permeability. It is also necessary for the activity of certain enzymes as cofactor. When magnesium is deficient in the diet of experimental animals, tetany is found to result.

Although the magnesium content of ordinary diets is almost as much as calcium content, the body store of magnesium is much less than that of calcium, most of which is in the bone (25 g as Compared to 1200 g). The greater requirement of magnesium relative to the amount present in the body is because of poor absorption.

Sulphur

Sulphur is an important constituent of the amino acids methionine, cystine and cysteine (these are called sulphur amino acids) and substances such as Coenzyme A and glutathione. Sulphate ions are present in the cells. Mucopolysaccharide chondroitin sulphate in the cartilage contain sulphur.

Methionine is an essential amino acid but cystine can be formed from methionine in the body. These two amino acids are the chief sources of sulphur in our diet but foods such as onions, garlic, cauliflower and cabbage contain sulphur in the inorganic form.

Trace elements

The body contains other inorganic constituents which are present in much smaller amounts because of which they are called 'trace' elements or elements found in traces.

Iron

The chief among the trace elements is iron. The total body stores of iron amount to about 3-4 g. Most of the iron present in the body is found in the blood or liver. Haemoglobin of blood is a compound of 'heme', an iron compound 'globin', a protein. The chief use of iron in the body is for the synthesis of haemoglobin. It is also required for the activities of certain enzymes as cofactor. The function of haemoglobin is to carry oxygen from the lungs to the tissues. It does this by forming a temporary loose association with oxygen resulting in the formation of oxy-haemoglobin. The oxygen is liberated in the cells and oxy haemoglobin becomes haemoglobin again. Because of this property of haemoglobin the requirements of the body for oxygen are met by a relatively small volume of blood (about 5 litres). If, for instance, water had to act as oxygen carrier,its volume would have to be much greater and its circulation would have to be much faster in order to cope with the demands of the cells for oxygen. The average adult man uses up about 11 litres of oxygen per hour. This means that each litre of blood carries about 2 litres of oxygen per hour. The efficiency of haemoglobin as a carrier of oxygen can be imagined from these figures.

The iron content of common foods is shown in Table 10. Leafy greens, jaggery or brown sugar, raisins, egg yolk and liver are some of the better sources of iron. Among food grains, bajra is a good source. Although cereals are not particularly good sources they are consumed in such large amounts that a substantial portion of iron in the diet is derived from cereals. On the other hand, spices such as mustard, cumin seeds, fenugreek, celery seeds and coriander contain liberal amount of iron but they are consumed in such small amounts that they may not make significant contribution to our dietary iron.

The absorption of iron like that of calcium is affected by oxalate and phytate in the diet and its protein quality and quantity. Most of the iron in the food is in the ferric form. Ferric form of iron has to be reduced to ferrous form before absorption and ascorbic acid is required for this purpose. An excess of calcium in the diet, intestinal parasites like hookworm are believed to prevent the absorption of iron. Diets containing large amount of milk which is a rich source of calcium may result in anaemia unless they also included liberal amount of iron. It is now well established that not all the iron in the food is available to the body because of various factors that affect iron absorption. Several studies have shown that heme iron, that is, the iron in myoglobin the muscle pigment is the most available form of iron.

Iron absorbed by the intestine is transported by the blood as a complex with a protein named transferrin is mostly deposited in liver for haemoblobin synthesis. Iron is stored mainly in the liver as haemosiderin from which free iron is released for haemoglobin synthesis. Haemoglobin synthesis requires vitamins such as Vitamin E, folic acid and vitamin B12, pyridoxine and ascorbic acid. Therefore, the synthesis of hemoglobin will be affected by lack of iron, protein, and the vitamins involved in the process. Since the haemoglobin synthesis is affected by a large number of nutrients the haemoglobin content is taken as a general index of nutritional status. Anaemia is found when the diet lacks one or other of the nutrients needed for haemoglobin synthesis.

The red blood cells which contain haemoglobin is formed in the bone marrow. The cells formed are first large in shape, irregular in size and contain no haemoglobin (megaloblasts). As they mature, they become smaller in size, circular in shape and contain haemoglobin. At this stage they also contain nucleus and are called normoblasts. The nucleus is then expelled and the cells are now fully mature red cells called erythrocytes. In the healthy individuals, circulating blood contain mostly erythrocytes as the cells mature before they leave the bone marrow. But in certain type of anaemia, normoblasts and megaloblasts are also found. In certain other cases, the cells are fully mature but much smaller than they are in healthy individual and contain less haemoglobin. Sometimes the cells are fragile and have a short life span.

In healthy individuals blood contains 13–15 g haemoglobin per 100 ml. This may be decreased to values as low as 5 g per 100ml in conditions of nutritional deficiency or disease. A low level of haemoglobin in blood is called anaemia. Anaemia is found when the diet lacks one or other nutrients needed for haemoglobin synthesis. It is also found in infections and disease conditions when diets are apparently adequate. Sometimes the efficiency of bone marrow to form red blood cells is affected. This often happens with excessive intake of antibiotics and certain drugs. In certain other conditions the red cells are rapidly destroyed or haemolysed. Such destruction is found when there is a chronic poisoning with metals such as lead and arsenic. Under such conditions the requirement of nutrients required for synthesis of haemoglobin is increased. Under extreme conditions even a liberal supply of the same may fail to restore haemoglobin synthesis to normal level.

Red blood cells are continually being destroyed and new cells being formed. The iron released in the former case is stored in the spleen and used again for haemoglobin synthesis. Otherwise we would need much more iron than we do at present.

Anaemia is associated with decrease either in the number and size of the red blood cells or their haemoglobin content or defect in their maturation. When the anaemia is due to lack of iron or pyridoxine the cells are smaller in size(microcytic) and have low haemoglobin content (hypochromic). This type of anaemia is called microcytic, hypochromic anaemia. In other conditions such as calorie or protein deficiency, the size and haemoglobin content are not altered but the number of cells is reduced. This condition is called normocytic, normochromic anaemia. In deficiency of Vitamin B12, folic acid and Vitamin E, the number of cells is decreased and the cells are large in size (macrocytic). This condition is known as macrocytic megaloblastic anaemia. The characteristics of different types of anaemia are summarized in **Table 14**.

As the body effectively utilizes iron from old red cells, it requires only enough iron to replace losses through faeces, sweat, urine, etc. so that our requirements are relatively small. However, we need much more in the diet because only a small portion of the iron is absorbed. Only one sixth of the iron in foods is estimated to be absorbed on an average in the western diet. In Indian diets containing more oxalate and phytate and less of protein and vitamins the absorption may be even less. About 15 mg of iron is considered sufficient in the west whereas the ICMR recommends about 20–30 mg for the adult. Although common diets in this country provide this amount, iron deficiency anaemia is very common. The liver stores of iron in Indians are relatively low according to Prof. Ramalingaswami at the All India Institute of Medical Sciences, New Delhi. This may be partly because of dietary factors and perhaps also because of the widespread incidence of intestinal disorders both of which may reduce the absorption of iron. The haemoglobin content of different groups of subjects is shown in **Table 15**. It can be seen from the same that haemoglobin content is low in both lower and upper classes as compared to normal values reported for western subjects. The anaemia found in lower classes is due generally poor diets deficient in most of the nutrients. That in the upper classes could be due to a deficiency of iron combined with excessive consumption of milk, sugar and fat to the exclusion of iron rich foods.

Copper

Copper is another mineral which is required by the body in small amounts. About 1–3 mg per day is considered sufficient. Ordinary diets usually supply this. The body contains about 0.1 g. A deficiency of copper results

Table 14. Classification of different types of Anemia.

Cause	Characteristics	Descriptive term and treatment
Deficiency of Iron	Decrease in size and haemorrhages content of red cells.	Microcytic, hypochromic, responding to iron
Calories	Decrease in number of red cells and presence of immature cells(normoblasts)	Normocytic, normochromic, responding to nutritional improvement
Proteins		
Folic acid	Decrease in number of red cells and presence of large immature cells (megaloblasts)	Macrocytic, megaloblastic, responding to treatment with the appropriate vitamin or intrinsic factor
Vitamin B12		
Vitamin E		
Pyridoxine	Decrease in size and haemorrhages content of red cells	Microcytic, hypochromic, not responding to iron but responding to pyridxine.
Vitamin C	Decrease in number of red cells and presence of normoblasts and megaloblasts	Normocytic or macrocytic, and normochromic, responding to vitamin C.
Non –dietary factors:		
Deficiency of intrinsic factor	As in Vitamin B12 deficiency	Pernicious, intravenous injection of vitamin B12 or administration of intrinsic factor
Toxic agents (antibiotics, sulpha drugs)	Reduced synthesis of red cells	Aplastic, generally but not always responding to increased supply of nutrients.
haemorrhages	Loss of blood cells due to bleeding flowing injury, surgical operations or internal hemorrhages	Post hemorrhagic, generally, but not always responding to increased supply of nutrients
Chronic poisoning with lead, arsenic etc.	Decrease in life span of red cells due to their destruction	hemolytic
Intestinal parasites such as hook worm	As in iron deficiency	Microcytic, hypochromic treated by the elimination of parasites.

in anaemia although its role in haemoglobin synthesis is not known. As milk is deficient in both iron and copper, milk diets are found to produce anaemia. In children treated for anaemia, administration of some copper along with iron is found to be more effective. 'Tonics' used for the treatment of anaemia often contain some copper and a deficiency of the same is believed to be responsible for the hair turning brittle. Copper is a cofactor of many metabolic processes. Mitochondrial electron transport system which generates major part of ATP has components that contain copper. It is common knowledge that excessive amounts of copper are toxic. The practice of coating copper vessels with tin has been in vogue to avoid copper

Table 15. Hemoglobin content of blood in different groups.

Age	Hemoglobin (g) in 100 ml of blood		
	Urban Baroda		
	Lower Class[1]	Upper Class[1]	Western Subjects[2]
New Born	17.3	19.6	21.8
1-2 years	9.2	11.2	11.8
2–5 years	9.5	11.4	12.5
7–11 years	9.6	11.8	13.0
Adult men	12.7	13.5	15.0
Adult women*	10.1	11.5	13.5

[1] On the basis of data obtained in the Biochemistry Department of Baroda University.
[2] From Hawkins, W.W. 1964 in "Nutrition" edited by Beaton, G.R. and E.W. McHenry, Vol.
   Chapter 6, 24 p., Academic Press.
* The levels are about 1 percent less in pregnant and lactating women.

toxicity in foods. The use of improperly coated vessels for acid foods may result in chronic copper poisoning.

Cobalt

Cobalt is part of the compound cyanocobalamin or vitamin B12. Ruminant animals such as cows, in which the bacteria in the rumen synthesize this vitamin need cobalt in the diet. Cobalt is not likely to be required by man if the diet provides enough vitamin B12. However, administration of cobalt has been found to help in the treatment of certain types of anaemia.

Iodine and Fluorine

Iodine and fluorine are two trace elements whose role in nutrition has been receiving increasing attention.

Iodine is part of the molecule thyroxin the hormone manufactured by the thyroid gland which is important for several body functions. The two thyroid hormones secreted by the thyroid glands are thyroxin and triiodotyronin. The amino acid tyrosine is the precursor of biosynthesis of these two hormones. The biosynthesis of thyroxin takes place through a number of stages. Iodine is first trapped by the thyroid as iodide and later incorporated in the thyroxin molecule. The capacity of the thyroid to take up iodine can be judged from the fact that the concentration of Iodine in the thyroid is about 40,000 times that in the plasma. The iodine in thyroid combines with tyrosine to form iodotyrosine which is further converted to thyroxin. A defect in any one of these steps can affect the synthesis of thyroxin.

When the supply of iodine in the diet is deficient or its utilization by the thyroid is defective, the gland is enlarged and nodular growth called goiter may result (See plate). Apart from the development of goiter, impaired thyroid function result in low rate of metabolism and arrested growth. In areas where goitre is endemic there is a high percentage of feeble-mindedness and deaf-mutism because of adverse effects of deficiency of fetal growth.

In some regions both the soil and the water have a low iodine content. This is particularly true of mountain valleys where glaciers have removed most of the top soil containing iodine over the centuries. Some examples are regions of the Himalayas and Alps. The foods, produced in such regions are also low in iodine as might be expected. About 10% of the world's population is estimated to live in such regions in which goitre and deaf-mutism are endemic. In this country about 45 million people live in goitre areas and about 10 million of them are having clinical symptoms of iodine deficiency. Children are born with thyroid malfunction as the supply of iodine to fetus is poor when the maternal diet is poor in iodine. Iodine deficiency in the mother, therefore, has serious consequences for the child.

The incidence of cretinism and deaf-mutism in a community is found to be decreased when the supplies of iodine are increased. This is usually done by adding potassium iodide or iodate to salt in the ratio 1:10000. Addition in the form of iodate is preferable in the humid regions where the salt becomes moist and the iodine in iodide is likely to sublime. As a person can be expected to consume about 10 g of salt, this will provide about 100 micrograms of iodine. About 50–75 micrograms of iodine are found to be sufficient to prevent iodine deficiency. The distribution of iodised salt is common practice in the West. In this country, for the distribution of iodised salt to people living in the goitre belt about 200000 tons of the same will be required annually. National Iodine Deficiency Disorders Control Programme (NIDDCP) has been formed by the Government with a goal to reduce the prevalence of iodine deficiency disorders below 10 per cent in the entire country by A.D. 2012. The number of iodised salt manufacturing units has been increased substantially to meet the demand of iodised salt to achieve this goal.

Although the iodine content of plant foods depends on that of soil and water, some plants have the capacity to absorb more iodine than others. Spinach is one such plant and contains 20 microgram of iodine per 100g. Sea weeds, algae and marine fish living on algae are rich sources of iodine. The cod fish is particularly a good source.

Even when the diet is reasonably adequate in iodine goitre and thyroid malfunctioning may occur because of other reasons. Some plants contain the compounds like allyl isothiocyanate which interfere with the efficient utilization of iodine for the formation of thyroxin. These compounds are called goitrogens. Goitrogens are found in rape seeds, yellow turnip, cabbage and ground nut skin. But they are not consumed in such large amount as to affect thyroid function in man. Only experimental animals which are fed these foods as major component of diet develop deficiency symptoms. But in areas where cattle graze on goitrogenic weeds children consuming large quantities of milk may develop the disease. In most cases the effects of goitrogens are corrected by increasing dietary intake of iodine.

Viral infections acquired from contaminated drinking water have also been believed to precipitate deficiency of iodine. In some people one or other steps involved in the formation of thyroxin is affected because of genetic factors. Majority of such cases can be corrected by increasing the dietary intake of iodine.

The increasing use of atomic energy for potentially harmful as well as peaceful purpose has increased the level of radiation in atmosphere. In areas where this is high some of the milk and other foods are likely to become radioactive. The presence of radioactive substances in the body is harmful. However, radioactive iodine is not retained in the body if there is an adequate supply of non-radioactive iodine. If iodized salt is made available in such regions, it will help reduce the risks of radiation.

Fluorine

Although it has not been demonstrated that fluorine is essential for life, it has been found to play useful roles in the structure of teeth and bones. Whether or hot it is essential it seems desirable to have some fluorine in the diet in order to maintain a satisfactory skeletal structure.

Interest in fluorine was aroused by the observation that in regions where the fluorine content of water is high, the teeth are 'mottled' i.e. they have below normal calcification. In some areas the teeth are covered by a chalky layer at first and gradually acquire a yellow stain. It was also found that the incidence of dental caries is less in areas where the drinking water contained moderate amounts of fluorine, and more in areas where the water contains little or no fluorine. These observations suggested that water deficient in fluorine is associated with an increased incidence of dental caries whereas that containing excessive amounts is responsible for mottled and chalky teeth. In the latter case the bone is also sometimes found to be chalky and changed in structure.

Plants vary in their fluorine content even when grown in the same soil because of differences in their ability to absorb it. Cereals, spinach and potatoes supply moderate amounts (0.5–1.2 ppm). Tea is a particularly rich source of fluorine. Salt obtained from the sea contains moderate amounts. Because of variations in the fluorine content of the diet and drinking water, the total fluorine intakes may vary from 10–25 microgram per kg of body weight.

As mentioned earlier, bone matter is composed primarily of hydroxyapatite crystals of calcium phosphate. Part of the water in these crystals may be replaced by fluorine resulting in the formation of fluorapatite crystals. The moisture content of the bone is thereby reduced and the bone becomes harder and less susceptible to demineralization or excessive loss of calcium from the bone. With excessive fluorine they become brittle.

Osteoporosis is a disease found after middle age characterized by the demineralization of the bone. The prevalence of osteoporosis is less in areas where the water contains more fluorine. Treatment with fluorine is claimed to help in recovery from the disease. An adult consumes about 1–1.5 mg of fluorine derived from both food and water. The fluorine content of water may vary from below 0.25 ppm (parts per million) to above 8 ppm. The association between the level of fluorine in water and the condition of teeth and bones is shown in **Table 16.** Dental fluorosis and osteo-fluorosis are found in regions where the water contains more than 8 ppm of fluorine. It has also been found in regions where water contains 2.5–5 ppm but this may be due to some extra fluorine contained in sea salt. It would appear then that fluorine levels above 8 ppm may not be desirable ordinarily, whereas those above 3–5 ppm may not be desirable in areas where the salt is obtained from the sea. In this country symptoms such as mottled teeth are found even with relatively low levels of 3–5 ppm.

Excessive amounts of fluorine are toxic and may result in gastroenteritis, nephritis and liver damage. But this toxicity is found only when the intake is several times more than the amount consumed ordinarily, as is the case when water contains more than 8 ppm of fluorine. In such regions the supply of de-fluorinated drinking water is desirable.

In western countries the high incidence of dental caries is a serious problem. In some communities more than 50% of children of the school-going age are found to have several 'filled' teeth or artificial teeth. This is partly due to the increased consumption of sugar, sweets and soft drinks between meals. When the teeth are not brushed after a meal, bacteria act

Table 16. Fluoride content of water in relation to dental caries and fluorosis[1]

Fluoride content of water (parts per million)	Factors found in association
Negligible	Increased prevalence of dental caries
1-2	Reduced prevalence of dental caries
2-3	Appreciable prevalence of mottled teeth (dental fluorosis)
3–8	Increased prevalence of fluorosis
8 and above	Skeletal fluorosis or osteofluorosis

[1] afterNikiforuk, G and Grainger, R.M. 1964 in Nutrition edited by Beaton, G.H. and E.W. MacHenry, Academic Press, New York.

on the carbohydate residues in the teeth and break them down into organic acids which can corrode the enamel on teeth. Sugar is a good medium for the growth of such bacteria.

As stated earlier, a liberal amount of fluorine in water is found to prevent the incidence of dental caries. This is believed to be achieved in several ways. Some of the hydroxyapatite crystals are replaced by fluorapatite crystals which are not easily corroded by acids. The fluoride may also form a thin film on the surface of the teeth and act as a barrier against the action of acids. It also inhibits the action of bacteria which act on carbohydrates.

Because of the beneficial effects of fluorine on the prevention of dental caries, fluoridation programmes have been taken up in many areas in the west where the water has low levels of fluorine. The amount of fluorine added is usually adjusted so as to raise the level of fluorine in water to 0.50–0.75 ppm. Fluoridation at this level has not been found to have any harmful effects.

Topical application of fluorine over the teeth has been found to have beneficial effects. This has been exploited by manufacturers of fluoridated tooth pastes. The use of the same may not serve any purpose when fluorine supply in water is adequate and when reasonable care is taken of dental hygiene.

Selenium

Our understanding of Selenium in nutrition has grown during the past 25 years. Selenium has been implicated in the protection of body tissues against oxidative stress and defence against infection. Selenium is present in the body tissues as selenoproteins. Selenium is conjugated with sulphur amino acids of tissue proteins. There are distinct selenium containing enzymes which includes glutathione peroxidase and thioredoxin reductase. These are involved in controlling tissue concentration of highly reactive oxygen containing metabolites. These metabolites are essential at low concentration for cell mediated immunity against infections but highly toxic if produced in excess. Selenoenzymes protect against the damaging effects of hydrogen peroxide or oxygen rich free radicals.

Other minerals

Other elements such as, manganese, zinc, molybdenum also play a role in nutrition but they are needed only in very small amounts which are provided by ordinary diets. Zinc deficiency has been occasionally found in the Middle East due to diets rich in phytate and the habit of eating clay which interferes with its absorption. As mentioned earlier, zinc has a greater affinity for phytate than calcium.

Chapter 5

Vitamins

After the identification that carbohydrates, fats, proteins and minerals are the major components of the diet, experimental animals fed diets composed of these constituents in reasonable proportions failed to thrive. Similar findings had been made much earlier on children in Paris who were fed artificial milk composed of these constituents when milk supplies were interrupted due to war conditions. In the case of animals, growth was found to be restored by the addition of small quantities of yeast extract and butter fat to the diets fed. Both these substances were believed to contain unknown nutrients needed by the body in minute amounts. These unidentified nutrients were termed vital amines or vitamins, now called vitamins. All the known vitamins have now been isolated and their chemical structures identified. Many of them are synthesized commercially and are available at cheap rates. **Table 17** gives some of the important landmarks in the history of vitamins.

Some vitamins are soluble in fat but not in water whereas others are soluble in water but not in fat. They are, therefore, classified as fat-soluble and water-soluble Vitamins. The first vitamin discovered in the former category was called vitamin A and those in the latter category collectively as water-soluble B. When more water-soluble vitamins were discovered they were referred to as B1, B2 B6, B12, etc.

When more new vitamins were discovered in both categories they were referred as vitamins C, D, E, etc. Now most of the vitamins are known by a word which denotes either their chemical nature or function. Designation of vitamins by the letters assigned to them continues, however, as the role of a particular vitamin in the body can be served by more than one substance. For instance, ascorbic acid and dehydro-ascorbic acid can both serve as vitamin C.

Table 17. Vitamins[a].

Vitamin	Observations leading to discovery	Other observations	Isolation[b]	Commercial production
Vitamin A	Failure of animals and children to thrive on purified diets	Capacity of butter fat and yeast to restore growth: separation of water soluble and fat soluble factors from egg yolk	From butter fat in 1914	From lemon grass oil and other substances
Vitamin D	Rickets in children lacking adequate exposure to sunlight	Curative effect of fish oil and sunshine. Presence of a nutrient other than Vitamin A in butter.	From fish oil in 1938	By irradiation of ergosterol
Vitamin K	Hemorrhages in chickens fed on purified diets containing ether extracted fish meal	Curative value of whole fish meal, hog liver fat.	From alfalfa in 1938	From quinines obtained from petroleum products
Vitamin E	Failure of reproduction in rats fed on experimental diets.	Curative value of wheat germ and other foods.		From quinones
Thiamine	Incidence of beriberi in people consuming polished rice. Polyneuritis in birds	Curative value of rice polishing	From rice polishing in 1934	From pyridine and thiazole which are synthesized chemically.
Riboflavin	Identification of a factor other than thiamine in yeast.	Presence of this factor in whey, liver and greens	From whey powdering in 1933	From alloxan which can be synthesized chemically. Also by microbial synthesis
Nicotinic acid	Association of pellagra with maize consumption and deficiency of free nicotinic acid in maize	Curative value of high quality proteins as well as nicotinic acid	From yeast and rice polishing in 1911. The vitamin was identified to be the same as nicotinic acid produced from nicotine.	From quinoline or beta picoline obtained from petroleum products

contd...

contd...

Vitamin	Observations leading to discovery	Other observations	Isolation[b]	Commercial production
Vitamin C	Scurvy in sailors living on diets not including fresh vegetables and fruits.	Curative value of lemons, sprouted beans and pine needle extracts.	From lemon juice in 1932	From L-sorbose which is produced by bacteria from sorbitol.
Vitamin B12	Value of liver in the treatment of pernicious anaemia	Curative value of liver and identification of intrinsic factor	From liver in 1948	By microbial synthesis
Folic acid	Factor present in greens and required for the growth of certain bacteria, respon of anemic women to yeast.	Response of certain types of macro cytic anemia to folic acid isolated from green leaves	From spinach in 1946	from para-aminobenzoylglutamic acid
Pantothenic acid	Presence in most foods of a factor required for microbial growth	Effects of deficient diet on experimental animals.	From liver in 1938	From beta- alanine and pantonic acid
Pyridoxine	Skin lesions in rats not responding to nicotinic acid or other nutrients.	Curative value of crude extracts prepared from rice bran	From yeast in 1938	From ethoxyace-tylacetone
biotin	Toxic effects of egg white fed to rats	Presence in egg white of avidin and in egg yolk of biotin	From boiled yolks of duck eggs in 1936.	From fumaric acid

[a] The information given is based on that given in the vitamin (1954), Vols. I–III, (ed). W.H. Sebrell Jt and R.S. Harris. Academic Press, New York and in A History of Nutrition (1957) by E.V. McCollum, Houghton Miffin Company, Boston.

[b] The vitamins were often isolated at about the same time from different sources by different teams. The dates and sources given are selective.

The first vitamin isolated out of the B group is vitamin B1 or thiamine. Other substances with a similar role were also called vitamins. But now we know that all such essential substances are not amines. Thiamine (meaning sulphur containing amine), came to be so-called because it contains sulphur.

Vitamins are necessary for the metabolic reactions in the body. Certain substances block the function of vitamins and are called antimetabolites or metabolic antagonists. For instance, egg contains avidin which blocks the function of biotin, a vitamin. Similarly, an enzyme which breaks down thiamine is found in some fresh water fishes. 'Clover' taken by cattle contains a substance which is a folic acid antagonist. Most of these substances get destroyed when the food is cooked. The presence of antimetabolites or a metabolic antagonist in foods, therefore, limits the availability of vitamins and increases their requirements. Some Vitamins are synthesized by the intestinal microorganisms. When we take certain drugs and antibiotics these organisms are destroyed resulting in decreased vitamin synthesis and increased requirements. Other bacteria present in the intestine utilize dietary Vitamins for their use and produce vitamin deficiency. Ordinarily, vitamins in the diet are bound to protein or fat. During digestion they get broken down and absorbed. Therefore vitamins present in undigested food are not available to the body. The body requirements of vitamins depend, therefore, on several factors. Also, people suffering from diseases such as tuberculosis or high fever may require more vitamins. In cold regions and at high altitudes the requirement of certain vitamins may increase.

Let us now discuss the individual vitamins.

Fat Soluble Vitamins

Vitamin A

As mentioned before, vitamin A was first isolated from butter in 1913 and subsequently from egg yolk and liver. It is present in considerable amount in milk, butter, egg, fish and liver. It is present in very high amounts in the liver of halibut,cod and shark. The oil from these livers is separated and used as cod and shark liver oils. The highest amount of Vitamin A is present in the liver of the polar bear.

Vitamin A is not found in Plants. But many plant materials including dark green leafy vegetables and yellow and red vegetables and fruits contain substances called carotene which can be converted to vitamin A in the intestine. If the diet contains carotene in sufficient amounts we can get this vitamin without supply of ready made preformed vitamin A. Those who do not take milk, egg, butter and ghee should include enough of greens, vegetables and fruits rich in carotene in their diets. Even those who take these foods generally get a considerable amount of vitamin A in the form of its precursor, carotene.

Vitamin A is present in several forms such as vitamin A alcohol (retinol), vitamin A aldehyde (retinal) and vitamin A acid (retinoic acid). Of this vitamin acid is only of partial value as it cannot cure or prevent night-blindness caused by deficiency of vitamin A but it can restore growth.

Carotene belongs to a class of pigments called carotenoids which are yellow or red in colour. Some of the carotenoids are alpha, beta and gamma carotenes, and cryptoxanthine. Beta carotene is the most important of these because it is the major carotenoid present in foods. Further alpha carotene and cryptoxanthin cannot be converted to vitamin A whereas; theoretically beta carotene can be fully converted to vitamin A. That is, 1 g of vitamin A in the form of retinol can be obtained from 1 g of beta carotene. However, such complete conversion does not take place in the body. Studies with experimental animals and in man suggest that for obtaining 1 g of vitamin A 2.6 g of beta carotene may be necessary.

Before techniques were available for the chemical analysis of vitamin A the amount of vitamin A in food was determined from the amount required to abolish growth inhibition in rats. This amount is called an international unit (i.u.), 0.6 microgram beta carotene or 0.3 microgram vitamin A (retinol) is being considered equivalent to one international unit. However, it is becoming more usual to express in terms of micrograms and international units. It used to be the practice to express the vitamin A value of the food by adding up its carotene and vitamin A contents expressed as international units, but since the net amount of vitamin A available to the animal depends on how much of it is derived from carotene and how much from vitamin A, it is better to express the carotene and vitamin A contents separately.

Carotenes are present in green leafy vegetables and yellow and red fruits and vegetables. Hundred years before vitamin A was discovered carotene was isolated from carrots but its relation to vitamin A was discovered only in 1920.

Table 18 gives the carotene and vitamin A content of some foodstuffs.

The vitamin A absorbed from the intestine is stored largely in the liver and to some extent in the kidneys. In animals such as the rats carotene is not absorbed from the intestine. But in some other animals and man carotene is also absorbed from the intestine and is present in blood and adipose tissue giving it a yellowish tinge. Similarly carotenepresent in the cow's milk is responsible for its yellow tinge whereas buffalo milk which does not contain carotene and is white.

Certain amount of fat is required for the absorption of carotene in the intestine. If vitamin A is present thoroughly in emulsified form, fat is not required. Otherwise it is required for the absorption of vitamin A. Bile

Table 18. Selected foods as sources of carotene or vitamin A.

Carotene* μg per 100g	Leafy vegetables	Roots, bulbs and tubers	Other vegetables	Fruits	Other foods
Less than 60	-	Potato, sweet Potato, onion	Cauliflower, Cucumber, ladies Fingers, runner beans	Bor, apple, water-Melon, pine-apple, guava, grapes	Rice, ragi, white Maize, ground-nut, mutton, blackgram raisins
60–120	-	-	Brinjal, drum-stick, green mangoes, peas	Wood apple	Wheat, seasame seeds, milk-greengram
120–300	-	Yams	Bitter gourd, cluster beans, field beans, French beans, green tomatoes	Jack fruit, White melon	Bajra, yellow maize, bengalgram, redgram
300–600	-	-	Tender redgram, capsicum	Tender tomatoes, ray an, phalsa	soyabean
600–1800	Cabbage, mint	-	Yellow pumpkin	Papaya oranges, rock-melon	Egg, ghee, butter Hydrogenated oil
1800–3000	Mustard green Paruppukeerai, Ponnangani	Carrot	Kankoda	Some varities of mangoes	-
3000–6000	Amaranth, spinach, fenugreek	-	-	-	-

contd...

Carotene* µg per 100g	Leafy vegetables	Roots, bulbs and tubers	Other vegetables	Fruits	Other foods
Greater than 6000	Coriander leaves, colocasia leaves, drumstick leaves, curry leaves	-	-	Alphonso and ratnagiri mangoes	Liver, red palm oil.

* vitamin A in the case of foods of animal origin and hydrogenated oil..

salts which aid such emulsification are essential for the absorption of all the fat-soluble vitamins. The absorption of vitamin A is also affected in intestinal disorders. Since vitamin A is fat-soluble, the consumption of oils such as castor oil and paraffin oil which are not absorbed may interfere with its absorption, especially if they are consumed soon after a meal. Repeatedly heated fats which are also not well absorbed may have Similar effect.

For the efficient conversion of carotene to vitamin A and for the absorption, storage, transport and utilization of vitamin A, a satisfactory supply of protein seems to be needed. Animals fed a low protein diet are unable to utilize carotene well. Even when vitamin A is given, its utilization is defective in protein deficiency. Children suffering from kwashiorkor may fail to absorb vitamin A given orally unless their protein status is improved. In normal children, if vitamin A is given by injection, the serum level of the vitamin increases but comes back to normal as the surplus vitamin is removed from the serum and stored in the liver. In kwashiorkor serum levels fail to come down suggesting a defect in storage. Utilization of available vitamin also seems to be affected as some who had died of kwashiorkor and who had become blind on account of vitamin A deficiency were found to have plenty of vitamin A in the liver.

Vitamin A helps the body to fight against infections and is necessary for the proper development and function of the skin, eyes, bone and the nervous system.

Effects of vitamin A deficiency

Vitamin A is essential for the functioning of the mucus membrane which is found in the epithelial tissues of the eyes, the tear-glands and respiratory, gastro-intestinal and urogenital tracts. In deficiency, the mucus membrane atrophies and the secretion of mucus decreases or ceases. This results in a series of changes in the eye, the dryness of conjunctiva (conjunctivitis) being the earliest change observed. Gradually the cornea also becomes dry and lustreless (corneal xerosis). The corneal epithelium is normally transparent. The deposits resulting from the changes in the conjunctiva may result in the formation of pigmented spots on the same called Bitot's spots. A thin film may develop over the whole of the cornea making it opaque and decreasing its sensitivity.

Normally, the cornea is supplied by nutrients through lymph and secretions of the tear-glands and the above changes result in a poor supply of nutrients. This results in the rupture of the blood capillaries in surrounding tissues resulting in corneal vascularization. The above changes are followed by the softening of the cornea (keratomalacia) and ulceration, associated with necrosis. This is a serious condition and must be treated promptly with massive doses of vitamin A by injection. Otherwise, rupture of the cornea may result causing irreversible changes such as the extrusion of the lens and infection of the whole eye ball. The role of vitamin A in the formation of mucus secreting cells which makes the epithelial linings of the eyes, lungs and such other sensitive areas of the body are now well established. The mucus secreted by these cells offers resistance to infections thereby protecting the linings of the lungs, eyes and such other sensitive areas. This is the reason why in vitamin A deficiency lung and eye infections are common.

One of the major functions of vitamin A is in vision in dim light or what is known as dark adaptation of the eyes. The retina of the eye contains a pigment called rhodopsin which is made up of retinal and a protein called opsin. When light falls on the retina rhodopsin breaks into retinal and opsin. When this happens a retinal potential is formed in the retina which is picked up by the optic nerves and conducted to the visual centres of the brain. When not illuminated opsin and retinal combine together to form rhodopsin. The make and break of rhodopsin is a process involved in vision in dim light or what is known as dark adaptation of the eyes. In vitamin A deficiency the supply of the pigment rhodopsin is limited and this affect vision in dim light. In vitamin A deficiency the person is unable to see objects in dim light and this condition is known as night blindness.

Bone development is also affected in vitamin A deficiency. The bone contains substances called mucopolysaccharides for the synthesis of which vitamin A is required. As mentioned earlier, bone is formed in three stages. First, Some cells form a fibrous network embedded in a 'cement' or ground substance. This substance is made of complex compounds called mucopolysaccharides derived from carbohydrates and proteins. Vitamin A is also necessary for the dissolution of cartilage and bone and the remodeling of the bone. In vitamin A deficiency the bones become short and thick and irregular in shape. In the very young animal the full development of the skull and vertebrae are affected resulting in pressure on the brain and spinal cord.

In vitamin A deficiency the skin becomes rough and dry and horny plugs are formed around the roots of hair and hair follicle giving rise to a condition called phrynoderma. This is particularly seen around the elbows and knees. The horny plug is due to the deposition of keratin and the condition is referred to as hyper follicular keratosis. The oily secretions of the skin are diminished in this condition. However, phrynoderma has often been found in this country in the absence of vitamin A deficiency also and has been attributed to a deficiency of essential fatty acids. In animal studies, both deficiencies are found to produce somewhat similar skin changes.

When rats are given a diet totally lacking in vitamin A, reproductive performance is affected. Either no pregnancy occurs or pups are born with congenital abnormalities including blindness and die soon after birth.

The requirements of vitamin A are believed to vary with age and body-weight. The amounts recommended by the FAO are shown in **Table 19**. In poor Indian diets most of the vitamin A has to be derived in the form of carotene. As carotene is not converted fully to vitamin A in the body, carotene requirements may be six times as much according to the FAO expert Committee.

However, three to four micrograms of carotene appear to be as effective as one microgram of Vitamin A in studies carried out by the author's laboratory at Baroda so that four times the amount of vitamin A recommended may be adequate if taken as carotene. Vitamin A requirements are between 300–700 micrograms for most age groups so that a carotene supply of 1200–2800 micrograms per day should be adequate. This is supplied by about 30–50 g of fresh dark green leafy vegetables. Fifty to seventy grams may be necessary if cooking losses are taken into account as about a third of the carotene present in foods is lost during cooking.

In feeding trials, about 30 g are found to be adequate for normal vitamin A status in the case of pre-school children and fifty gram in older subjects.

As against a requirement of about 1000-1500 microgram of carotene, ordinary diets in this country provide only about 600 microgram. In many regions the supply is much less. It is not surprising that symptoms of vitamin A deficiency, particularly, eye symptoms and night-blindness are widely prevalent in this country. The same can be prevented and cured by

Table 19. Dietary allowances for vitamin A[2].

Age		Recommended intake (µg)	
		Vitamin A[1]	carotene[2]
0-6	months	300–400	1200–1600
6–12	"	300	1200
1	year	250	800
2	years	250	800
3	"	250	800
4–6	"	300	1200
7–9	"	400	1600
10–12	"	575	2300
13–15	"	725	2900
16–19	"	750	3000
Adults	"	750	3000

[1] according to amount in breast milk for the youngest age group and FAO Expert Committee recommendation for other ages.

[2] assuming that 4 µg of carotene are equivalent to 1 µg of vitamin A. This is 6 ug according to the FAO committee.

taking regularly vegetables and fruits rich in carotene. Another important factor governing vitamin A deficiency is adequacy of protein intake. It has been observed that symptoms of vitamin A deficiency exist in protein malnutrition among children. Serum proteins are involved in the transport of vitamin A to the various tissues where Vitamin A is utilized. The transport of vitamin A is thus affected when serum proteins level go down.

Prevalence and prevention of vitamin A deficiency

Vitamin A deficiency continues to be a problem in India and most of the cases of blindness is acquired in the post weaning period primarily due to vitamin A deficiency. keratomalacia which may result in blindness is found more often in children suffering from severe kwashiorkor especially in regions such as Tamil Nadu. Their diets are seriously deficient in both protein and vitamin A. Children in Tamil Nadu suffering front keratomalacia are also found to show photophobia. This may be due to concurrent deficiency of riboflavin as well.

In Gujarat and other similar regions young children show less vitamin A deficiency than adolescents and pregnant mothers. This may be because their diets here are not different from those of adults, but only restricted in quantity and may contain 250–300 microgram of vitamin A as against 60 microgram in rice-eating areas. Their serum level of vitamin A is about 20 microgram per 100 ml as against 5–10 in very poor children in rice-eating areas. They do show, however, milder symptoms.

Severe vitamin A deficiency must be treated promptly with massive doses of vitamin A to prevent irreversible changes in the eye. But milder symptoms can be easily cured and serious deficiency prevented by the regular consumption of leafy vegetables and other carotene-rich vegetables and fruits. Alternatively other concentrated sources of vitamin A should be made available. Vitaminised oil can be distributed to children and mothers. In studies carried out at Baroda vitamin A added groundnut oil was given to the mothers who were asked to add a teaspoon of the oil (giving some 300 microgram of vitamin A) to food consumed by the child (roti, rice, conjee, etc.). Night-blindness is common in adults and pregnant women in this country. The deficiency of vitamin A in pregnancy seems to be partly physiological as the condition improves after delivery without dietary improvement.

It is unfortunate that we have the highest incidence of blindness in this country, most of it caused during childhood by vitamin A deficiency. This tragedy could be prevented by the simple and expedient cultivation and consumption more of green leafy vegetables.

About 60% of the poorer sections of the population in this country are found to suffer from some degree of vitamin A deficiency. There is now a worldwide awareness of the need for preventing this, particularly blindness and night-blindness caused by vitamin A deficiency. It is particularly important to ensure that young children who do not get enough milk, eggs, etc. are given daily one or other of the carotene-rich foods such as leafy vegetables, carrots, yellow pumpkin, papaya, mangoes, etc. The vegetables can be boiled and mashed so as to make them suitable for very young children. Alternatively, oil enriched with vitamin A should be made available for young children by the Panchayats and municipal bodies and used in feeding programmes where they are in operation. In some areas, young children are given massive doses of vitamin A once or twice a year.

Hypervitaminosis A

Excessive consumption of vitamin A results in hypervitaminosis. In hypervitaminosis the skin becomes rough and thick and the bones become soft and fragile. In the case of the young, bone development is affected. Excess vitamin A interferes with the utilization of vitamin K in the body. Vitamin K is necessary for the clotting of blood and hence there is an increased tendency for bleeding in hypervitaminosis A. Hypervitaminosis A has resulted in death in arctic explorers due to the consumption of polar bear liver or seal liver which may contain more than 4500 microgram of vitamin A per gram.

Ordinary diets based on natural foods do not result in hypervitaminosis A as the symptoms are found only when the amounts consumed are about hundred times those consumed normally. Prolonged ingestion of less generous amounts (say, ten times the required amount) may also result in hypervitaminosis A. This has happened when children are given shark or halibut liver oil in place of cod liver oil in the belief that the two are similar while, in fact, the former contain much more vitamin A (2500–3600 microgram/g) than the latter (300 to 1800 microgram/g).

Vitamin D

Rickets, a disease involving gross malformation of the skeleton was common in young children living in cold climates. As early as the 18th century cod liver oil was used as a traditional folk remedy for rickets and has been used by physicians for more than a hundred years. Early in this century, it was found that rickets produced in, puppies by a poor diet could be cured by a factor isolated from cod liver oil. This factor was first isolated from butter and named vitamin D.

An association was also suspected in the last century between the prevalence of fog and lack of sunshine in industrial cities such as London and the incidence of rickets. Severely rachitic children were found to be cured by subjecting them to ultraviolet light. Certain foods when subject to ultraviolet radiation were also found to cure rickets. Subsequently, it was found that certain sterols present in the animal body (7-dehydrocholesterol) and in yeast and fungi (ergosterol) possess vitamin D activity When irradiated. As vitamin D is necessary for proper bone calcification, it was called calciferol (to signify an alcohol promoting calcification). Cholecalciferol(Vitamin D3) is formed from 7-dehydrocholesterol present in the skin during exposure to sunlight and ergocalciferol (vitamin D2) is formed from ergosterol with Ultra-violet irradiation.

As vitamin D can be synthesized in the body with adequate exposure to sunlight it is not generally needed in the diet. However, when such exposure is restricted because of living in dark, poorly ventilated houses, a deficiency may result. Deficiency is often found in young children who are kept indoors most of the time. It was also found in Muslim women in the Middle East and elsewhere because of the custom of 'purdah' (veil).,

As mentioned before, calcium is required for the development of bone. Vitamin D is required for the absorption of calcium from the intestine as well as the proper utilization of both calcium and phosphorus for bone development. As it is difficult to separate vitamin D from foods and estimate it, it was usual to estimate the amount present in a food by its capacity to restore bone development in rats in which bone growth is arrested by feeding a diet severely deficient in calcium or phosphorus. Vitamin D activity, therefore, came to be measured in terms of international units (i.u.). Now that vitamin D can be chemically estimated and 1 microgram of the Vitamin is found to be equal to 40 i.u.

In foods vitamins A and D are often found in association with each other. The vitamin D content of selected foods is shown below:

Vitamin D	(i.u. per 100 g)
milk	1–4
butter	30–100
egg, whole	50–60
egg, yellow part	150–400
fat fish	200–1800
shark liver oil	1300–5000
cod liver oil	8000–30000
halibut liver oil	20000–400000

In general, plant foods have no vitamin D activity although vitamin D like activity is suspected in two plant species which do not form part of our diet. People living predominantly on plant foods must, therefore, get either adequate exposure to sunlight or synthetic vitamin D. In vitamin D deficiency the utilization of both calcium and phosphorus are impaired and losses of phosphorus through the kidney are increased. The latter may result in low serum levels of phosphorus. When the diet is deficient in calcium as well, serum calcium levels may also be decreased resulting in,tetany. In severe cases this may end in death.

As mentioned earlier, bone mineral is deposited over a network of collagen fibres held in place by the ground substances. Because of this, bone combines great hardness with tensile strength. In vitamin D deficiency, the amount of bone mineral deposited is reduced. In young children, the ends of the long bones are cartilaginous and their gradual replacement by true bone is also affected in vitamin D deficiency. Because of these factors, the shape, structure and strength of bone are affected.

Children suffering from rickets are recognized by rather obvious symptoms such as bow legs, flat feet, pigeon chest and beaded ribs. Bead-shaped 'swellings' appear in the ribs on either side of the chest bone so as to resemble a rosary (chain). This is called the rachitic rosary. They are pot-bellied, lethargic, apathetic and irritable on touch. Often, a recovery occurs after the age of four or five years, but some of the symptoms such as bow legs and flat feet may remain.

As mentioned earlier, the parathyroid hormone which has an important role in bone metabolism and calcium homeostasis needs vitamin D for its action. The biological action of vitamin D2 and vitamin D3 are at two levels. One is at the level of calcium absorption by the intestinal mucosal cells and the other is at the level of calcium deposition on the bones. It is now well established that both the effects are mediated by the biologically active forms of Vitamin D2 and vitamin D3. Vitamin D2 and vitamin D3 undergo activation process by 25 hydroxylation in the liver to form 25-hydroxycholecalciferol and 25-hydroxy ergocalciferol. These two compounds are the biologically active forms of Vitamin D. These two compounds and parathyroid hormone regulate calcium absorption by the intestinal mucosa and calcium deposition on the bone and desorption from the bone. The homeostatic mechanism mediated by the above two vitamin D metabolites and parathyroid hormone maintains the calcium level in the blood within a narrow range.

A major amount of phosphorus in plants is present as phytate. Phytate is not absorbed in the intestine. In the intestine some of the phytate is broken down by an enzyme called phytase. Vitainin D seems to facilitate the activity of phytase.

The body contains calcium and phosphorus approximately in the ratio of 2:1. The requirement for the two may be of the order of 1:1 as relatively more phosphorus than calcium is lost from the body. The utilization of either calcium or phosphorus is not efficient when their ratio deviates appreciably from this value. Vitamin D helps in their utilization in spite of an unbalanced ratio.

Requirements

It is not known how much vitamin D is required by the body. About 400–800 i.u. are considered sufficient for young children. However, breast milk contains much less than this and breast-fed children do not normally show deficiency if they have adequate exposure to sunlight. The requirements, if any, are less in older age groups.

As sunlight is plentiful in India a supply of vitamin D may not seem a problem except when mothers do now allow their children to play outdoors in the sun. Although severe vitamin D deficiency results in rickets, no abnormalities of the bone are evident with mild deficiency, but skeletal growth and maturation are slowed down and the bone of a three-year old, for instance, may look like that of a 2 to 2.5 year old on an X-ray examination. Such retarded bone development is found in many young children.

Vitamin D deficiency is also found in pregnant and nursing mothers who observe purdah and do not get enough sunlight. No vitamin D deficiency is usually found in older children as they manage to spend enough time outdoors.

Rickets used to be more common in Britain, particularly Scotland. It has now practically disappeared due to the fortification of milk and other foods with vitamin D. However, both rickets and osteomalacia(rickets in adults) have been found occasionally in persons of Pakistani or Indian origin presumably because of changes in their living habits and exposure to sunlight. In Germany, osteomalacia was found in older adolescents and young men who had to work long hours in factories without adequate exposure to sunlight during World War II.

Hypervitaminosis D

In order to eradicate rickets which was highly prevalent in Britain, the practice of fortifying foods such as milk, breakfast foods, bread, etc. was introduced. It can be seen from the data given earlier that the vitamin D content of fish oil differs from species to species. The unwary mothers often substituted halibut or cod liver oil which contains much more vitamin D for shark liver oil. This resulted in an overdose of vitamin D. If this is also associated with an excessive intake of calcium, serum calcium increases and calcium is deposited in soft tissues such as the kidney, heart, eyes and abdomen. The joints become swollen and stiff and muscular movements difficult and painful. In such cases a diet devoid of vitamin D and low in calcium should be promptly introduced.

Resistant rickets

Rickets caused by excessive loss of phosphate in urine may also occur because of hereditary factors. Such cases may fail to respond to ordinary treatment. This condition was called resistant rickets. Very high doses of vitamin D are found to help in this case.

Vitamin K

The discovery of vitamin K followed the observation that hens, fed a purified diet died of haemorrhages and this could be prevented by the addition of alfalfa to the diet. The curative factor was isolated from alfalfa and found to be present in many greens especially in spinach. It was called vitamin K because of its role in the coagulation (spelt koagulation in European languages) of blood. It is synthesized by microorganisms.

Normally, blood flows in the body without clotting as otherwise normal circulation is not possible. But when bleeding occurs at any site because of injury, the blood clots and the bleeding is stopped. The clot is made of fibrin, a protein which is deposited as fine threads to form a network. The formation of fibrin from its precursor fibrinogen requires thrombin. Thrombin is formed from prothrombin and this process requires calcium and vitamin K. Thus vitamin K is essential for the clotting of blood.

As vitamin K is synthesized in the intestine by the intestinal microflora a deficiency of vitamin K is seldom found. However, deficiency may occur because of either poor absorption or synthesis. The latter occurs following treatment with sulfonamides and antibiotics. Poor absorption is found in diarrhoea and liver disease because of deficiency of bile salt which are needed for the absorption of fat soluble vitamins. Vitamin K deficiency is sometimes found in newborn children (especially premature children). This can be prevented by giving vitamin K to the mothers a few days or hours before delivery. Alternatively, vitamin K is given by injection to the mothers just before delivery (Or to the child soon after birth). A small percentage of the children (0.1–1%) die of haemorrhage caused by vitamin K deficiency and this can be prevented to a large extent by following the above procedures, preferably by treating the mother. However, indiscriminate administration of synthetic vitamin K (K3 or menadione) to the newborn infant is found to result in jaundice. This is not found when natural forms of the vitamin of either plant (K1) or bacterial (K2) origin are used.

Vitamin E

During the course of certain experiments, animals fed a diet containing protein, lard, carbohydrates, minerals, butter and yeast could grow but failed to reproduce. Reproduction became normal when lard was replaced by vegetable oils suggesting that some nutrient not present in lard is provided by the vegetable oils. This substance was later isolated from wheat germ oil and called vitamin E.

Vitamin E has been named tocopherol meaning an alcohol necessary for child bearing. Different forms of vitamin E have been identified; alpha tocopherol is the most important of these from the nutritional standpoint as it is more completely utilized by the body.

It is not yet known definitely how vitamin E functions in the body. As an antioxidant it may prevent the uncontrolled oxidation of fatty acids in cells, especially those in the cell-membranes. Thus it may be important for preserving the integrity of cells.

In experimental animals subjected to deficiency of vitamin E many symptoms are found including haemolysis of blood (rapid destruction of red blood cells due to changes in the cell membrane), muscular dystrophy (wasting of muscle), and infertility in the male and unsuccessful pregnancy in the female due to the failure of fetuses to develop.

A deficiency of vitamin E severe enough to affect reproductive performance has not been found in man. However, an increased tendency for the blood to haemolyse resulting in haemorrhage and death have been found in some newborn and premature infants and this is associated with low blood levels of vitamin E.

Blood levels of vitamin E are found to be relatively low in malnourished children either because of poor intake or poor absorption. They are also low in conditions affecting the absorption of fats generally. Haemolytic anemia attributed to vitamin E deficiency has been reported in the Middle East.

In the presence of vitamin E, vitamin A oxidation is also prevented and thus vitamin A is protected from destruction.

Fats of vegetable origin are rich sources of vitamin E. Vegetable oils and oils of food grains may contain 50–100 mg per l00g but coconut oil contains only 8 mg. Wheat germ oil contains 260 mg/100 g. The chief sources in the Indian diet are thus vegetable oils other nuts, oilseeds and whole grains. However, when vegetable oils are refined some vitamin E may be lost. Many dark green leafy vegetables contain 0.5–1.5 g of fat per 100 g (0.5–1.5 mg of vitamin E). Requirements are estimated to vary between 10–30 mg and found to depend on the amount of polyunsaturated fatty acids in the diet. Thus the requirement may be less with diets containing less fat, specially unsaturated fat.

Amount in ordinary diets

The average western diet is estimated to contain about 15 mg of vitamin E. The poor Indian diet may be expected to contain a similar amount, About 20 g of oil would provide 10 mg and 400 g of food grains is expected to contain 6–8 g of fat and containing 3-4 mg of vitamin E. However, rice contains less fat and in areas such as Tamil Nadu, oil consumption is only about 5–10 g so that the diets may provide less than 5 mg of vitamin E. This is also the case in tribal people such as the Bhils of Gujarat state who hardly Use any cooking fat. It may be even less in Kerala where coconut oil is consumed. No information is available on the vitamin E status of these different groups. Serum levels in children and pregnant women are somewhat lower than values reported in the west.

An appreciable prevalence of more than a mild deficiency must be ruled out as haemolytic anaemia of the type associated with vitamin E deficiency has not been reported. This may be because the diets are low not only in vitamin E but also in fat. Vitamin E is stored in the muscle and adipose tissue. High concentrations are found in the uterus and testes.

Because vitamin E deficiency was found to impair reproduction in experimental animals, abortions were sought to be treated by vitamin E supplements but generally without any effect. A deficiency of vitamin E has also been believed to be one of the factors responsible for heart disease and prevention and treatment of this disease with vitamin E supplements have been attempted, but the results are conflicting. However, in view of the demonstrated effects of deficiency in other species it would seem desirable to include in the diet adequate quantities of whole grains, oilseeds or their oils and leafy vegetables.

Water soluble Vitamins

As mentioned earlier, yeast extract was found to contain nutrients vital for body functions. At about the same time rice polishings were found to contain a factor capable of preventing and curing beriberi. Funk who obtained this in the pure state called it the anti-beriberi factor. Subsequently, it came to be called vitamin B1 or thiamine. Later, other vitamins have been identified and isolated from yeast extract and other sources.

Thiamine (Vitamin B1)

Beriberi is a disease associated with the exclusive consumption of highly polished rice. It is widely prevalent in many regions of Asia. In a small country such as Philippines 25000 deaths used to occur annually due to this disease. A naval medical officer of Japan was the first to suspect that beriberi is a deficiency disease caused by some deficiency in the diet. However, he believed the deficiency to be due to lack of good quality proteins. Some time later, Eijkman, a physician working in the Dutch East Indies (Indonesia), found that polished rice caused polyneuritis in birds and that this could he prevented by feeding whole rice or by adding the rice polishings. His colleagues found the prevalence of beriberi in man to be associated with the consumption of polished rice. The vitamin was later isolated from rice polishings and obtained in crystalline form. Other scientists were able to synthesize thiamine which is now manufactured commercially.

Thiamine is important for the metabolism of carbohydrate in the body. The most important function of thiamine is the synthesis of thiamine pyrophophate (TPP) a coenzyme required in the metabolism of carbohydrates. As stated earlier, glucose is converted to a series of compounds in the body resulting in its slow oxidation by stages. Pyruvic acid is an important compound in this series and this compound requires thiamine pyrophosphate for its further metabolism. In thiamine deficiency, pyruvate fails to get oxidized and is converted to lactic acid which accumulates in the tissues. As carbohydrate is the major fuel source utilized by the body and the only fuel used by the brain, the importance of thiamine can be well imagined.

The thiamine content of selected foods is shown in **Table 20**. Whole grain cereals and legumes are the major sources of thiamine in the diet. Most of the thiamine is found in the outer layer of grains much of which is removed during milling. Highly milled rice and refined flour are poor sources thiamine. Parboiled rice is a much better source as the thiamine diffuses from the outer layer into the inside portion of the grain during parboiling and hence not removed on milling. Legumes are generally very good sources and animal foods including milk are relatively poor sources. During the fermentation of products such as 'idli' thiamine content is found to increase appreciably.The bacteria involved in 'idli' fermentation synthesize the vitamin required for its growth.

The requirement of thiamine depends on various factors such as carbohydrate and energy intakes. Some amount is also synthesized by intestinal bacteria but this is not sufficient to meet the required amounts in most individuals. The requirement is estimated to be of the order of 0.3-0.4 mg per 1000 Calories and the FAQ recommends an allowance of 0.4 mg per 1000 Calories. Ordinary diets consumed by the poor which do not include much of pulses provide about 0.8 mg per 1000 Calories in regions where food grains other than rice are used as staple. Diets based on parboiled rice provide about 0.65 mg and those based on polished rice, 0.30 mg per 1000 calorie. Upper class diet based on polished rice provides more because of the greater consumption of foods such as pulses, vegetables, milk, etc.

Thiamine deficiency is found in regions where highly polished rice is consumed and used to be found to some extent in Andhra Pradesh and to a much greater extent in the Philippines. In both regions the incidence seems to be declining. It was also found in the west with the advent of refined flour but now the refined flour used for making bread in most western countries

Table 20. Thiamine, riboflavin and nicotinic acid content of selected food stuffs.

	mg per 100g			mg per 1000 Calories		
	Thiamine	riboflavin	Nicotinic Acid	Thiamine	Riboflavin	Nicotinic Acid
Wheat	0.45	0.17	5.5	1.3	0.49	15.9
Maize	0.42	0.10	1.8	1.2	0.30	5.3
Rice: Parboiled	0.27	0.12	4.0	0.8	0.34	11.4
Handpounded	0.21	0.16	3.9	0.6	0.46	11.3
Polished	0.06	0.06	1.9	0.2	0.20	5.5
Bajra	0.33	0.25	2.3	0.9	0.65	5.4
Jowar	0.37	0.13	3.1	1.0	0.37	6.4
Kodri	0.33	0.09	2.0	1.0	0.30	6.5
Refined flour	0.12	0.07	2.4	0.3	0.20	6.8
Bengalgram (dal)	0.48	0.18	2.4	1.3	0.48	6.5
Redgram (dal)	0.45	0.19	2.9	1.3	0.57	8.6
Black gram (dal)	0.42	0.37	2.0	1.2	1.08	5.8
Greengram	0.47	0.39	2.1	1.4	0.80	4.1
Soyabean	0.73	0.39	3.2	1.7	1.17	7.4
Sesame	1.01	0.34	4.4	2.0	060	7.8
Groundnut	0.90	0.13	19.9	1.6	0.23	35.1
tapioca	0.05	0.10	1.4	0.3	0.60	8.9
Potato	0.10	0.01	1.2	1.0	0.1	12.0
Brinjal (egg plant)	0.04	0.11	0.9	1.7	4.6	37.5
Onions	0.08	0.01	0.4	1.6	0.2	8.0
Fenugreek leaves	0.04	0.31	0.8	0.8	6.3	10.3
Spinach leaves	0.03	0.26	0.5	1.1	10.0	19.2
Amaranth leaves	0.03	0.30	1.2	0.7	7.0	26.6
Milk						
Cow	0.05	0.19	0.1	0.7	2.8	1.5
Buffalo	0.04	0.10	0.1	0.3	0.8	0.8
Egg	0.10	0.40	0.1	0.6	2.3	0.4
Mutton	0.18	0.14	6.8	0.9	0.7	35.2
Chicken	0.05	0.09	11.0	0.4	0.8	92.0
Sheep liver	0.36	1.70	17.6	2.4	11.3	117.3
Fish (pomfret, white)	-	0.15	2.6	-	1.7	28.8
Yeast, dried (brewer's)	6.0	4.00	40.0	18.7	12.5	125.0

is fortified with thiamine. However, even in the West thiamine deficiency is found in people given to excessive consumption of alcohol.

Thiamine deficiency results in several disorders. The most common disorder is beriberi characterized by several symptoms, Some of them are loss of appetite and nausea. Numbness, soreness, heaviness and weakness of the legs and other muscles are common findings. General weakness and shortness of breath are commonly experienced. Paralysis of the leg muscles results with severe deficiency. The subject becomes depressed,irritable and confused and experiences vague fears and uneasiness.

Beriberi is classified as wet beriberi and dry beriberi. In the former, oedema is prominent. In the latter, there is neuritis and the heart may also be affected. One form often changes into the other.

Normally, the breast-fed infant is well-nourished and healthy and mortality in breast-fed infants is very low. However, when the maternal diet is poor in thiamine the breast milk is also poor and the infant develops infantile beriberi characterized by several symptoms such as palpitation of heart, vomiting, oedema, wasting and aphonia (crying without producing audible sound). The condition often results in death.

Generally, even in poorly nourished communities, mortality before the age of six months is low as the breast-fed child is usually a healthy child, whereas mortality after weaning, specially between 1–3 years of age is quite high. In regions where polished rice is the staple, mortality before 4-5 months of age is quite high because of the prevalence of infantile beriberi.

Beriberi can be prevented by the under milling of rice or the use of parboiled rice and adequate consumption of pulses. It is more common in Andhra Pradesh where polished rice is consumed than in Tamil Nadu or Kerala where the poor people consume parboiled rice. In rice consuming regions, it would be desirable to include other grains such as wheat and bajra along with rice. This is already being done to some extent.

In certain countries rice and refined flour are fortified with thiamine and other nutrients and beriberi has been completely eradicated in these countries. But in India the presence of many rice mills and flour mills all over the country, and the fact that most of the food consumed is locally produced and does not pass through a central distribution system, makes such fortification difficult. It would seem more practicable to popularize the consumption of parboiled or under milled rice and the inclusion in the diet of other cereals such as wheat and bajra.

Riboflavin (Vitamin B2)

As mentioned earlier, yeast extract when added to purified diets was found to have restored survival and growth and the factors responsible in yeast extract were collectively called water soluble B. The first factor isolated was thiamine. It soon became evident that other factors essential for metabolism are also present in yeast. These factors are now collectively referred to as vitamins of the 'B' complex group. Thiamine is destroyed more easily than riboflavin and this led to the identification of the latter as a separate substance. Riboflavin was obtained in a concentrated form from whey as a yellow pigment with green fluorescence. A similar substance was obtained from yeast. This was termed variously as vitamin B2, yellow enzyme, lactoflavin, etc. Since the substance contains the sugar ribose, it was finally termed riboflavin. Like many other vitamins riboflavin is now synthesized commercially.

Riboflavin is necessary for the metabolism of fat and carbohydrate. It plays an important role in enzymes involved in tissue respiration. Flavin Adenine Dinuleotide (FAD)and Flavin Mononucleotide (FMN) are coenzymes of many ezymes of carbohydrate and fat metabolism. Both these coenzymes have riboflavin as part of their structures and hence in deficiency of riboflavin, carbohydrate and fat metabolism will be sluggish.

Table 20 shows the riboflavin content of selected foods. Animal foods are by far the best sources of riboflavin. Among plant foods leafy vegetables are good sources. The diets based on vegetable foods riboflavin tend to be a limiting nutrient. But the riboflavin content of such diets can be increased by a more liberal intake of greens and the frequent use of sprouted and fermented foods as the vitamin is found to be synthesized during sprouting and fermentation.

The amount of riboflavin required depends on the protein content and calorie value of the diet. About 0.4 mg per 1000 calories is found to be required and the FAO recommends 0.5 mg per 1000 calories as a desirable amount. The poor Indian diets provide per 1000 calories 0.3, 0.5 and 0.6 mg if based on milled rice, parboiled rice and mixed grains respectively. These amounts would be less if cooking losses are taken into account.

A deficiency of riboflavin results in several clinical symptoms such as changes in lips, tongues corners of lips and eyes. The lips become dry and chaffed (cheilosis), the tongue becomes red and shiny (glossitis) and develops fissures with yellowish colour(fissured tongue). The angles at the corners of the mouth become ulcerated (angular stomatitis) (See plate). The exposed part of the eye-ball is covered by a delicate membrane called the conjunctiva which is continued forward on to the inner surfaces of the lids. In riboflavin deficiency the conjunctiva becomes red and inflamed and eye-lids appear swollen and matted together with a sticky substance (conjunctivitis). They also become abnormally sensitive to light. Intrusion of the small blood capillaries into the cornea is also found (corneal vascularization).

Some of these symptoms in the mouth and tongue are also found in other deficiencies (for instance, of nicotinic acid) and in association with non-dietary factors (e.g. amoebic and other infections which may perhaps increase requirements). However,when the diets are deficient in riboflavin and many of the symptoms occur together it would be reasonable to conclude that they are caused by a dietary lack of the vitamin.

Symptoms of riboflavin deficiency are common in India because of the lack of animal foods rich in this vitamin. About 80% of adolescent boys and pregnant women are found to show symptoms of deficiency in the mouth and lips. The deficiency symptoms are found to clear gradually with an improved diet and more rapidly with supplements of 10–15 mg of riboflavin per day. In studies carried out in Baroda deficiency symptom were found to clear in most of the children fed a good lunch containing leafy vegetables and sprouted and fermented legumes for a period of 6 months.

Nicotinic acid

Nicotinic acid was first prepared from nicotine in 1867 but its physiological role remained unknown till much later. The curative value of rice-polishing in beriberi led to a search for the factor involved. Nicotinic acid was identified in the same but it was found to have no value in the treatment of beriberi.

A disease known as pellagra (rough skin) associated with the consumption of maize was known in South Italy as early as the 18th century and was suspected to be due to the poor protein quality of the diet. The disease was also suspected to be due to infection and the presence of toxic factors in maize. In the 19th and early part of the 20th century the disease was found in association with maize consumption in the U.S.A. In the early studies, tryptophan or good quality proteins were found to be effective. Yeast and lean meat were found to contain the pellagra-preventive factor.

A similar disease was produced experimentally in dogs by Chittenden in 1917 and Goldberger in 1928. This disease, characterized by black tongue, was found to be prevented and cured by the administration of nicotinic acid or its amide.

Pellagra is characterized by lesions of the skin (dermatitis). Symmetrical butterfly-shaped patches on the cheeks are found typically. A glossy tongue is often found as in the case of riboflavin deficiency. Diarrhoea and mental changes (dementia) are common and the disease came to be called the disease of 3 D's (dermatitis, diarrhoea and dementia) and was particularly more prevalent in alcoholics. It was found later that the disease could be cured and prevented by consuming a good protein diet including milk, meat, legumes etc. Subsequently, it was recognized that maize is deficient in the amino acid tryptophan which can be converted to nicotinic acid in the body. Although maize contains nearly as much nicotinic acid as other grains, most of it is believed to be in a bound form not absorbed by the intestine. Nicotinic acid was, therefore, believed to be the chief deficiency in maize diets and the administration of large amounts of the vitamin was found to help in curing pellagra. However, the more severe cases were not found to respond to the nicotinic acid alone and a good protein diet was found to be necessary. Moreover, nicotinic acid is present in bound form not only in maize but also in other grains and the absence of pellagra in association with the consumption of other grains needs explanation. Also, ordinary cooking procedures are found to convert some of the bound niacin to the free form. Maize is also deficient in lysine and methionine and has a relative deficiency of isoleucine caused by excess leucine resulting from antagonism.

In animal studies carried out at Baroda the addition of lysine to maize was not only found to promote greater weight gain than that of nicotinic acid but also found to result in improved niacin status. The beneficial effects of lysine supplementation to maize have also been found in several human studies. These observations suggest that lysine rather than tryptophan is the first limiting amino acid in maize and that the poor niacin status associated with maize consumption is at least in part due to its poor protein quality. It is likely that the deficiency in maize responsible for pellagra is a complex one of amino acids as well as nicotinic acid. It is also probable that the excessive consumption of alcohol along with poor maize diets combined with the consumption of maize grits instead of whole maize precipitates the deficiency as pellagra is much less frequent among people consuming whole maize as a staple diet in India. Bhils, a tribal people whose diets are based exclusively on white maize do not show a high incidence of pellagra in them. On the other hand, they show extensive incidence of clinical symptoms of vitamin A and riboflavin deficiencies. Their nutritional status is not found to differ from either that of people in the same region consuming jowar or a mixture of rice, wheat and bajra in Tamil Nadu, Uttar Pradesh and Gujarat. The relative rarity of pellagra in maize-consuming people in India contrasts with the reports of the association between maize consumption and pellagra. In this connection, it must be noted that maize was often consumed in the west in the form of hominy prepared from maize grits (decorticated or degerminated meal), which contain only the endospermic portion of the grain. Maize grits contain less of niacin and tryptophan (1.8 mg and 70 mg per 1000 Calories) as against 5.0 and 100 mg per 1000 Calories provided by whole corn.

In India pellagra-like symptoms have been found occasionally in people subsisting on highly polished rice. This may be because such rice, especially after it is washed, cooked, and the cooking water discarded, contains only small quantities of vitamins. It is also found that severe undernutrition can cause symptoms resembling those of pellagra. More recently pellagra has been reported in people consuming jowar. This was formerly attributed to the excessive amount of leucine present in jowar, in contrast to nicotinic acid deficiency in maize. However, neither the leucine content of jowar, nor its nicotinic acid content are appreciably different from those of maize as can be seen from the data given in **Table 21.**

It would appear, therefore, that the etiology of pellagra is complex and may involve a deficiency of calories, protein, amino, acids, and nicotinic acid. It would also appear from certain studies that the requirement of nicotinic acid may be increased with an amino acid imbalance.

In the body, nicotinic acid and nicotinamide are converted to nicotinamide adenine dinucleotide or NAD. NAD is essential for the activities of many respiratory enzymes. Nicotinic acid and its amide have, therefore, a vital role to play in metabolism.

Sources of niacin

Yeast, liver, lean meat, pulses and nuts are good sources (Table 20). Sprouting and fermentation are associated with about 50% increase in nicotinic acid. A 100% increase is found when grain legumes are fermented after sprouting.

Trigonelline which is found in coffee, cereals and fenugreek is partially converted to nicotinic acid during roasting.

The tryptophan content of the diet should also be taken into account while considering the niacin value of foods. For instance milk and eggs are not rich sources of niacin but they contain fair amounts of tryptophan. The biochemical pathway of conversion of tryptophan to nicotinic acid in the body has been well established. About 60 mg of tryptophan are considered to be equivalent to 1 mg of niacin.

The requirement of nicotinic acid depends on the tryptophan content of the diet, body weight and calorie intake and the availability of the vitamin

Table 21. Free nicotinic acid.

	Raw	Pressure cooked	Alkali treated	Lysine	Methio nine	Isoleu cine	Leucine	Tryp tophan
	(mg/100 g)				(g/100 g)			
Maize	0.03	0.33	1.78	0.18	0.12	0.23	0.83	0.04
Jowar	0.04	-	1.86	0.20	0.14	0.30	0.65	0.03

Values taken from the following sources:
Rajalakshmi R., K Nanavati and A. Gumastha. 1964. *J. Natur Diet.* 1.276.
Belavady, B. and C Gopalan. 1965. *Ind. J. Biochem*3.1.44.
Harper, A.E, B.D. Punekar and C.A. Elvehjem. 1958. *J. Natur.* 66,163.

present in the diet and is believed to be of the order of 4–8 mg per 1000 kcalories after taking into account the amount that can be derived from tryptophan. More than this amount is found to be supplied by most diets in this country. Diets based on maize and jowar provide about 5.0 mg per 1000 Calories and those based on milled rice, parboiled rice and a mixture of grains provide 6.0, 12.0 and 10.0 mg taking, into account the tryptophan content of the diet.

Vitamin B12

As mentioned earlier, anaemia is associated mainly with a deficiency of iron and B-vitamins and usually responds to liver which is a good source of both.

In Britain, some persons having macrocytic anaemia failed to respond to oral supplements of liver and other rich sources of B-vitamins. This type of anaemia was called pernicious anaemia. But they were found to show a response to injections of liver extract. Subsequently, a factor isolated from liver, was found to promote the growth of certain microorganisms. This factor was called cobalamine as it contains an amine group as well as cobalt. It is now known that this vitamin is synthesized by certain microorganisms. Neither plants nor animals have the capacity to synthesize this vitamin and only certain microorganisms have the capacity to do so. Such microorganisms are found in the rumen of ruminant animals. The vitamin synthesized by these organisms is absorbed by the animals and we get our supply of the vitamin from animals through milk, eggs and other foods of animal origin. It is now known that pernicious anaemia is caused by a failure to absorb vitamin B12.

Vitamin B12 was previously called as the animal protein factor or cow manure factor as it is present in animal foods, cow dung and urine. The vitamin is also synthesized in man by microorganisms in the large intestine but the vitamin synthesized is bound to a protein. The large intestine lacks enzymes necessary for liberating the vitamin from the protein-vitamin complex and, therefore, the vitamin synthesized in the same is not believed to be available. People living on diets composed mainly of plant foods are likely to suffer from a deficiency of this vitamin. However, about 100 ml of milk or its equivalent in the form of butter milk can supply about 0.2-0.7 microgram. If this is completely absorbed it should be sufficient to prevent a deficiency of the vitamin. About 1 microgram of this vitamin is generally believed to be desirable.

Functions of Vitamin B12

Vitamin B12 is a coenzyme in few enzymes of fat and carbohydrate metabolism. In the beta oxidation of odd chain fatty acids propionyl CoA is the end product. This compound is converted to methyl malonyl CoA which is converted to succinyl CoA by the enzyme methyl malonyl CoA mutase which require Vitamin B12 as a coenzyme. The conversion of homocysteine to methionine does take place in humans and Vitamin B12 is involved as a coenzyme.

Vitamin B12 is involved in many important functions of the body. Along with folic acid vitamin B12 coenzymes are involved in 'one carbon' transfer reactions of biosynthesis of nuleic acids and proteins. Deficiency of Vitamin B12 affects the maturation of red blood cells and is associated with megaloblastic anaemia. Symptoms such as mental confusion and degeneration in the spinal cord have sometimes been found with a deficiency of this vitamin. Thyroid deficiency is believed to affect the absorption of vitamin B12 and the vitamin is practically absent in the serum of cretins. In some studies carried out in the west, the addition of vitamin B12 to deficient diets has been found to promote weight gain. However, studies in this country have generally failed to reveal a beneficial effect of vitamin B12 supplementation on growth rate. Also, megaloblastic anaemia of the type attributed to vitamin B12 deficiency is quite rare in this country, although common diets do not include much of animal foods. The very low requirement of about 1.8 microgram per day and the heat stability of this vitamin may be attributed to this. However, consumption of milk in vulnerable group like pregnant women in vegan society is important as milk is the only dietary source for them.

Even when the diet contains enough vitamin B12 a deficiency may occur because of poor absorption. The gastric secretion contains a substance called the intrinsic factor which is necessary for the absorption of this vitamin. When this is lacking, anaemia results. This type of anaemia, called pernicious anaemia, fails to respond if only vitamin B12 is given orally. It is treated by the oral administration of the vitamin along with the intrinsic factor or by injections of the vitamin.

It is not known how the intrinsic factor helps in the absorption of B12. It is believed to get bound to B12 and thus protect it from destruction by microorganisms in the intestine and release it at the site of absorption.

The intrinsic factor of one species may not help in the absorption of B12 in another species. However, hog and man have similar intrinsic factors and that obtained from hog-liver is used for the treatment of pernicious anaemia in man.

A deficiency of intrinsic factor seems to be hereditary to some extent. Pernicious anaemia is not found in either India or among the Bantus in South Africa. Although their diets contain low amounts of B12 they do not suffer from B12 deficiency.

In this country B12 deficiency does not seem to be a serious problem. It has been suggested that drinking water may contain some B12 because of previous contact with sewage. Even rain water has been reported to contain B12 derived from dust particles in the air which contain microbes synthesizing the vitamin. People such as vegans in Britain do not take any foods of animal origin including milk. Yet the majority of these people are found to maintain satisfactory B12 status and their general health is not different from that of the rest of population. In a few vegans, however, severe deficiency symptoms were found, and this has been attributed to the excessive intake of folic acid which results in an increased requirement of B12.

Folic acid

Some pregnant women in Mumbai who were found to show macrocytic anaemia which failed to respond to liver extract (presumably containing vitamin B12 but not folic acid), showed a response to yeast. Their diet which consisted mainly of polished rice produced anaemia in monkeys. Yeast was, therefore, believed to contain a factor not hitherto identified.

The above observations were made in 1931 by a British doctor Lucy Wills. About a decade later, spinach was found to contain a factor necessary for the growth of a certain species of microorganisms. This factor was found to cure anaemia in chicks. Since it was isolated from leaves and is acidic in nature it was named folic acid (acid in foliage). Liver and leafy vegetables are the major sources of folic acid in our diet. Yeast is also a rich source.

Folic acid is converted in the body to tetrahydrofolic acid which act as a cofactor in 'one carbon' transfer reaction of body metabolism which includes the synthesis of nuleic acids. It is necessary for the maturation of red blood cells. It is also essential for many other important reactions in the body (such as those involving the sulphur amino acids. The actions of folic acid and vitamin B12 are interrelated. Deficiency of folic acid leads to defective DNA synthesis in cells. Tissues most affected are those with greatest cell turn over. Example is the cells of the haematopoietic system which generate red blood cells.

A deficiency of folic acid results in macrocytic megaloblastic anaemia which resembles pernicious anaemia caused by a deficiency of B12 but does not involve neurological symptoms. Diarrhoea and gastrointestinal disorders and glossitis are also found. Although macrocytic anaemia in pregnancy caused by folic acid deficiency was first identified in this country it has also been found in other countries. Anaemia is common in pregnant women who respond to treatment with iron but not to folic acid or B12 and is of the microcytic hypochromic type. Further, the levels of vitamins in the milk of Indian mothers are rather low as compared to

Western values but that of folic acid is quite satisfactory. It is believed that the requirement of folic acid is increased during pregnancy. According to studies in Hyderabad supplementation with folic acid during pregnancy increases the birth weight of the child. It is possible that the apparent deficiency of folic acid during pregnancy is due to the vitamin being stored in the liver for future use during lactation. A similar phenomenon is observed in the case of vitamin A and although pregnant women often show symptoms of vitamin A deficiency they clear up spontaneously after the child birth.

Whatever is the folic acid status in pregnancy, it would be desirable for pregnant women to take generous amount of leafy vegetables which provide not only folic acid but also other important nutrients. Lack of folic acid at a critical stage of conception is found to be the important cause of neural tube defects in the neonates. A high prevalence of neural tube defect is reported in India especially in the poor sections of population.

Deficiency of folic acid is associated with elevated blood homocystiene levels which is reported to be a risk factor in cardiovascular diseases. Methionine, the essential amino acid is converted to homocysteine by demethylation which requires tetrahydrofolic acid as a cofactor. Methionine Folate cycle depicted in **Fig. 7** (chapter 8) is a classical example of 1 carbon metabolism where tetrahydrofolic acid act as a carrier of 1 carbon units such as methyl, formyl and formamino groups from substrates to product. Therefore, deficiency of folic acid leads to disturbances in metabolism of 1 carbon transfer reactions.

ICMR committee has made a recommendation of 100 microgram of folic acid per day as the requirement. However, taking into account of cooking losses and absorption higher levels of 200–400 microgram per day is considered as safe level.

Pantothenic acid

Williams and his associates demonstrated in 1933 the presence in most foods of a substance required for the growth of yeast and other microorganisms. They named it pantothenic acid meaning an acid present everywhere. The vitamin is found to be required by all animal species and microorganisms studied.

Pantothenic acid is part of coenzyme A which is involved in the formation of active acetate from pyruvate and, therefore, in the metabolism of carbohydrates, fats, and amino acids.

In rats, a deficient diet results in growth retardation, impaired reproduction, and in the case of black rats, premature greying of hair. The adrenal cortex is also affected. In man a deficiency is rare with ordinary diets as it is present in liberal amounts in plant and animal foods and can also be synthesized by microorganisms in the intestine. Wheat and jowar contain 1–1.5 mg per 100 g, and milk, about 0.4 mg. Liver, kidney and brain are good sources. Ordinary diets provide 5–10 mg and this amount is usually adequate.

When an experimental deficiency was introduced by feeding artificial diets practically free from the vitamin, with or without the addition of a metabolic antagonist of the vitamin, the subjects showed personality changes such as irritability and restlessness. Periods of sleepiness and sleeplessness were found to alternate. The symptoms were found earlier in the group receiving the metabolic antagonist. Muscle cramps, impaired coordination, vomiting and loss of sensitivity in the extremities were found in another group of subjects. In this country, 'the burning feet syndrome' in which a burning sensation is experienced in the lower limbs has been attributed to a deficiency of pantothenic acid and has been reported to respond to treatment with the same.

Biotin

During the course of investigations on the nutritive value of diets based on eggs, raw egg white was found to be toxic to rats and chicks and the toxicity could be prevented by adding yeast extract or liver. Egg white was found to contain a substance called avidin (antivitamin) which inactivates vitamin 'biotin' present in liver and yeast. Biotin is a coenzyme of carboxylase an enzyme involved in the synthesis of fatty acids. It is found to be essential for the growth of certain microorganisms. Adult volunteers who were fed large quantities of raw egg white experienced fatigue, loss of appetite and muscle pain. Anaemia, changes in the heart beat and increase in serum cholesterol were also found. These symptoms have not always been found probably because the vitamin is synthesized in the body and the amount synthesized may vary.

Yeast, liver, pulses and nuts and some vegetables (e.g. cauliflower) are the major sources of biotin in our diet. 0.1–0.2 mg per day of the vitamin is found to cure the symptoms of deficiency so that this amount is quite sufficient.

As enough of the vitamin is synthesized by intestinal bacteria a deficiency is rare unless the diet contains excessive amounts of antivitamin. Whole eggs do not ordinarily produce deficiency as the vitamin is present in egg yolk. However, deficiency has been found in some individuals who consume more than a dozen raw eggs daily in the belief that they are good for health. Cooking destroys the avidin present in egg white.

Vitamin C

Scurvy, a disease now known to be caused by a deficiency of vitamin C has been recorded since early times. It has been mentioned in the papyrus (1500 B.C.) and by Hippocrates (about 406 B.C.) and Pliny (1st century B.C.). It was a scourge in the crusades. The long voyages in the fifteenth century including the one undertaken by Vasco de Gama resulted in substantial losses of life in Sailors due to scurvy. Cartiers' sailors would have met a similar fate in 1536 if not for timely treatment by the Red Indians who used a tea made of swamp spruce. Scurvy grass, water cress and oranges were known for their therapeutic value. Lime juice was found to have a prophylactic value in the British Navy. This was confirmed by the British Naval surgeon Lind in 1753 and followed by the introduction of antiscorbutic substances such as lemons, oranges and sprouted beans in the British Naval rations in 1795. Yet, a century later many American soldiers lost their lives due to scurvy during the civil war (1860–65) and it was not till 1890 that steps were taken to ensure a supply of vitamin C in army rations. Infantile scurvy was first described in 1650 and identified as distinct from rickets in 1883. The incidence increased in early 20th century following pasteurization of milk.

Vitamin C was termed ascorbic acid because of its protective action against scurvy and acid nature. It is also present in the oxidized form as dehydroascorbic acid. Ascorbic acid is synthesized from glucose in many animals but not in man and primates.

Fresh fruits and vegetables are the major sources of ascorbic acid. Dry legumes contain small amounts (1–8 mg per 100 g) which increase enormously during germination. Sprouted cereals are found to contain 5–10 mg per 100 g and sprouted legumes 50–75 mg. The ascorbic acid content of selected foods is shown in **Table 22**. Some substances such as chillies, mango and amla (Indian gooseberry)retain their ascorbic acid activity even in the dry form. However, chillies are consumed in such small amounts that their value as a source of ascorbic acid is negligible. Amla is the richest source of ascorbic acid. Amla contains about 400 mg of this vitamin per 100 g. Ascorbic acid is one of the heat labile vitamins and rapidly lost due to oxidation by exposure to air at room temperature. The oxidation is speeded up by heat and prevented or reduced by cold storage. The losses of ascorbic acid during cooking depend on the methods employed. Vegetables should be cooked rapidly under cover to minimize the time and degree of exposure to air. The losses are less when they are cut into larger pieces than when they are finely chopped. Cooking along with dals and addition of tamarind juice, lemon juice or sour butter milk during cooking or even towards the end of cooking reduces losses as an acid medium prevents oxidation (**Table 23**). Root vegetables should be boiled with their skins to reduce losses. The vegetables should be scrubbed and washed before cutting and should be

Table 22. Common vegetables and fruits as sources of ascorbic acid.

Foods containing the amount indicated (mg per 100g).

	Less than 10	10–25	25–50	50–100	100–150	More than 150
Leafy Vegetables	Chowli, curry and tamarind leaves	Mint, ponnan-ganni & manathakkali	Spinach, paruppukeerai	Beetgreens, colocasia leaves, fenugreek	Amaranth, cabbage, coriander leaves, radish tops.	Agathi, parsley & drum stick leaves, chekkurmanis, kuppakerai.
Root Vegetables	Carrots, colocasia, elephant Yams	Potato, radish, sweet potato.	Tapioca, turnips	Beet roots	-	-
Other vegetables	Bottle-ash & snake-gourds, pumpkin, cucumber peas, field beans	Brinjal, cow-peas, pink and French beans, tender redgram	Tomatoes(raw-ripe) cluster & runner beans, parwar	Bitter-gourd, cauliflower, capsicum, knolkhol	drumstick	-
Fruits	Apple, most bananas and mangoes, grapes, water meloan, chiku, jack fruit, wood apple.	Phalsa, jambu, rayan, sakkarteti, pomegranate	Grape –fruit, Sweet lemons, Oranges, pineapple	Bor, papaya	-	Guava, alma, cashew fruit
Other foods	Dry legumes	Liver, some varieties of fish	Sprouted legumes, mango powder, tamarind pulp	-	chilies	-

* values for dry and sprouted legumes and tamarind pulp obtained by analysis.

Table 23. Losses of ascorbic acid with different methods of cooking.

Foodstuff	Ascorbic acid content (mg per 100g)		Otherwise[2] Cooked
	Raw	Cooked by Ordinary method[1]	
Spinach	26	7	13 (a)
Drumstick	211	145	183 (b)
Drumstick flowers	129	83	93 (c)
Fenugreek leaves	75	10	69 (d)
Drumstick leaves	171	-	106 (e)

1 A little oil was heated in a pan, the chopped vegetable tipped in, stirred and cooked under cover with water added.
2 After correcting for the vitamin content, if any, of the material added.
   (a) The chopped leaves were added to mug dal the latter was three-fourth cooked and the mixture cooked to completion.
   (b) The leaves were boiled in water, mashed, tamarind juice added and the mixture brought to boil.
   (c) Tamarind juice was added immediately on cooking and the mixture brought to boil.
   (d) 100 g of chopped leaves were boiled in 100 ml water and the vitamin content determined in the liquid extract.
   (e) Buttermilk thickned with dehusked bengalgram flour and the mixture boiled for a munute.

cut just before cooking. The surplus water used for cooking may be used up in soups and gravies. The losses are found to vary not only with the method of cooking but also with the vegetable used. The losses are greater in an alkaline medium and less in acid medium. Under identical conditions of cooking, vegetables such as drumstick, ladies fingers, string beans and tender red gram are found to show much smaller losses than cabbage and spinach as can be seen in **Table 24**. Thus the final ascorbic acid consent of the diet as consumed may vary widely both because of differences in the methods of cooking and the kind of vegetables purchased.

Table 24.   Retention of ascorbic acid in different vegetables[1].

vegetable	Ascorbic acid content (mg per 100 g)		% retention
	Raw	Cooked[2]	
Tender redgram	23	22	96
Ladies fingers	6	5	83
String beans	29	25	86
Cabbage	106	10	9
Spinach	26	7	27
Drumstick	211	145	69

1 Data abstracted from R. Rajalakshmis and Bhanu B. Kothari. 1964. Ind. Dietet. Assoc. Vol. 2, No. 1.
2 A little oil heated in crucible, the chopped vegetable tipped in, stirred and cooked under with a little water added.

Preserved foods such as jams, jellies and pickles may retain a considerable portion of the vitamin C present if prepared by proper methods. Fruits such as papaya used for making jam should be crushed and sugar and lemon juice added immediately. Fruit used for serving as such or for fruit salad may be sliced into a bowl containing sugar and lemon juice. This not only conserves vitamin C but also markedly improves the flavour. The fruit should be kept covered under cold conditions.

Boiled infusion prepared from drumstick leaved is found to contain liberal amounts of ascorbic acid (about 1 mg per gram of leaf used) and can be given to infants and others as a substitute for orange juice as the leaves are to be had for the picking in most areas.

Ascorbic acid is a component of all cells and plays a role in a number of important functions not all of which have been identified. In rats the highest concentration is found in the adrenals (about 300 mg per 100 g), the next highest being found in the brain (50–60 mg), liver (20–30 mg) and kidney (15–20 mg).

Vitamin C and collagen synthesis

It was mentioned earlier, that the first step in the formation of bone is a fibrous network. This network consists largely of a protein called collagen. More generally speaking, collagen is found in 'connective tissue' or tissue which holds together different tissues or organs including the walls of the blood vessels. Ascorbic acid is essential for the formation of collagen. Collagen is a fibrous protein which is rich in the amino acid hydroxyproline. In the synthesis of collagen a non-fibrous protein chain is formed which has proline residues in the polypeptide chain. In the final stage of collagen synthesis the proline residues of the polypeptide chain are hydroxylated to hydroxyproline to form the fibrous collagen. Ascorbic acid acts as a hydrogen donor in this hydroxylation reaction. A deficiency of ascorbic acid impairs collagen formation and retards healing of bone fractures and wounds. In Vitamin C deficiency the blood capillaries become fragile and haemorrhages occur. The first symptoms of deficiency to be experienced are weakness, fatigue, loss of appetite and swollen gums which bleed profusely on touch (bleeding gums). The joints become swollen and painful and the skin becomes dry and rough.

Vitamin C and intestinal absorption of iron

As mentioned earlier ascorbic acid is involved in the reduction of ferric iron to ferrous iron before it can be absorbed by the intestine.

Vitamin C and cardiovascular system

Vitamin C helps in the prevention of clogging of arteries thereby making the blood flow through the arteries smoother.

Vitamin C and immune system

The immune system which involves the T-cells and the white blood cells protect the body from foreign substances and toxins which enters the body system resulting in diseases. Vitamin C is necessary for the proper functioning of these cells.

Vitamin C and steroid biosynthesis

The biosynthesis of the adrenal steroids involves hydroxylation of the basic steroid nucleus at various positions. Vitamin C is necessary for these hydroxylation reactions and adrenal glands is rich in vitamin C.

In the West, scurvy has generally been found in children brought up on bottle milk and elderly adults living alone and not taking proper diets. In this country and in tropical countries generally, frank scurvy is quite rare. Symptoms such as bleeding gums are found, but they may be due to a variety of causes. The blood levels of the vitamin are generally not deficient as can be seen from **Table 25.**

Requirements

Most mammals synthesize ascorbic acid and do not need it in the diet. Exceptions are men, monkeys, apes and guinea pigs. Guinea pigs require a large amount of ascorbic acid in relation to body weight. Among the birds, the bulbul is found to require the vitamin and stops singing when deprived of the same. The minimum requirement of ascorbic acid is found to be of the order of 10 mg in adult man but larger amounts are usually recommended. The British Medical Council has recommended 30 mg, the Indian Council of Medical Research, 50 mg and the National Research Council of The United States of America 70 mg. Many nutritionists believe that these allowances are exaggerated, and about 15 mg would appear to be sufficient in view of the satisfactory vitamin C status of individuals getting this amount or less

Table 25. Ascorbic acid content of serum or blood in different groups of subjects.

Age (years)		Material analyzed	Ascorbic acid content (mg per 100 ml[1])	
			Lower class	Upper class
2–5		Serum	0.34	0.66
7–11		Serum	0.36	0.70
20–40	women	blood	0.49	0.55
Pregnant	"	blood	0.62	0.70
Lactating	"	blood	0.41	0.58

[1] Values obtained in the Biochemistry Department of Baroda University.

in their diets. However, as ascorbic acid is found to increase the absorption of iron and iron deficiency anaemia is widely prevalent in this country, there may be other beneficial effects of taking larger amounts of the vitamin.

Ascorbic acid requirement is believed to be related to body weight so that children require less. This may be responsible for the fact that infantile scurvy is rare as the relatively smaller amounts needed by them may be supplied by occasional consumption of fruits, but even this is rare in most cases.

Generally, pregnancy and lactation are believed to increase vitamin C requirements. But scurvy is seldom found in pregnant and nursing mothers in spite of the fact that their vitamin C intake is not increased during this period. However, rich sources of the vitamin such as oranges and lemons may help stimulate appetite and reduce the nausea of pregnancy.

The requirement of the vitamin C is believed to be increased during treatment with drugs, exposure to cold, infections, prolonged fever, etc.

Massive doses of vitamin C (1–10 g per day) have been advocated on the ground that they ward off viral infections including the common cold and a wide variety of metabolic disorders including rheumatism, asthma and cancer. The evidence on this point is controversial and beneficial effects have been claimed for doses varying between 100 mg and 10000 mg. On the other hand, studies on experimental animals suggest that very large doses may result in the formation of kidney stones and a disturbance of carbohydrate metabolism. No such effects have been found in man, but the withdrawal of such large doses is found to precipitate scurvy even when the diet is reasonably adequate with regard to vitamin C. Even a fruit and nut diet of the sort which might have been consumed by our evolutionary ancestors would not provide much more than about one gram per day.

Vitamin B6

B6 group of vitamins include pyridoxine, pyridoxal and pyridoxamine. Phosphorylated forms of these vitamins act as coenzyme in transamination and decarboxylation reactions in the metabolism of amino acids. These reactions are involved in the biosynthesis of biologically important compounds such as neurotransmitters serotinin, dopamine, taurine, gamma amino butyric acid(GABA),norepinephrine and histamine. GABA is present only in the brain and has function in the regulation of electrical activity in the brain. When there is a deficiency of vitamin B6 the formation of GABA is affected resulting in convulsions. Clinical deficiency symptoms of vitamin B6 include peripheral neuritis, anaemia, glossitis and dermatitis. Evidence of Vitamin B6 deficiency has been reported in young women in India particularly during pregnancy.

Dietary sources rich in vitamin B6 include meat, fish, poultry, pulses, nuts and wheat. Other cereals, potato and banana are moderate sources. Considerable amount of this vitamin is lost during cooking. Certain percentage of Vitamin B6 present in cereals, legumes, fruits and vegetables is in the glycosylated form which is not biologically available to the body.

As the major function of vitamin B6 is in the metabolism of amino acids the requirement of this vitamin depends on the protein intake. It has been observed at the studies in NIN, Hyderabad that when dietary protein was increased from 30 to 100 g vitamin B6 requirement is increased from 1.25 to 1.4 mg per day.

Chapter 6

Digestion, Absorption and Metabolism

Nutrients such as protein, fat and carbohydrate cannot be assimilated as such and have to be broken down into simpler Substances and resynthesized in accordance with the composition of the body. For instance, proteins are not utilized as such but broken down into amino acids and assimilated to the body tissues where they are recombined to form body proteins. Similarly carbohydrates are converted to sugar and fat broken down to fatty acids and glycerol before they are assimilated. Vitamins and minerals are released from the complex molecules to which they are often bound.

Digestion essentially involves the breakdown of complex substances progressively to simpler units which can penetrate the walls of the intestine and into the blood stream. From the blood the absorbed nutrients are assimilated into the body tissues. The 'giant' molecules are converted progressively to simpler substances. For instance, complex starches are converted to simpler starches, dextrin, maltose and glucose. Proteins are progressively converted to proteoses (soluble proteins), polypeptides (containing several units of peptides), peptides (combination of a few amino acids) and finally to amino acids.

The processes of ingestion, digestion and absorption of food and excretion of undigested food take place in the alimentary canal or digestive tract comprised of the mouth, gullet, stomach, the small intestine and large intestine. The small intestine consists of the duodenum, jejunum and ileum and the large intestine consists of the colon, caecum and rectum. The parts of the alimentary canal are shown in **Fig. 4**.

Food is ingested through the mouth, digested partly in the stomach and mainly in the small intestine although some digestion of starch may

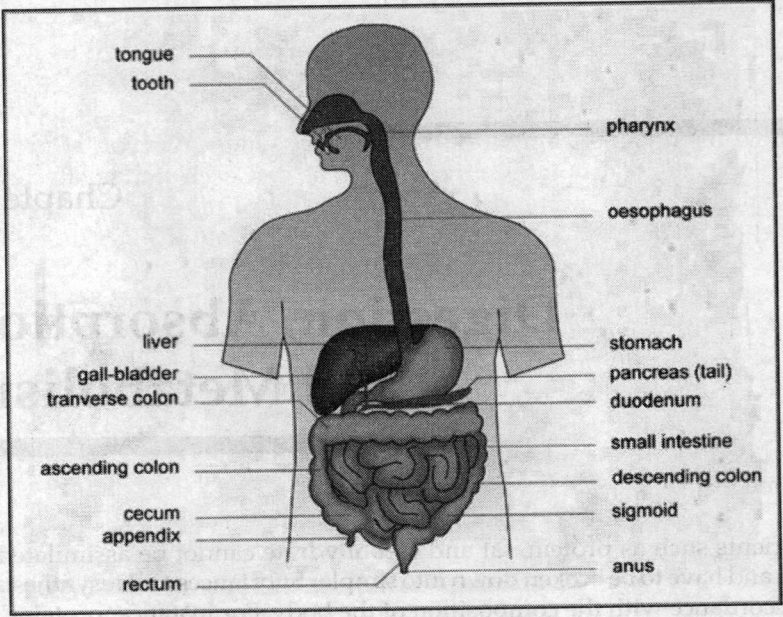

Figure 4. Digestive System.

take place in the mouth. Most of the nutrients are absorbed from the small intestine. The undigested residue is concentrated in the large intestine where it is broken down by bacteria and excreted from the rectum through the anus.

The process of digestion is the breaking down of the nutrients in food to simpler soluble substances which can pass through the walls of the alimentary canal at the site of absorption. This process is effected by enzymes. Food can also be digested chemically outside the body. For instance, acid and heat treatment can digest carbohydrate and protein but the enzymes digest the food at body temperature and do not require a high temperature for their action. As a matter of fact, they are destroyed at high temperatures. The enzymes also act slowly at a regulated rate so that the absorption of food can proceed efficiently in a streamlined fashion.

Food does not become nutrient until it enters the blood stream from the alimentary canal which can function to some extent as a sort of customs barrier regulating the entry of substances according to the needs of the body. The functions of the alimentary canal, starting from the act of chewing and swallowing, and ending with the evacuation of feces or unabsorbed residue from food and digestive juices is controlled to a large extent by the autonomous nervous system. However, swallowing and defecation are partially under voluntary control. The traffic in the intestine is strictly one-way, although food may occasionally be vomited from the stomach. But once the food leaves the stomach and enters the intestine, no Reversal of the direction of traffic takes place. However, a small amount of the intestinal juices may enter the stomach during the contraction of the intestine.

The enzymes of the digestive system, like enzymes in any other system show remarkable team work. For instance, the conversion of protein to amino acids takes place in different steps and each step is effected by a particular enzyme. The digestive enzymes like most other enzymes are highly specific in the sense that each enzyme acts only on a specific substance and brings about a specific transformation.

Ordinarily, enzymes can effect a metabolic reaction in either direction. But the digestive enzymes, effect metabolic reactions only in one direction in the body. Although it would appear that some of them do not lack the capacity to work in the other direction outside the body, they are not found to do so inside the body. If this were not the case, the process of digestion would be partially reversed.

The intestine not only digests food but is also a metabolically active site. As stated earlier, the conversion of carotene to vitamin A takes place during the passage of the former through the intestine. Similarly, fatty acids may be converted to triglycerides in the mucosal cells of the small intestine. The bacteria in the intestine, as mentioned earlier, make a significant contribution to the vitamin nutrition of body.

The digestion of food involves not only nervous control but also control by hormones. For instance, the hormone glucagon can suppress the secretion of gastric juice. The texture, quantity and quality of the food consumed also influence digestive functions.

The passage of food through the small intestine is accomplished by a series of local contractions and relaxations, somewhat analogous to the manual squeezing after washing of a long fabric to get rid of surplus water; But the analogy is far from complete as the contraction and relaxation occur in alternation at all sites simultaneously.

To digest food the way the body does a large factory would be needed. The body gets sufficient factory space from the elaborate architecture of the alimentary canal whose length (32 feet) is more than five times the height of man. The small intestine alone is more than 20 feet in length because of the many folds in it. These folds provide more working space for carrying on the activities of digestion, absorption and synthesis just as an irregular coast-line provides more room for fishing

Digestion in the buccal cavity

The digestion of starch begins in the mouth where saliva is secreted. The saliva secreted in the mouth also serves other functions. It makes the food moist and makes it easier for the same to be ground into a paste. Moisture is necessary for taste sensitivity and dry foods would have no taste if not for saliva. The food mixed with saliva forms a slimy paste which is easier to swallow. The saliva also keeps the mouth clean and if it is not secreted in enough quantities, the mouth begins to feel dry and smell foul. The throat is also kept moist by saliva which facilitates the action of the vocal cords. Speaking is difficult when the throat is dry. Starch is converted to dextrin and maltose by the enzyme amylase in saliva. The saliva also contains a small quantity of lipase. Amylase can function only in alkaline medium and this is provided by saliva. As it cannot function in an acid medium its activity stops when the food gets mixed with hydrochloric acid secreted in the stomach. A small quantity of starch is partially digested in the mouth. When food is chewed and swallowed hastily, digestion in the mouth will hardly have any practical significance.

Digestion in the stomach (Gastric digestion)

From the stomach the masticated food enters the stomach. The stomach wall consists of two types of cells namely the chief cells and the parietal cells. The chief cells secretes pepsinogen and the parietal cells secretes hydrochloric acid. These are the two major components of the gastric juice. The gastric hydrochloric acid has two functions. Pepsinogen is converted to its active form pepsin by gastric hydrochloric acid. The second function of gastric hydrochloric acid is to provide acidic pH required for the optimum activity of pepsin. The masticated food is subjected to digestion by the enzymes of the gastric juice. Pepsin is an endopeptidase which breaks the peptide linkages present in the inner portions of the protein chain in a random manner to form smaller fragments called proteoses and peptones. The gastric juice of young mammals contains rennin, an enzyme which curdles milk. It is not found in the adult animal. However, milk protein can be digested in the absence of rennin. Its presence and role in the gastric juice of the human infant seem to be a matter of controversy.

The gastric juice also contains mucin which forms a coating on the walls of the stomach and protects them against attack by pepsin and hydrochloric acid. Mucin can combine with hydrochloric acid and make it unavailable for pepsin. Heavy secretion of mucin may, therefore, impair protein digestion by pepsin.

In some individuals the amount of hydrochloric acid secreted is small and this condition is called hypochlorhydria or hypoacidity. In some individuals hydrochloric acid is altogether absent and this case is called achlorhydria or anacidity. In many individuals, the secretion of hydrochloric acid is excessive in which case the condition is called hyperacidity or hyperchlorhydria.

Digestion in the intestine

The partially digested food called chyme passes from the stomach into the duodenum of the small intestine where it is subjected to digestion by the intestinal juice. The intestinal juice is made up of three different secretions namely pancreatic secretion, secreted by the pancreas, intestinal secretion, secreted by the intestinal gland and the bile secreted by the liver. The bile secreted by the liver is stored in the gall bladder from where it is transported to the small intestine. The pancreatic secretion contains the enzymes trypsinogen and chymotrypsinogen,alpha amylase,lipase and carboxy peptidase. Enterokinase of the intestinal juice converts the inactive trypsinogen and chymotrypsinogen to active trypsin and chymotrypsin. These two enzymes break the proteoses and peptones to still smaller fractions of polypeptides. Carboxypeptidase hydrolyzes the polypeptides sequentially from the end which has the free carboxyl group in the polypeptide chain. The intestinal juice also contain the enzyme amino peptidase which hydrolyzes the polypeptide chain from the end which has the free amino group. By the combined action of these enzymes the proteins are completely broken down to amino acids.

The digestion of starch continues in the duodenum where alpha amylase hydrolyzes the long chain of starch to smaller chain called dextrin. Dextrin is further broken down to the disaccharide maltose. The maltase enzyme present in the small intestine hydrolyzes maltose to glucose thereby completing the digestion of starch. In the digestive juice is present sucrase and lactase. The former hydrolyzes sucrose to glucose and fructose and the latter hydrolyzes lactose to glucose and galaxies. Lactose is important for the digestion of lactose present in the milk. Generally this enzyme is present in children up to the age of 5 but as they grow up the activity of this enzyme comes down. Children who have deficiency of lactase need to be fed lactose free milk or other substitute like soy milk.

As mentioned earlier, cellulose is not utilized except by ruminant animals in which the microorganisms present in the rumen secrete the enzyme cellulase. However,cellulose plays a useful function by acting as a mechanical stimulant to the intestine. Such mechanical stimulation increases the secretion of intestinal juices, provides bulk to the diets and contributes to the feeling of fullness and makes the evacuation of bowels easier.

The fat present in the food need to be emulsified and dispersed in an aqueous medium in order that the lipase of the small intestine can act on it.

The bile salts secreted by the liver and present in the small intestine act as an emulsifying agent in the digestion of fats. Individuals who have liver disorders have limitation of bile secretion by liver and hence fats are poorly digested. Bile is necessary for the absorption of fatty acids and fat soluble vitamins. When the secretion of bile into the duodenum fails which may happen due to a variety of reasons bile pigments and salts accumulate in the blood resulting in jaundice. The bile is not only a secretion which helps digestion but also the means by which substances synthesized in the body and not wanted are disposed off, particularly those which are not excreted in the urine. Some examples are bile salts, bile pigments, some hormones, cholesterol, etc. However, a portion of these substances may be reabsorbed from the small intestine.

The products of fat digestion by lipase are 1,2-diglycerides,2-monoglycerides, glycerol and fatty acids. Fat digestion is never complete in that one gets a mixture of the above substances as a result of digestion.

The digestive juices and their components and action are shown in **table 26.** Vitamins and minerals are often bound to proteins in foods. They are liberated from this complex and then absorbed. Minerals such as calcium and iron have to be ionized before they are absorbed.

The bacteria in the intestine play a vital role in nutrition. As mentioned earlier, they synthesize several vitamins needed by the body. The bile contains bile salts and hormones which are often present in combination with other substances. The bacteria in the intestine convert bile salts to free acids and the conjugated hormones to the free form, and make it possible for them to be reabsorbed.

About 8 litres of digestive juices are secreted every day into the digestive tract. They contain valuable nutrients such as protein, fat, calcium, bile salts, etc. Most of these nutrients are reabsorbed from the intestine. If not for this, we should require nutrients in much greater quantities. The digestive juices continue to be secreted, although at a reduced rate, even when the body is fasting. This explains the fact that even if a person has not taken any food for some time, he may vomit and lose liquid or have diarrhoea.

The unabsorbed residue which enters the large intestine contains not only undigested food, but also the unabsorbed substances from the digestive juices. Here the excess water is absorbed. The fecal matter expelled from the large intestine is quite different in character from the matter which leaves the small intestine. This is because of the action of bacteria in the large intestine which act on the food. By the time the feces are evacuated most of the nitrogen in the residue has been assimilated by the bacterial cells so that it consists mostly of dead bacterial cells. The action of bacteria on undigested food may result in the formation of flatus. The fecal matter enters the rectum after removal of water and is evacuated from there through the anus. When the evacuation is irregular because of faulty habits, or when there is excessive absorption of water resulting in the formation of hard stools or loss of muscle tone by the rectum, constipation results.

Table 26. Digestion in the alimentary canal

Part of the alimentary canal	Digestive juice secreted	Components of secretion	Digestion of		
			Carbohydrate	Fat	Protein
Mouth	Saliva	Amylase	Starch converted to dextrin and maltose	-	-
		maltase	Maltose converted to glucose	-	-
Stomach	Gastric juice	hydrochloric acid	A small portion of maltose hydrolyzed by hydrochloric acid	-	-
		renin			Milk curdled
		pepsin			Proteins converted to proteoses and peptones
duodenum	Bile	Bile salts and pigments	-	fats emulsified	
	Pancreatic juice	amylase	further conversion of starch to maltose		
		lipase	-	fats broken down to fatty acids and glycerol	
		trypsin and chymotrypsin	-	-	Proteoses converted to polypeptides and peptides
Jejunum	Intestinal juice	Peptidases	-	-	Some polypeptides converted to amino acids.
		amylase	Starch digestion completed		
		Lactase	Lactose converted to glucose and galactose		

contd...

contd...

Part of the alimentary canal	Digestive juice secreted	Components of secretion	Digestion of		
			Carbohydrate	Fat	Protein
		Maltase	Maltose converted to glucose		
		Sucrose	Sucrose converted to glucose and fructose		
		Lipase	-	Fat digestion completed	
	-				
		Erepsin	-	-	Peptones, poly peptides and peptides converted to amino acids.
Large intestine	Mucus: negligible amounts of other substances	Excess water and some salts absorbed and unabsorbed residue acted on by bacteria and excreted as faeces			

Digestion and absorption are quite efficient in the normal individual. The feces contain less than 2-3% of the carbohydrate and 5–7% of the fat ingested. About 10% of the protein ingested is lost through the feces with the kinds of diets consumed in the west, but when the diets are based mainly on vegetable sources of foods as much as 20% may be lost as the protein bound to cellulose is not completely digested. About 5% of the calorie value of the diet is lost in the feces in western diet but 5–10% in the diet ordinarily consumed in this country.

When there is haemorrhage any where in the alimentary canal some blood is also through the feces which may not always appear 'bloody' as the blood may be acted on by digestive enzymes or bacteria depending on the site of haemorrhage.

When toxic substances are ingested the intestine acts to some extent as a barrier against their absorption and the body tries to get rid of the unwanted substance by vomiting and diarrhoea which are frequently found in food poisoning (examples: copper poisoning or bacterial cholera), However, when the toxic material is present in excess their entry into the blood stream cannot be prevented altogether so that poisoning results.

The efficiency with which absorption takes place is affected in a number of conditions. For instance when the intestine is infested with parasites such as hook worms or *Entamoeba histolytica* (the organism which causes amoebic dysentery) absorption is affected. In this and other similar conditions the wall of the intestine, becomes inflamed and ulcerated and this also results in malabsorption. Ulcers in the stomach or duodenum affect the absorption of vitamins.

In conditions such as kwashiorkor and severe marasmus, the intestine atrophies (shrink) and the secretion of intestinal enzymes and absorption of nutrients are affected. The effects are less severe in marasmus. Absorption is also affected in conditions such as sprue and diarrhoea. In kwashiorkor excessive losses of nitrogen may take place as the nitrogenous compounds secreted through the intestinal juices are not efficiently reabsorbed.

In the case of several nutrients such as glucose, absorption has often to take place against a concentration gradient. Normally when solutions of the same substance (say salt) differing in concentrations are separated by a thin permeable membrane provided the membrane is permeable to both the solvent (water) and the solute (salt), water molecules from the weaker solution move into the stronger solution whereas salt molecules from the stronger solution move into the weaker till the two concentrations become equal. If this were true of transport across the intestine we should be loosing nutrients such as glucose as their concentration in the blood is usually greater than that in the content in the intestine which has therefore to pump these nutrients into the blood against a natural concentration gradient just as we pump water from a lower level to a higher level against pressure gradients. When transport takes place in this way against a concentration gradient, it is called active transport as distinguished from ordinary diffusion.

The substances absorbed across the intestine into the lymph or blood are supplied to the tissues and used for energy, for the synthesis of enzymes, hormones and other cellular constituents like body fat and tissue proteins. The end products of metabolism and the nutrients not utilized are excreted through the urine (if they are water-soluble), feces, sweat and expired air. Nutrients are also lost through discarded cells on the surface of the skin and intestine and in the form of hair and nails.

The functions of the alimentary canal are also affected by psychological factors. For instance, worry and mental depression may depress the secretion of digestive juices. Tension may result in the excessive secretion of hydrochloric acid and result in gastric hyperacidity.

The nutritive value of food to the body thus depends not only on its chemical composition, but also on the extent to which it can be digested and absorbed as well as the extent to which nutrients are lost through the various channels. This in turn will depend on many factors such as the type of food eaten, secretion of the various digestive enzymes which depend on factors such as psychic stimulation afforded by food, nutritional status of the individual and emotional factors.

Hunger is the response of the body to the need for food. It is aroused by factors such as the sugar content of blood, emptiness of the stomach, etc. The chief factor is believed to be the response of the central nervous system to a reduced level of glucose in the blood. Some people believe that the relative rates at which fat is utilized from and deposited in the body tissues may be related to *hunger*. When the former is more than the latter, a supply of food from outside is called for.

Appetite is the pleasurable anticipation of food aroused by hunger or by memories of the same. Appetite is influenced by the pleasantness or otherwise of the surroundings and the appearance and flavour of the food.

Apart from the general need for food, one may also get 'hungry' for particular foods. Children and rats given free choice of a wide variety of foods are found to choose their foods in such a way that the resulting diet is a balanced diet. However, this capacity appears to depend on sound nutritional habits in early life. In civilized man, food intake is not always regulated by body needs and other factors such as food habits play a role. Thus a decrease in energy requirements is not always followed by a decrease in food intake. If this were the case we should not have problems such as over-weight.

Metabolic fate of nutrients in the body

The nutrients absorbed from the intestine are transported by the blood to the tissues of various organs of the body. The nutrients enter the cells of the tissues from the blood. The membranes of the cells are highly specialized and have the transport systems for specific substances into the cells. Inside the cells the nutrients enters various channels of chemical reactions catalyzed by enzymes. These channels of enzyme catalyzed reactions are called metabolic pathways and the intermediate compounds formed in these pathways are called metabolites. These intricate pathways can be compared to the railway networks of a huge country. There are junctions in these pathways and the intermediate compounds can be diverted to different directions from these junctions. The extent to which the intermediate compounds are channelled to a particular metabolic path depend on several factors and most of it is decided by the body requirement, age, environmental factors, metabolic state and diet. The endocrine system and the hormones and the hormones secreted by the endocrine glands act as signals for the rate at which a particular pathway should operate. The level of hormones in the blood is regulated by the brain mediated by the hypothalamus of the brain. The hormones are secreted in extremely small concentrations. The question now is how these low concentrations of hormones can bring about changes of metabolic fate of large amount of nutrients that flows through the metabolic channels. This question is answered by the concept of metabolic amplification cascade operating in the cell.The concept was enunciated by Nobel Laureate Earl Sutherland. According to this concept the hormones do not act directly affect the rate of enzyme activity. In between the hormones and the targeted enzymes there is a series of intermediate signals and in each of these intermediate step there is amplification of hormonal effect. Compounds like cyclic-AMP(C-AMP) have vital role in this amplification cascade and they are known as second messengers.

Metabolic fate of carbohydrates

Sugars such as glucose,fructose and galactose formed as a result of digestion of dietary carbohydrates are absorbed by blood and transported to the cells of various tissues where they are oxidized for energy purpose as discussed in chapter 2. Glucose the major sugar in the circulating blood is the immediate source of energy in tissues such as skeletal muscle, heart muscle and brain. However, there is distinct difference in the pathways of glucose oxidation in skeletal muscle and heart muscle. The skeletal muscle predominantly utilizes glucose by glycolysis generating 2 molecules of ATP per one molecule of glucose. The 2 molecules are formed from ADP and inorganic phosphate by a process known as substrate level phosphorylation which does not involve oxygen. There is profuse breakdown of glucose to lactic acid by glycolysis in exercising skeletal muscle and the ATP generated is used up in the process of muscular contraction. ATP is broken down to ADP and inorganic phosphate and the energy released is used for muscular contraction. ADP so formed is reconverted to ATP by substrate level phosphorylation utilizing the energy released when glucose is broken down by glycolysis.

The cardiac muscle utilizes glucose predominantly by aerobic process which involves oxygen resulting in complete oxidation of glucose to carbon dioxide and water. This involves glycolysis and Krebs Cycle and generates 38 molecules of ATP for each molecule of glucose utilized. Pyruvic acid formed in glycolysis enters the mitochondria of the cell where it is converted to acetylCoA and then to carbon dioxide and water in the Krebs Cycle. The cardiac muscle depends on this mechanism of energy production from glucose for meeting the requirement of ATP for pumping blood to skeletal muscle and other tissues.

ATP is an inhibitor of rate limiting key enzymes of glycolysis where as ADP is an activator of these enzymes. The ratio of ATP to ADP is called the energy charge of the cells. When the energy charge is high as in resting muscle the rate of glycolysis goes down and when the energy charge is low as in exercising muscle the rate of glycolysis goes up.

In many of the steps of Krebs cycle coenzymes NAD and FAD are reduced to NADH2 and FADH2 by dehydrogenation reactions. The reduced coenzymes are oxidized back to their original state by the electron transport system which transports hydrogen to molecular oxygen by a series of hydrogen carriers located in the mitochondria. When the electron transport operates a series of redox systems are generated in the mitochondria with the development of redox potential. The potential energy available in this process is used to synthesize ATP from ADP and inorganic phosphate. The transduction of redox potential energy into chemical energy of ATP is known as oxidative phophorylation. ATP generated in this manner is vital for the contraction and expansion of heart muscle and to pump blood to skeletal muscle during physical activity. Electron transport and oxidative phosphorylation are coupled phenomena. In a coupled state these two processes are complementary to each other. The higher the rate of oxidative phosphorylation the higher is the rate of electron transport. However, in an uncoupled state electron transport will proceed in the normal rate but transduction of energy by oxidative phosphorylation is blocked. In uncoupled state dissipation of energy takes place without the generation of ATP. Agents that can bring about uncoupled state are known as uncouplers. There are naturally occurring and artificial uncouplers. The hormone thyroxin produced by the thyroid gland and thermogenin* a protein present in the brown adipose tissue are naturally occurring uncouplers the increased levels of which result in thermogenesis.

As mentioned earlier, the metabolic route of carbohydrates is decided by various factors and these aspects are discussed in the following sections.

In normal human subjects the blood sugar level is maintained at 70–110 mg per 100 ml blood (some schools recommend 80–120 mg).This level of glucose is a net balance of glucose utilized for energy purpose and that channelled to other metabolic route and the glucose that enters the blood primarily from the diet. When the dietary carbohydrate intake is high the sugar level in the blood tends to go up and this increased blood sugar stimulates the pancreas to produce more insulin. Insulin regulates glucose metabolism at two levels, namely the level of glucose uptake by the cells and and at the level of rate limiting key enzymes of glucose metabolism such as glycolysis, glycogen synthesis and lipogenesis. When there is high physical activity the rate of glycolysis is increased by stimulation of the key enzymes of glycolysis by insulin and in this process glucose is drawn from the blood. The increase in the rate of glycolysis provides for the increased demand for ATP at high physical activity. Conversely, in a well fed but physically inactive state there is only moderate utilization of glucose by glycolysis. More of glucose is drawn from the blood for glycogen synthesis in muscle and liver where it is stored.

When there is a restriction of dietary carbohydrate as in the case of fasting the blood sugar level tends to go down below the normal level. Insulin secretion by pancreas is reduced in this condition as a result of which rate of gycolysis decreases thereby maintaining the blood sugar level at normal level. The breakdown of glycogen stored in muscle and liver sets in under this condition. Glycogenolysis is the breakdown of glycogen to glucose which is controlled by the hormone glucagon secreted by alpha cells of pancreas. Lower levels of glucose in the blood stimulate the pancreas to secrete more of this hormone. Glucagon increases the rate of glycogenolysis,that is the breakdown of glycogen stored in muscle and liver to glucose. The key reaction of glycogenolysis catalyzed by the enzyme glycogen phosphorylase is up regulated by increase in glucagon level. Cyclic AMP acts as second messenger in the regulation of this enzyme by glucagon.

Aspects of glucose metabolism under various situations and hormonal regulation of diversion of glucose to various metabolic channels has been dealt with in the foregoing sections. The actions of two pivotal hormones

*Ricquier, D. and F. Bouillaud. 2000. *Biochem J.*, **345(2)**:161.

insulin and glucagon are antagonistic to each other in the regulation of carbohydrate metabolism. Insulin is hypoglycemic (tend to reduce glucose level in the blood) and glucagon is hyperglycemic (tend to raise the glucose level in the blood). This is a classical example of homeostatic mechanism of diversion of metabolites to different routes according to the needs of the body in various situations.

Non-fuel functions of carbohydrates in the body

The carbon skeleton of glucose is used for the synthesis of several other body constituents such as the following:-

Non-essential amino acids

As mentioned earlier non-essential amino acids can be synthesized in the body by the biosynthetic pathways of these amino acids. Intermediates of carbohydrate metabolism especially keto acids like pyruvic acid and alpha ketoglutaric acid can be transaminated to alanine and glutamic acid. Glutamic acid can also be formed by the fixation of ammonia to alpha ketoglutaric acid catalyzed by the enzyme glutamate dehydrogenase. The reverse of this reaction also provides the route for the oxidation of glutamate for energy purpose.

Connective tissues of joints are made up of collagen a fibrous protein and Mucopolysaccharide chondroitin sulphate. For the strength of connective tissues of joints chondroitin sulphate which is an oligosaccharide made up of glucosamine needs to be formed from glucose in the tissues.

Glycolipids like cerebrosides are constituents of nerve cell membrane and glucose provides the carbohydrate part of glycolipids. Glycoproteins are proteins containing carbohydrate part. Mucin is a glycoprotein present in mucus of respiratory and digestive tract and act as a lubricant and protective agent.

Metabolic fate of dietary fat

The products of dietary fat digestion namely 1,2-diglyceride, 2-monoglycerides and free fatty acids enters the mucosal cells of the small intestine where the are reconverted to triglycerides and passed on to the circulating blood through the lymphatic system. The triglycerides along with cholesterol and phospholipids combine with serum proteins to form micelles of different densities. They are lipoproteins with varying protein content. The lightest and the largest of them are called chylomicrones. In the order of density the chylomicrones are followed by Very Low Density Lipoprotein (VLDL), Low Density Lipoprotein (LDL)and High Density

Lipoprotein (HDL). Cholesterol associated with VLDL and LDL are referred to as bad cholesterol because elevated serum concentration of these lipoproteins correspond to incidence of coronary artery disease. Cholesterol associated with HDL is referred to as good cholesterol and correspond to lower rate of coronary heart disease. The chylomicrone remnants are endocytosed into liver and hydrolyzed into their component parts and the protein part is recycled

From the liver the fats are mobilized to various tissues where they are oxidized for energy purpose. The mobilization of triglycerides starts with the action of lipoprotein lipase to form free fatty acids and glycerol. The free fatty acids are transported to tissues by the blood in combination with albumin. Glycerol formed from the fat is converted to glycerolphosphate in liver and kidneys and then to glucose by gluconeogenesis.

In certain pathological conditions there is a limitation of this enzyme resulting in fat accumulation in the liver. This condition is known as fatty liver.

The oxidation of free fatty acids takes place in the mitochondria of the cells. Carnitine acts as the carrier of fatty acids into the mitochondria. Fatty acyl carntine which enters the mitochondria of the cell is broken down in the mitochondria releasing free fatty acid and carnitine. The released carntine is recycled for the transport of fatty acids into the mitochondria.

In the mitochondria of the cell fatty acids undergo a series of reactions called beta oxidation catalyzed by a multienzyme system called fatty acid oxidase which require NAD and FAD as coenzymes. The reduced coenzymes NADH2 and FADH2 enter the electron transport chain where they are converted back to their original state by molecular oxygen and transduction of energy as ATP. The result of beta oxidation is acetylCoA which enters Krebs Cycle (chapter 2) resulting in its further oxidation to carbon dioxide and water.

Oxidation of fatty acids yield more energy per carbon atom than does oxidation of carbohydrate. The net result of oxidation of 1 mole of oleic acid (C18) will be 146 moles of ATP as compared to 114 from an equivalent number of glucose carbon atoms.

The sources of body fat are diet and endogenous synthesis in adipose tissue. When there is excessive intake of carbohydrate especially in the form of carbohydrates with high glycemic index like sucrose, acetylCoA formed in the carbohydrate metabolism can be diverted to fatty acid biosynthesis. The key regulatory enzyme of in fatty acid biosynthesis namely acetylCoA carboxylase is up regulated by insulin and hence high carbohydrate intake promotes fat accumulation in adipose tissue.

The accumulated fat in the adipose tissue is mobilized during starvation. The triglycerides in adipose tissue are hydrolyzed by hormone sensitive lipase which is stimulated by the hormones epinephrine and norepinephrine. The fatty acids liberated are transported by blood as albumin complex to tissues such as heart,liver and muscle where they are oxidized for energy purpose as discussed above. Cyclic AMP acts as second messenger in the amplification cascade of action of these hormones in fat metabolism.

AcetylCoA formed from fatty acids can also be diverted to biologically important compounds such as cholesterol, phopholipids and steroid hormones. Major part of cholesterol in the body is synthesized in the liver by the pathway of cholesterol biosynthesis established by Konrad Bloch who was awarded Nobel Prize in Chemistry in 1964.

Metabolic fate of protein

The amino acids absorbed from the blood are supplied to the cells in different tissues and the tissue proteins are either synthesized or renewed.

The amino acid sequence of the proteins synthesized in the body is determined by the genes corresponding to different proteins and the rate of synthesis of each of these proteins is under genetic control. The dietary amino acids thus gets incorporated into tissue proteins,the proteins of the blood and body fluids, the various enzyme systems of metabolism and protein hormones. Amino acid oxidation provides a major source of energy in liver,muscle,kidney and small intestine. Amino acids can be transaminated or deaminated to the corresponding keto acids like alpha ketoglutaric acid from glutamic acid and oxaloacetic acid from aspartic acid which are intermediates of carbohydrate metabolism. These keto acids join the major pathways of carbohydrate metabolism for their further oxidation to carbon dioxide and water with the generation of ATP. Ammonia produced when amino acids are oxidized is converted to urea which is excreted in the urine. Under certain situations these intermediates can be converted to glucose by the process of gluconeogenesis. Gluconeogenesis is one of the mechanisms by which blood sugar level is maintained in conditions of starvation.

The amino acids derived from the diet join the free amino acid pool of the body tissues and diverted to metabolic fate as discussed in chapter 2. The extent to which the amino acids are diverted to different pathways is decided by the body requirement in various situations.

Vitamins and minerals

The iron absorbed is stored in the form of ferritin or haemosiderin in the liver and is used up as needed. As mentioned earlier calcium is deposited in the skeleton. Vitamin A is stored in the liver and also in the kidney. Carotene is stored in the liver as well as in adipose tissues.

The body has only limited stores of the B-vitamins which must, therefore, be regularly consumed. Vitamin C is distributed in all the tissues and the tissues become under saturated when the vitamin is deficient in the diet.

The vitamins absorbed are often stored in the bound form as protein-vitamin complexes.

Some of the ways in which the nutrients absorbed by the body are utilized are shown in **Table 27.**

Table 27. Utilization of nutrients in the body.

Nutrient	Form in which absorbed	Form in which stored	Chief sites of storage	Chief compounds synthesized	Other functions
carbohydrates	Glucose, fructose, and galactose	Glycogen and fat	Liver, muscle and adipose tissue	Non-essential amino acids, fatty acids, glycerol, glycogen and mucopoly saccharides	Oxidized as fuel source
Fat	Fatty acids, glycerol	Fat	adipose tissue	Glucose, phospholipids, sterol hormones, vitamin D, proteolipids, lipoproteins.	Oxidized as fuel source
Protein	Amino acids	Protein	Tissues	Enzymes and tissue protein, hormones, glucose, lipo proteins, proteo lipids	Used for tissue building and renewal; oxidized as fuel source
Calcium	Calcium, iron	Hydroxyapatite crystals of calcium phosphate	skeleton	-	Skeletal development, regulation of cell permeability and irritability, cofactor in enzymes
Phosphorus	Phosphate ions	Phosphates	Skeleton	High energy compounds such as ATP and nucleic acids	Skeletal development. ATP acts as a reservoir of energy
Magnesium	Magnesium ion	Magnesium phosphate	Skeleton and soft tissues	-	Enzyme cofactors, regulation of cell permeability and irritability
Iron	Ferrous iron	Ferritin, haemosiderin	Liver and spleen	Hemoglobin myoglobin	Component of certain enzymes.
Iodine	iodine ion	Inorganic iodide as well as thyroglobulin	Thyroid gland	Thyroxine	-
Carotene Vitamin A	Carotene or vitamin A	Carotene or vitamin A ester	Carotene in liver and adipose tissue vitamin A in liver and kidney	Rhodopsin	Involved in growth, vision, reproduction, bone formation etc.

Vitamin D	Free as well as esterified form	Liver, kidney, adrenals, bone	Dihydroxy cholecalciferol	Regulation of calcium and phosphorus metabolism; stimulation of para thyroid gland; involved in citrate metabolism
Vitamin K	Free and esterified form	Liver and spleen	Coenzymes for respiratory enzymes prostaglandins	Blood coagulation
Vitamin E	Vitamin E	Liver		Act as antioxidant; necessary for blood formation-vitamin
B-Vitamins	Free form	Liver	Enzyme cofactors	Metabolism of carbohydrates, proteins and fats
vitamin C	Ascorbic acid and dehydro ascorbic acid	Distributed throughout the body; concentrated in pituitary gland, adrenals, brain. liver and kidney	Ascorbic acid and dehydroascorbic acid	Wound healing; oxidation-reduction systems; detoxification; hydroxylation of amino acids

Chapter 7

Formulation of Dietary Allowances

We have seen in the previous chapters the different nutrients required by the body their functions and recommended daily allowances. In practical nutrition it is important to know the adequacy of ordinary diets in terms of meeting these requirements. For instance, does the fact that we need vitamins or protein mean that we should take vitamin tablets and special protein foods? We cannot answer such questions without knowing how much we require and how much is supplied by the diet.

The first step in recognizing the need for a nutrient is the recognition that the deficiency of a particular nutrient results in disease. For instance, the consumption of polished rice was found to be associated with beriberi and the disease found to be cured by rice polishing. Subsequently the specific factor was identified as thiamine and methods worked out for the estimation of thiamine in foodstuffs. The next step was to find out the amount of thiamine provided by the diets of healthy individuals and the minimum amount on which an individual can subsist without developing beriberi.

How does one go about finding how much of these nutrients are needed? Many approaches have been made by nutritionists and it is beyond the scope of this book to discuss them adequately. They can be only indicated briefly in this context. One approach is to investigate the effects of the deficiency of a particular nutrient in man and to determine the amount of the nutrient that can prevent or reverse these effects. The subjects are fed diets containing graded amounts of the nutrient ranging from nil to generous amounts and adequate in other respects. The amount needed for maintaining a satisfactory nutritional status or for clearing the deficiency symptoms is taken to represent the amount needed. The growth, performance and tissue composition of experimental animals fed specific diets have been used as indices for the adequacy of these diets. Their extrapolation to man presents problems but they may give a reasonably good idea of the comparative value of different foods or diets with regard to protein, carotene, calcium, iron etc. Also, vitamin requirements are found to compare in different mammalian species when considered in relation to energy requirements in the case of B vitamins, and in relation to body weight, in the case of vitamin A.

Assessment of nutritional status

This takes us to the question of assessment of nutritional status. Nutritional status is judged in terms of criteria such as general appearance, health and well-being, physical stature, physical stamina, work performance and activity level, presence or absence of clinical deficiency symptoms, composition of urine, blood and tissues, radiological assessment for skeletal status and so on,

Body measurements

Physical stature and body build are recognized as indices of nutritional status even by the layman. Measurements of height, weight and the circumference of head, chest, abdomen and hip are all used. An individual who is tall and heavy for his age is likely to have been well-nourished on the whole during the period of growth though there is no guarantee that he would be free from specific deficiencies. Recent changes in weight can tell us whether or not he is eating satisfactorily. In the case of a child changes in height can give an idea as to whether growth and skeletal development are proceeding satisfactorily.

Height is affected by prolonged undernutrition and weight by both recent and prolonged undernutrition. The ratio of weight to height is also used as a measure.

The growth of the trunk may be less affected by undernutrition than the growth of the long limbs so that the ratio of sitting height to standing height may be more in undernourished children. Similarly, the ratio of arm circumference and chest circumference to head circumference is decreased as head growth is preserved but the arms tend to be extremely thin. The ratio of chest circumference and abdominal circumference may be affected in conditions characterized by pigeon chest and pot belly. Body measurements may give us an idea about the nutritional status of a population group and thereby some idea of the adequacy of the diets consumed.

In the case of population groups such as young children or school boys suspected of not getting specific nutrients in the required amounts, the effect of nutritional supplements on body growth can tell us whether the diet is satisfactory or not. For instance, if a high protein supplement promotes better growth in young children than one low in protein, it may signify that the diet is perhaps not having the required amount of protein. If it does not, then we would be justified in concluding that the diet is already adequate in protein, provided, of course, it is not seriously lacking in other nutrients. If the diet is also lacking in other nutrients supplementation with protein may have no value.

In experimental animals, a simple way to find out how much of a particular nutrient is needed is to feed different amounts of the nutrient to different groups of subjects, generally young animals, and determine the minimum amount needed for good growth. For instance, if a diet containing only 5% protein produces a weight gain of about 5 g per week, and that containing 20% protein, a weight gain of about 15 g we would conclude that a 5% protein diet is not enough for the growing animal. If, on the other hand, we find that the weight gain is not further increased when the protein content of the diet is further increased to 25% we would conclude that it is unnecessary to have more than 20% protein. In this approach, it is necessary to see that only one of the nutrients is varied in amount and that the diet is satisfactory in other respects. A similar approach can be made for comparing the nutritive value of different foods or different diets used by man by feeding them to young animals and comparing their growth rates.

Prevention and cure of deficiency symptoms

Similarly, the amount needed to cure or prevent deficiency symptoms can be determined by feeding different amounts of nutrient. This type of study can be carried out in both animal and human subjects. In the animal, deficiency symptoms can be induced by feeding a deficient diet and the amount necessary for their disappearance determined. Alternatively, the minimum amount that will prevent the appearance of these symptoms can also be determined by giving different amounts of the nutrient.

Similar studies can be carried out on human subjects exhibiting deficiency symptoms and the amount needed for the disappearance of deficiency symptoms determined. Occasionally, groups of healthy subjects have volunteered to take a diet deficient in some particular nutrient. This method is more reliable as malnourished subjects found to be showing deficiency symptoms as a result of faulty diets are likely to be consuming diets deficient in more than one nutrient, whereas experimental diets used with volunteers are adequate except with regard to the nutrient under study. This type of experimental approach also helps to identify the clinical symptoms and subjective feelings caused by a particular deficiency. Studies using this approach have been carried out on the effects of a deficiency of calories, protein and vitamins.

Balance studies

While growth can be used as one of the criteria for determining dietary requirements with younger animals and children, this cannot obviously be done with adult subjects. Other approaches have been made in the latter case. One of these is to carry out balance studies. In these studies the amount of the nutrient eaten by the subject is compared with that excreted by him, mainly through the feces and urine. The losses from the skin, hair and nails are generally considered too small to worry about. For instance, we can estimate the protein content of food and feces during 24 hour intervals, by estimating their nitrogen content. The nitrogen content of urine will give us an idea of the amount of protein used up by the body during this period. Suppose the figures obtained are as follows:

Nitrogen in diet	...	10 g
Nitrogen in feces	...	1 g
Nitrogen in urine	...	9 g

Then the amount of nitrogen taken in food is equal to the amount excreted through the urine and feces. In other words, the body is neither gaining nor losing nitrogen assuming that sweat and other losses are not appreciable. Such a subject is considered to be in equilibrium or in balance. Suppose, in the above example, the figure for dietary intake were 13 g, then the subject is consuming more than what is excreted and storing some protein in the body, even if we allow for some loss in sweat etc. (say 1.5 g) and he is said to be in positive balance. Suppose, on the other hand, the dietary intake were 8 g, then he is excreting more than he eats and at least 2 g are used up from tissue stores and such a subject is said to be in negative balance. The three situations can be compared with a man living on his income, saving from his income or going into debt.

Whether or not the money-saving habit is beneficial to man, a continued positive balance with regard to nutrients is not necessarily helpful in the case of adult subjects. For instance, a positive balance with regard to energy results in obesity.

Generally, in the case of protein, calcium, iron, etc. an adult needs only the amount needed for maintaining balance but in the case of children, in addition to this, an extra amount will be needed for the formation of new tissue and for the increase in the concentration of many nutrients in the body as can be seen from the following data:

—	Total		Per kg body weight	
	Newborn child	Adult man	Newborn child	Adult man
Body weight (kg)	3.5	70	-	-
Water (kg)	2.4	42	0.7	0.6
Nitrogen (g)	66.0	2000	18.8	28.6
Sodium (meq)	243.0	5150	69.4	73.6
Potassium (meq)	150.0	4050	42.8	57.8
Calcium (g)	28.2	1320	8.1	18.8
Iron (mg)	320.0	4350	91.4*	62.1

* This value becomes very low at one year of age and increases thereafter
  According to E.M. Widdowson, in Mineral Metabolism, Vol III. edited
  by Comar and Bronner.

In a balance study involving fecal collections it is necessary to make sure that the same are derived from the food consumed during the period of study. The feces excreted on any particular day are likely to be derived from food consumed during the previous day or earlier. The interval between the consumption of food and the excretion of the undigested residue may vary in different individuals and during different periods in the same individual. Usually, some colouring matter or 'marker' is given along with food at the start and end of balance studies. The appearance of the colour in the feces determines the point at which feces collection should be started or terminated.

Balance studies are usually subject to some error. The amount of nutrient consumed is determined by estimating it on an equal portion of the food consumed. This may be over-estimated if some of the food is spilled or left over by the subject. It may be under-estimated if some of the food consumed is not represented in the collection. The former is more likely in animal subjects and both, in the case of human subjects.

Such direct balance studies cannot be carried out with fats and carbohydrates. Here the problem is complicated and the only approach we can make is to study changes in weight in relation to the total calorie content of the diet. Weight may not always indicate an increase or decrease in the amount of energy stored by the body as changes in weight may occur due the retention or loss of water which has no energy value. Generally, an individual maintaining a steady weight may be expected to be in energy balance.

In the case of balance studies with regard to water-soluble vitamins such as vitamin C the amount in the feces is not usually determined as it is assumed that most of the vitamin is absorbed and the analyses are made of only urine and diet.

In the case of fat-soluble vitamins such as vitamin A or carotene, balance studies are rather complicated because of some destruction in the intestine. Moreover, some of the carotene is converted to vitamin A in the intestine.

While carrying out balance studies, nutrients lost through sweat, hair, nails and cells discarded from the body are generally ignored. Losses through these channels may be considerable in the case of nutrients such as nitrogen, iron, sodium and potassium. These must also be taken into account in determining the amounts needed.

Balance studies have also been used to determine the requirements of amino acids. The amount of a particular amino acid needed for achieving nitrogen balance on a diet providing generous amounts of other amino acids is determined. Balance studies also help to determine the availability of a nutrient in a food. For instance, the amount needed for achieving nitrogen balance is more with maize protein than with milk protein as less of the former is utilized.

The basic assumption in balance studies with regard to nutrients such as protein or calcium is that the amount required for equilibrium represents the minimum amount required by the subject. This is not always the case as the amount required for balance may depend on amounts ordinarily consumed by the subject. An adult habitually taking 100 g of protein will be in negative balance with regard to nitrogen when put on a diet containing 50 g of protein. On the same diet, one habitually consuming 35 g of protein may show a positive balance whereas another habitually consuming 50 g may show a neutral balance.

Sometimes, the subject is given a diet free from the nutrient under question and the amount lost through the feces and urine after an initial period of adaptation determined. The same is considered to represent the minimum metabolic requirements. But the losses from the body during a period of deprivation are variable, being greater during the initial stages of deprivation and reaching a minimum value with the progress of the deprivation period. However, neither the initial heavy losses nor the minimum value reached may represent the amounts lost with the normal diet.

In the case of the water soluble vitamins, a state of saturation, when almost the entire vitamin ingested is excreted in urine is taken to indicate that the tissues are 'saturated' with the vitamin. In other words they cannot hold any more of it.

In spite of the above limitations balance studies have helped to make rough estimates of the requirements of different nutrients and to make enlightened guesses about desirable amounts. They have greater validity

if the diets fed are not too different from those ordinarily consumed by the
the subject.

Biochemical status

The amounts of nutrients which will maintain normal concentrations
of the same or substances formed from them in blood and urine is also
determined for use in developing dietary standards. For instance, protein
nutrition can be assessed in terms of the amounts of different proteins such
as albumin and globulin, or the total amount of proteins in the serum. In
subjects adequately nourished with regard to protein, the serum is found
to contain about 4-5 g of albumin per 100 ml. Similarly, the composition of
blood with regard to haemoglobin and of serum with regard to vitamin C,
calcium, iron, vitamin A, carotene, etc. are determined in order to assess
the nutritional status of a subject.

Similarly, the composition of urine with regard to water-soluble
vitamins and metabolic end products of nutrients is used as a criterion. In
the case of the water soluble vitamin, it is assumed that spill-over in the
urine means that the body has a supply greater than demand of the vitamin.
However while liberal amounts of a vitamin in the urine may be taken as
indicating a satisfactory nutritional status with regard to the same, low
levels of the vitamin do not necessarily indicate deficiency. For instance,
many subjects, in whom urine levels of vitamin C are low, blood levels are
not deficient. Many other biochemical criteria including some which have
been recently developed are being used.

Other criteria

In animal studies it is also possible to analyse the liver, bone, etc. The
former can be analysed for protein, iron, water soluble vitamins and
certain enzymes which are affected by nutritional status. The bone can be
analysed for ash and calcium contents. The whole body of the animal is
also analysed and this is referred to as carcass analysis. The amount needed
for maintaining a satisfactory composition of the tissue studied is taken to
indicate requirement.

X-ray examination of the hand, spine and long bones is used for the
assessment of skeletal status and to detect signs of skeletal retardation,
rickets, osteomalacia, osteoporosis etc. If the bones show good growth and
calcification one must presume that the amounts of calcium and phosphorus
in the diet are adequate.

Work performance under standard conditions, performance on
psychological tasks, etc., are also now used as indices of health and well-being.

The epidemiological approach

A common sense approach is to find out the amounts of nutrients in the diets of apparently well-nourished individuals. In the case of adults we assume that the health and performance of the individuals under question cannot be further improved by increasing the nutrients in the diet. In the case of children a satisfactory growth is considered as indicating a satisfactory nutritional status. In this case, we assume that the growth rate obtained is optimum and that a further acceleration of growth is not necessarily desirable. In spite of the limitations involved in such assumptions these approaches have reasonable validity if the individuals selected for defining our standards are reasonably healthy and functioning as efficiently as can be expected.

The amounts of nutrients present in the diet of apparently well-nourished individuals represent amounts which are sufficient but it does not always mean that they are necessary. A well-nourished individual in the west, for instance, may consume 100 g of protein and 1000 mg of calcium but we know that these amounts are much more than necessary. For the epidemiological approach to be valid, the subjects must be chosen from the population group for which dietary standards are being developed and must be subsisting on diets within the reach of the population. An individual in India living on liberal amounts of cheese, meat, etc. is not a practical model for dietary formulations even if he is well-nourished.

The above approaches can also be used for assessing the nutritional status of the community as a whole or of any segment of the population. In addition, birth weights, growth rate, infant and childhood mortality, maternal mortality, life expectancy and incidence of deficiency diseases are all used as criteria. If a population group scores well on the basis of these criteria, we can conclude that the typical diet consumed by the group is quite adequate.

In summary, we can say that the amount of a nutrient required is the amount that can enable an individual to maintain a satisfactory status with regard to that nutrient as judged by one or more of the above criteria.

Requirements and recommended amounts

Determining the amount of a nutrient needed is only the first step. The amounts of different nutrients recommended in dietary standards usually exceed those found to be needed for metabolic requirements. For instance 10mg of vitamin C are found sufficient to cure and prevent scurvy, but most authorities recommend amounts varying from 30 to 70 mg of this vitamin. Similarly, the minimum amount of protein required is found to be about 20–30 g for an adult man weighing 60 kg, but the amount recommended is often more than double this figure. An extra amount representing a margin of safety is added to allow for differences between foods with regard to availability of nutrients and between individuals with regard to the efficiency of utilization. Liberal amounts are recommended so that they will be adequate for more than 95% of the relevant population.

It is evident from the foregoing discussions that estimates of requirements vary depending on the criteria used the type of subjects, used, etc. Even after arriving at agreed estimates of requirements, one can arrive at different figures for recommended amounts in diet depending on the safety margin added. The amounts recommended must be taken as rough approximations and guides to practical nutrition and not as final and accurate ones. Also, in the case of several groups such as infants, expectant and nursing mothers and the aged, no extensive studies have been carried out and the amounts recommended are based on even more approximate estimates.

Also, requirements are likely to vary to some extent with environmental conditions such as temperature and with other nutrients present in the diet. For instance, thiamine requirement is reported to depend on carbohydrate intake and ascorbic acid requirement on folic acid intake, etc.

Conditions such as fever which influence metabolic rate and intestinal disorders which affect intestinal absorption and other conditions such as infections and metabolic disorders may increase nutrient requirement in different ways. Their detailed discussion is not possible in this context.

Organizations such as the FAO and WHO are concerned with the formulation of dietary and nutrient allowances which enable us to judge whether or not the diet of an individual or a group is generally adequate or inadequate with regard to a specific nutrient. Besides international agencies national organizations such as the British Medical Council in UK and the National Academy of Sciences in the U.S.A. have, also undertaken this task. In India, the Indian Council of Medical Research has also formulated dietary allowances. The author and her colleagues have also been engaged in getting information in this area and arrived at their estimates of calorie requirements for different age groups based on the heights, weights, activity levels and food intakes of well-nourished upper class subjects in this region. They have also come to the conclusion that a diet providing 8–10% protein calories would be desirable. These formulations and allowances recommended by the FAO and ICMR in respect of calories, protein and vitamin A have been discussed earlier. The requirements for other nutrients have been discussed in the appropriate context. They are summarized in **Table 28**. The amounts that can provide these nutrients are shown in **Table 29**.

Table 28. A summary of nutrient allowances suggested for different age groups.

Age (years)	Calories	Protein (g)	Vitamin A (μg) as Retinol according to FAO (1967)[1]	Carotene present report[2]	Calcium (mg) (FAO, 1962)[3]	Iron (mg) (ICMR 1971)[4]	Vitamins (FAO, 1967) mg per 1000 calories
1	900–1200	20–25	195–215	800–900	400–500	1.0 mg/kg	Thiamine: 0.4
2–4	1200–1600	28–35	210–225	850–900			
5–6	1400–1800	32–36	270–285	1100–1150			
7–10	1700–2000	32–41	345–360	1400–1450	500–600	15–20	Riboflavin: 0.55
11-12	1800–2400	36–45	450–465	1800–1850		25	
13–15 M*	2100–2800	44–56	630–645	2500–2600	600–700	25	
F*	2000–2700	41–53	525–555	2100–2200		30	
16–19 M	2200–3000	48–62	600–615	2400–2500	500–600	25	Niacin: 6.6
F	2000–2600	41–51	555–600	2200–2400		30	
Adults M	2300–3100	44–60	630–645	2500–2600	400–500	20	
F	1900–2500	36–50	540–600	2200–2400		30	

* M—Males : F—Females

[1] FAO/WHO Expert Group. 1967. Requirements of vitamin A, thiamine, riboflavin and niacin. *FAO Nutr. Meet.* Ser. No. 41. The amounts recommended by this source have been applied to the body-weights of Indians.

[2] Assuming 25% availability for carotene.

[3] FAO/WHO. 1962. Calcium Requirements. *FAO Nutr. Meet.* Ser. No. 30.

[4] "Dietary allowances for Indians". Gopalan, C. and B.S. Narasinghrao. 1971. Nutritional Research Laboratory. I.C.M.R.

Table 29. Diets suggested for different age groups.

Age (yrs)	Economic Level (a)	Cereals	Pulse (b)	Milk	Leafy vegetables	Root vegetables	Other vegetable (c)	Fruits (c)	Fats and oils (d)	Sugar + Jaggery (d)
1	I	100–150	50	200	5–10	25	25	25	10	25–40
	II	50–75	25	500–600						
2–4	I	150–175	50–60	150–200	25–50	25–50	25–50	50	15–25	25–40
	II	75–100	25–40	400–500						
5–6	I	175–200	50–60	100–200	50	25–50	50	50	25	25–40
	II	100–150	25–40	400–500						
7–10	I	250–300	60–70	100–200	50	50–100	50	50	25–40	25–40
	II	150–200	50	400–500						
11–12	I	275–375	60–75	100–200	50–75	50–100	75	50	25–40	25–40
	II	225–275	50	400–500						
13–15	I	300–450	75	100–200	50–75	50–100	75	50	25–50	25–50
	II	300–325	60–75	400–500						
16–19	I	375–475	75	100–200	50–75	50–100	75	50	25–50	25–50
	II	325–375	60–75	400–500						
20–40	I	375–550	75	100–200	50–75	50–100	75	50	25–50	25–50
	II	350–375	60–75	400–500						

Amount (g) per day

(a) I-low income, II-middle and high income.
(b) Groundnut and nuts can replace parts of the pulses and fats suggested.
(c) These are realistic amounts. More can be included if available.
(d) The amount would very with the calories provided by cereals and pulses.

Chapter 8

Nutrition in Relation to Genes— Nutrigenomics and Epigenetics

It is now well recognized that human beings have pre-disposition to their genetic make up. To understand this phenomenon in the right perspective it necessary to have a basic knowledge of the gene structure and the variations that occur in the gene structure due to several factors.

Chemical nature of genes

The macromolecule Deoxyribonucleic acid (DNA) is the genetic material of the living cell. The building blocks of this polymer are the purine and pyrimidine nucleotides. The nucleotides are linked together by phosphodiester linkages. There are four nucleotides in the DNA chain and the common structural parts of the nucleotides are the deoxyribose and phosphate. The basic difference among the four nucleotides is the composition of the purine and the pyrimidine parts.

The purines are adenine and guanine and the pyrimidines are thymine and cytosine. Therefore, the four building blocks of DNA chain are Adenine Mononucleotide Phosphate (AMP), Guanine Mononucleotide Phosphate (GMP), Guanine Mononucleotide Phosphate(GMP) and Cytosine Mononucleotide Phosphate(CMP). As the deoxyribose and phosphate parts of the nucleotides are common the four nucleotides are assigned the symbols A for AMP, G for GMP,C for CMP and T for TMP. There are 3 billion nucleotides in a single DNA chain and they are arranged in a certain sequence. The three dimensional structure of the DNA as depicted in the Watson and Crick model show that the DNA is a double helical structure. Each molecule of DNA consists of two strands of polynucleotide chains connected together by hydrogen bonds between complementary nitrogen bases. The complementary nitrogen bases are a) adenine and thymine and b) guanine and cytosine. A section of the entire DNA structure is shown in **Fig. 5.**

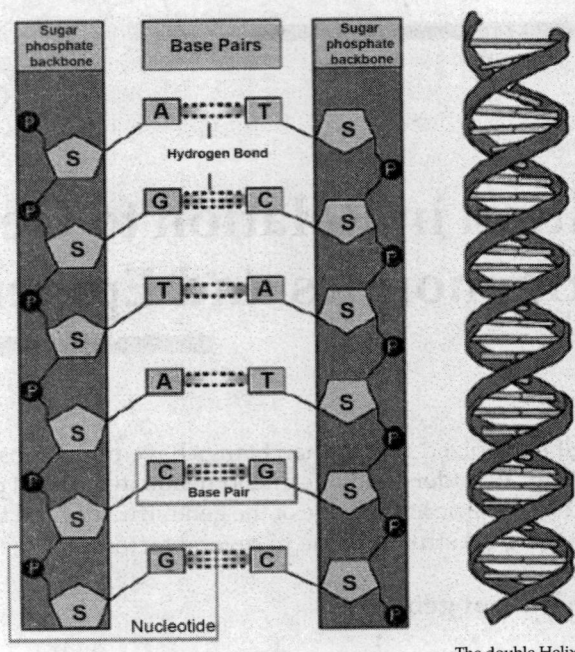

Figure 5. A section of DNA structure.
A - Adenine, T - Thymine
G - Guanine, C - Cytosine

The entire length of the DNA chain is divided into 23 segments in the case of human beings. Each segment is known as a chromosome. Thus there are 23 chromosomes in man. In genetics out of the 23 chromosomes 22 are known as autosomal and they decide the various physical features of the progeny where as the 23rd chromosome is the sex determining chromosome. Each chromosome is further segmented into genes. The genes are the working unit of the entire genome or the DNA.

Human genome project

Human Genome Project was a 13 year project with the goal:

a) identify all the 20,000–25,000 genes in human DNA (genome)

b) determine the sequence of the three billion nucleotide base pairs that make up the human DNA

c) Store this information in data bases.

The project completed in 2001 but the data will continue for many more years.

In molecular biology every protein that is synthesized in the cell is a product of gene expression. The sequence of the nucleotides in the genes decides the amino acid sequence of the protein that is coded by the gene concerned. The major metabolic reactions involved in the utilization of major nutrients vis-à-vis carbohydrate, fat and protein in various organs of the body discussed in chapter 6 are catalyzed by enzymes whose synthesis is guided by a specific gene or a group of genes. However, the aspects covered under the fate of major nutrients covered in Chapter 6 is only part of the myriad of enzyme catalyzed biochemical reactions that normally take place in the body. These biochemical reactions involving the biosynthesis of several functional substances are implicated in the normal functioning of specialized cells of the body. For instance, the compound dihydroxyphenylamine (dopamine) is synthesized in the substantia nigra the cells in the region of mid brain. Dopamine is synthesized by decarboxylation of dihydroxyphenylalanine(DOPA). Dopamine is involved in the brain function and defects in the synthesis of dopamine leads to Parkinson's disease. The exact aetiological reason of Parkinson's Disease has not been established although there are different theories attributing Parkinson's Disease to a latent virus, certain genes and environmental factors. Suffice it to state that the physiological functions of various organs of the body are closely connected to intermediates of specific biochemical reaction pathway catalyzed by enzymes. Disturbances in the normal physiological functions originate from defect in biochemical reaction rates. The rate of the myriad of biochemical reactions are determined by intracellular concentration of enzymes in the biosynthetic pathways. As mentioned earlier, the genes are the blue prints of the amino acid sequence of these enzymes and the expression of the gene in the normal manner maintains the concentration of the enzymes in consistent to the physiological requirement of the body. Defects in the gene function in terms of rate of expression or defective protein get manifested as various diseases and pathological conditions.

Single Nucleotide Polymorphism (SNP)

This is a phenomenon wherein on of the nucleotide base is replaced by another. For instance, in the base sequence AACTA, C can be replaced by T and in the complementary strand, TTGAT, G can be replaced by A as depicted in **Fig. 6**. This small variation in gene structure is known as Single Nucleotide Polymorphism (SNP). SNPs are scattered through out the DNA. SNP can be silent, harmless or harmful or have latent effect. They occur every 100–300 bases along the DNA. If the SNP is found close to a particular gene it acts as a marker for that gene. If the SNP happen

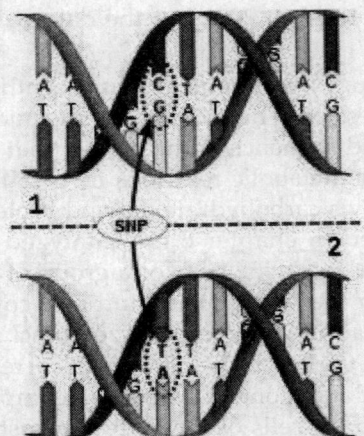

Figure 6. Single Nucleotide Polymorphism (SNP).

in the coding region of a gene it could alter the amino acid sequence of the protein coded by that gene. The protein(enzyme) so formed will be different from the normal enzyme and its activity will not be akin to the normal physiological function of the body where that enzyme is involved. The normal physiology will change as a result of which the health of the individual will be affected.

SNP as a risk factor

SNPs do not cause disease but can help the likelihood that someone will develop a particular disease under conditions like environmental factors, toxins, virus and contaminants in foods that are conducive for the expression of the altered gene. This will help nutritionist to design personalized diets that can help to preempt the individual from ill health caused if such genes are expressed. A few examples of altered protein structure as a result of SNPs are discussed below:

Apolipoprotein E (ApoE)

One of the genes associated with Alzheimer's Disease is the gene which codes for the protein apolipoprotein E. Alzheimer's Disease is a progressive brain disease characterized by progressive memory loss and cognitive functions of the brain. The disease develops due to the formation of a peptide amyloid plaques which has 36-46 amino acids. This peptide causes shrinkage of the cortex region of the brain and death of the cells. The connection between the nerve cells is lost in this disease. Early onset of this disease is inherited due to SNP on chromosome 21, 14 and 1. Late onset of Alzheimer's Disease develops after the age of 60 and the pre-disposing risk factor relates to ApoE gene found on chromosome 19.

ApoE gene consists of 3 genetic variations carried by alleles E2, E3 and E4. of which E3 is the most prominent. E4 version of ApoE gene increases the individual's risk of developing late onset of Alzheimer's Disease.

ApoE and atherosclerosis

ApoE is essential for the normal catabolism of triglycerides rich lipoproteins containing cholesterol. Inadequate catabolism of triglycerides and cholesterol is a risk factor in the development of atherosclerosis and cardiovascular disease. ApoE has been studied for its role in several biological processes including lipoprotein transport, Alzheimer's Disease and immunity. ApoE4 has been shown to greatly increase the risk of developing atherosclerosis. ApoE2 has been shown to increase the risk of a condition known as hyperlipoproteinemia type III. This condition is characterized by increased blood levels of cholesterol and triglycerides.

ApoE genotype testing can be done using blood samples of subjects. Knowledge of relative proportion of the three genetic variants of apoE is helpful in the selection of foods appropriate for people of the various categories in the contents of the three variants in the genes.

Nutrigenomics promises us the ability to tailor diets based on individual genetic make-up. Through the advances made in the Human Genome Project, SNP in important genes have been identified and their clinical association with many metabolic aberrations have been discovered and documented. Nutrigenomic test panel has been created that can be used to identify individual genomic differences in the laboratory. Correct interpretation of nutrigenomic test result will enable to recommend specific foods and food constituents that can modify the negative health effects of individual genetic profile offer great promise in personalized nutrition. Nutrients and phytonutrients in fruits, vegetables and various herbs used in foods can interact with genome causing changes in their expression thereby reducing the negative effects of individual genetic profile.

Epigenetics

Epigenetics refers to heritable changes in gene expression or phenotypic characteristics by mechanism other than changes in nucleotide sequence in DNA. In other words, epigenetic effects of gene expression do not involve SNP as discussed in nutrigenomics. The two classical examples of epigenic changes in genes are:

a) DNA methylation and b) Histone modification

Both these processes regulate gene expression without altering nucleotide sequence in DNA. These mechanisms can enable the effects on parents to be passed on to offspring. The genes in the chromosomes are normally in combination with a basic protein called histone. These basic proteins are called epigenetic marks. When the epigenetic mark sit on the gene the gene does not get expressed. The genes are silenced by the epigenetic marks. Histone modification is the process by which the histone loose its capacity to sit on the gene. One prominent histone modification is the acetylation by addition of acetyl group at the N terminal of the histone. Acetylation loosen the DNA histone combination. When this happens the gene starts expressing and the initiation of protein coded by this gene starts.

Addition of methyl group to the DNA occurs mostly on cytosine at the CG loci of the gene to convert cytosine to 5 methyl cytosine. 5 methyl cytosine behaves like a regular cytosine pairing with regular guanine. Some areas of the genome are more heavily methylated than others and highly methylated areas are less expressive.

The importance of DNA methylation in altering the physical characteristics of an organism was demonstrated in 2003 by Randy Jirtle and Robert Waterland. They conducted an elegant experiment on mice with a gene called agouti gene—a gene that gives mice yellow coat and tendency for obesity and diabetes. Jirtle and Waterland fed one group of pregnant agouti mice with a diet rich in folic acid and vitamin B12. Another group of genetically identical pregnant agouti mice got no such pre-natal nutrition. A third group was fed a diet supplemented with the phytoestrogen genistein present in soya bean. Folic acid and Vitamin B12 facilitate the addition of methyl group to the gene at the cytosine residues, methyl group being supplied by methionine by mechanism of C1 metabolism (methionine folate cycle) shown in Fig. 7. Supplementation of Folic acid and Vit B12 facilitated addition of more methyl groups to the agouti gene in the uterus thereby altering its expression without altering the genomic structure of

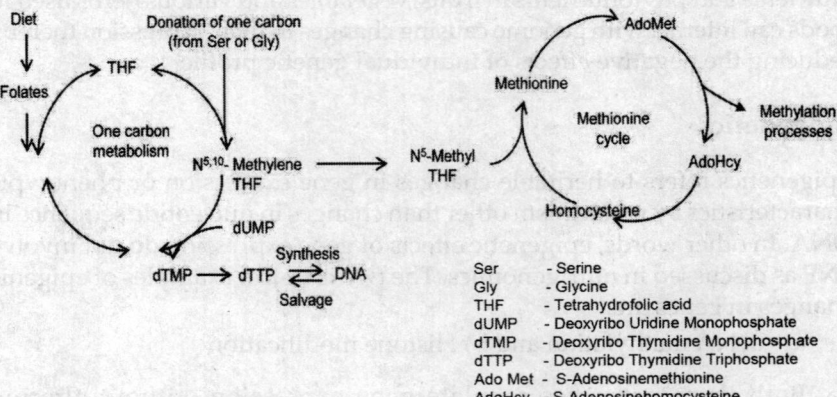

Figure 7. Methionine Folate Cycle.

the mouse DNA. Simply by furnishing B vitamins Jirtle and Waterland got agouti mothers to produce healthy brown pups with normal weight and not prone to diabetes and obesity. Similar results were obtained with genistein supplemented diet as depicted in Fig. 7a (*Courtesy:* Randy Jirtle).

Nutrients and other dietary components can reverse or change epigenetic phenomena such as methylation and histone modification resulting in altered expression of genes associated with development of pathological conditions starting from the embryonic stage to aging, diseases such as cancer, cardiovascular diseases, diabetes and brain disorders like Alzheimer's Disease. Nutrients and phytochemicals in foods can bring about epigenetic changes either by directly inhibiting enzymes or by limiting or increasing the availability of substrates.

There are many dietary components with epigenetic properties. Some of the components have been mentioned under phytonutrients in Chapter 14. A few other components with known epigenetic properties are shown below:

Lunasin – A small peptide of 43 amino acids is present in Soyabean. It inhibits the expression of oncogene, implicated in cancer.

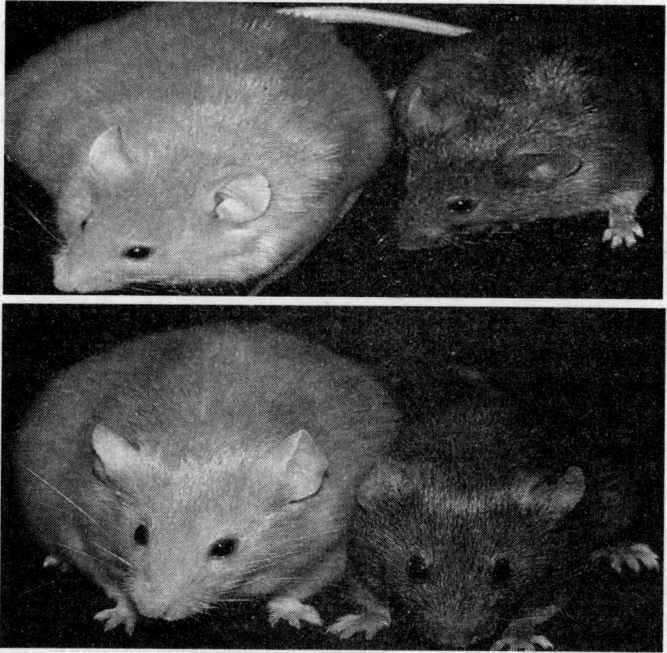

Figure 7a. Left Side of both photos—offsprings of mother fed normal diet, Top Right Side—offspring of mother fed normal diet with methyl donors, Bottom Right Side—offspring of mother fed normal diet with genistein. (*also see colour plate*)

Sulforaphanes – They are sulphur containing compounds present in Brassica family of vegetables. They inhibit histone deacetylation by the enzyme histone deacetylase (HDAC). HDAC removes the acetyl group from the N-terminal of the histone and this enzyme is inhibited by sulforaphanes.

EGCG – One of the polyphenols present in green tea. EGCG is implicated in demethylation of DNA.

Genistein – One of the isoflavones present in soyabean. Genistein is implicated in methylation and demethylation of DNA.

Resveratrol – A phenolic compound present in red grapes. Resveratrol affects NAD dependent histone deacylases involved in the regulation of protein called PGC-1 alpha. PGC-1 alpha is a member of transcription coactivators that plays a central role in the regulation of cellular energy metabolism. This protein is strongly induced by cold exposure which helps in thermogenesis so as to enable the body to adapt to cold environment. PGC-1 alpha stimulates mitochondrial biogenesis so that muscle metabolism turns more oxidative than glycolytic. PGC-1 alpha participates in the regulation of carbohydrate and fat metabolism in such a way as to enable the body to adapt to environmental cold stress.

Diet during early development can cause changes lasting into adulthood. Mother's diet during pregnancy and the diet taken during infancy can cause critical changes that is carried on to the adulthood. Animal studies have shown that methyl donating folate deficiency during late foetal or early post-natal development cause certain regions of the genome undermethylated for life. In the case of adults, diet deficient in methyl donors can still lead to decrease in DNA methylation but changes are reversible with resumption of normal diet.

Although the possibility of developing a treatment or devising preventive measures against a number of diseases by nutritional intervention is exciting, the current knowledge in the field is limited and further studies are needed to use this approach for maintaining health and preventing diseases.

Further Reading

Ann L. Yaktin and Robert Pool. 2007. Nutrigenomics and Beyond. Institute of Medicine, National Academic Press, Washington, D.C.

Kaput, J. and R.L. Rodriguez. 2004, Nutritional Genomics: The next frontier in the post-genomic era. *Physiological Genomics*, **16**:166–177.

Kaput, J. and R. Rodriguez (eds.) 2006. Discovering the path to Personalized Nutrition: In Nutritional Genomics. Wiley and Sons Inc., New York.

Jirtle, Randy. 2005. Epigenetics Means What We Eat, How We Live and Love, Alters How Our Genes Behave. *Science Daily*. Work of Prof. J. Randy Duke University.

Part II:
Foods

Chapter 9

Use of Food Tables

In the foregoing chapters we have discussed nutrients required by the body in relation to metabolic function and the desirable amounts in which they should be consumed. However, we do not get our nutrients in the form of pure proteins, carbohydrates, etc. and they have to be derived from foods such as bread, roti, rice, dal, snacks, vegetables and beverages. These, in turn, are composed of cereals, millets, legumes, vegetables, oils, milk, sugar, etc. The translation of foods consumed to their nutrient content is made possible by the availability of food tables which give the chemical composition of different foods on the basis of actual analysis in the laboratory. In this country, the most widely used tables are those published by the Indian Council of Medical Research*.

These tables generally give the amounts of different nutrients present in 100 g of the foodstuffs. A scrutiny of the tables enables us to recognize not only the nutrient content of individual foods but also the general chemical composition of food groups such as cereals, legumes, vegetables, meats, fish, etc. For instance, we find that cereals and millets are similar in that 100 g of the same have a protein content ranging from 7–13 g and energy value of about 350 Calories. Legumes have a similar calorie content but a higher protein content of 20–25%. Oil seeds are rich sources of protein, fat and calories. Vegetables have a low calorie content and high moisture content. Vegetable oils and refined sugar contribute only calories and not protein, vitamins or minerals. Thus food tables help us to recognize the general characteristics of different categories of foodstuffs.

These tables can also help us to recognize particularly good sources of different nutrients. For example, we can easily recognize from the

---

* Gopalan, C., B.V. Ram Sastri and S.C. Balasubramanian. 1972. Nutritive value of Indian foods, *National Institute of Nutrition*, ICMR, Hyderabad, India.

same that leaf greens contain liberal amounts of carotene, and milk, of calcium.

They also help us to recognize the deficiencies in individual foodstuffs or classes of the same. It is easy to see, for instance, that grains such as rice and vegetable oils (with the exception of red palm oil) have no carotene. Tables of amino acid composition tell us that cereals are deficient in lysine, whereas pulses are good sources of the same.

People concerned with assessing the nutrient content of foods should, therefore, familiarize themselves with the use of such tables. An intelligent use of such tables can help in the formulation of satisfactory meals.

The use of food tables involves an awareness of their limitations. First of all, it must be recognized that the figures given are based generally on analysis of casual samples and that the nutrient content of the same foodstuff may vary from sample to sample depending on factors such as genetic strain of seed (or animal), method Of cultivation (or farm management), processing and quality of soil or feed. For instance, the protein content of rice may vary from 6 to 10%. The variation is greater in the case of minerals and much greater in the case of vitamins. For instance, different samples of bitter gourd analyzed in the author's laboratory were found to contain 100-180 mg of ascorbic acid per 100 g. Similarly, the carotene content of amaranth was found to vary from 9000 to 11000 i.u. **Table 30** shows the composition of different hybrid strains of bajra from which some idea can be had of variations in the composition of food grains. Also, foodstuffs such as milk and curd vary very much in quality and degree of adulteration (**Table** 31). Some judgment must be exercised in guessing the degree of adulteration.

Table 30. Chemical composition of selected strains of hybrid bajra.

Sam-ple No.	Amount per 100 g									
	Protein (g)	Fat (g)	Carbo-hydrate (g)	Ash (g)	Calcium (mg)	Phos-phorus	Iron	Thia-mine (mg)	Ribo-flavin (mg)	Niacin (mg)
1	9.8	6.3	82.1	1.8	24.1	340	4.8	0.38	0.28	5.6
2	8.9	5.9	83.7	1.5	23.6	251	5.6	0.25	0.26	5.2
3	8.7	6.7	82.6	2.0	25.2	269	4.6	0.27	0.28	2.6
4	16.4	5.7	76.1	1.8	32.4	258	4.7	0.28	0.26	5.5
5	17.1	5.7	75.2	2.0	25.0	377	5.6	0.33	0.25	4.5
6	16.4	6.9	74.7	2.0	30.4	385	6.9	0.31	0.26	4.2
7	16.2	6.1	76.0	1.7	21.7	344	4.6	0.36	0.25	5.0
8	17.8	6.2	74.0	2.0	28.8	370	4.8	0.31	0.29	4.0
9	16.2	6.0	76.1	1.7	20.7	348	3.9	0.32	0.23	5.2

*   Data obtained in the Biochemistry Department of Baroda University.

Table 31. Composition of different market sample of buffalo milk[1].

Sample	Amount (g) per 100 g			Calories per 100 g
	Carbohydrate	Fat	Protein	
1	2.2	3.2	1.5	43
2	4.2	6.3	3.1	86
3	2.7	2.8	1.8	43
4	2.6	3.8	2.2	53
5	4.4	4.8	3.0	73
6	4.7	6.2	3.2	87
7	5.0	7.3	3.5	100
8	5.1	8.8	4.3	80
ICMR Food Tables	5.1	8.8	4.3	118

[1] Data obtained in the Biochemistry Department of Baroda University.

With practice, it is possible to taste the sample and make a guess about the water content. Similarly, cuts of meat vary very much in fat content and, therefore, in calorie value.

The aim of food tables is to give us an idea of the approximate nutrients of a particular foodstuff rather than its actual composition. Fortunately, in most cases the actual values are close enough to the average value expected for most practical purposes. However, in balance studies and the like, the food samples must be analyzed.

Also, it must be remembered that the values given in food tables do not take into account possible losses of nutrients during cooking. For instance, a considerable proportion of the water soluble vitamins in rice may be removed by washing and straining off the excess cooking water. Similarly, cabbage as cooked in most households is practically devoid of vitamin C by the time it is consumed. While calculating the vitamin content of foods, allowances must be made for such losses. The losses of ascorbic acid and carotene amount on an average to 33–50% depending on the method of cooking. The losses of thiamine may be of the order of 25%.

Another problem is that the presence of a nutrient in a particular foodstuff is no guarantee that all of it will be available to the animal body because of differences in absorption. This applies particularly to nutrient such as calcium, iron, carotene, protein and nicotinic acid. An awareness of factors governing absorption and the average proportions in which they are absorbed from different categories of foodstuffs is necessary. For instance, the amount of iron available from vegetable source is believed on an average to be 15% with wide variation on either side of this figure, and that of carotene from 25–80% perhaps with an average value of about

40–50%. The availability of lysine is affected by dry heat as in roasting and parching. The presence or absence of substances such as phytic acid and oxalic acid which are believed to interfere with mineral absorption must be noted. It is necessary to distinguish between 'good' and 'poor' sources of a nutrient on the basis not only of the amount of the nutrient present but also the proportion likely to be absorbed and utilized by the body.

Finally, it is not enough for a foodstuff to be rich in a particular nutrient, but its relevance from the practical standpoint will depend on the amounts in which it is likely to be consumed. Many spices are rich in protein and mineral content but they are not of much nutritional significance because of the small amounts in which they are consumed. For instance, 'ajma' (omum) is rich in iron (28 mg in 100 g) but one must consume more than 50g or half a cup of the same to meet the day's requirement of iron whereas one can hardly consume more than 2 g. The food tables published by the ICMR are the most extensively used in this country. Other tables include those published by McCance and Widdowson, the United States Department of Agriculture and the FAO.

Processing involves changes in nutrient content. Parboiled, hand-pounded and milled rice, for instance, differ in nutritive value, but in order to get an idea of the effects of processing, analysis must be done on samples derived from the same lot of paddy.

When the values show marked discrepancy, we should be able to exercise some discretion and choose what appears to be a more reasonable value on the basis of the food group to which the foodstuff belongs and a comparison of the values reported in different food tables.

When diet surveys are carried out, the data are often in the form of amounts of different food groups consumed. In this case it is sometimes convenient to use typical values for the different food groups. The author has arrived at average values for grains, vegetables, etc. consumed in Gujarat **(Table 32).** Similar values can be compiled for other regions. However such values should be used only when information on the specific foodstuffs consumed is not available.

In summary, one must learn to use food tables to get an idea of the average amounts of different nutrients present in different categories of food stuffs, to identify 'poor' and 'rich' sources of individual nutrients and to assess the nutritional adequacy of a given diet. But one must remember that the figures given are average values which vary from sample to sample, that the values do not allow for losses in nutrient content during processing and cooking, that the amount of nutrient present must be considered in relation to average amounts of the foodstuff likely to be consumed, and that the availability of nutrients may vary in different foodstuffs and sometimes, in the same foodstuff, on account of differences in absorption.

Table 32. Average nutrient content of different foodstuffs.[a]

Foodstuff	Approximate amount per 100g						
	Calories	Protein (g)	Calcium (mg)	Iron (mg)	Vitamin A (µg)	Ribo-flavin (mg)	% protein calories
Cereals	345	10	30	6.0	60	0.10	11
Pulses	345	24	80	8.0	60	0.40	28
Groundnuts	550	26	190	1.6	40	0.30	19
Leafy vegetables	50	4	250	15.0	4500	0.30	32
Other vegetables	40	2	40	2.0	180	0.06	20
Root vegetables	100	1.5	20	0.6	60	0.02	6
Milk (buffalo)[b]	80	3.5	210	0.2	30	0.10	17
Egg	170	13	60	2.0	600	0.18	31
Mutton	200	20	12[d]	2.0	10	0.27	40
Fowl	109	26	12[d]	2.0	30	0.27	95
Liver	130	20	12[d]	2.0	2800	1.70	62
Fruits[c] (i)	100				600 (iii)		3
Fruits (ii)	50	0.8	30		30 (iv)		6
sugar	400	0	0	0	0	0	0
Oil	900	0	0	0	0	0	0

[a] approximate averages of values given in the food tables published by the ICMR for commonly consumed foods in each group in Gujarat.
[b] values for calories, protein and vitamin A based on analysis of dairy milk in Baroda.
[c] (i) and (ii) fruits rich and poor in carbohydrate. (iii), (iv) fruits rich and poor in carotene
[d] These values are taken from the food tables published by the FAO.

Chapter 10

Cereals and Millets

Many grasses are known for their edible seeds. It is the seed or kernel of the grass that is used for food purposes. These are known as cereals and millets. They constitute a major foodstuff in the diet of man and the predominant item in the diet of the poor. The chief staples used in this country are rice (*Orysa sativa*), wheat (*Triticum aestimm*), jowar {*Sorghum vulgare*}, maize {*Zea mays*)and bajra (*Pennisetum typhoideum*). Ragi (*Eleusine corcana*) and kodri or varagu (*Paspalum scorbiculatum* L) are cultivated on a smaller scale (**Table 33**).

Cereals and millets are not only the chief sources of calories but also of most other nutrients. The per capita intake of cereals among the middle classes is of the order of 250 g, among the urban poor, 350–400 g and among agricultural 400–500 g.

Table 33. Food grain production in India during 2011-12.

Cereal	Production in 2011-12 (million metric ton)	% of total grain produced
Rice	103.0*	41.0
Wheat	90.0*	36.0
Jowar	6.0**	2.4
Maize	21.0*	8.4
Bajra	10.0**	4.0
Barley	1.7**	0.7
Ragi	2.0**	0.8
Small millets	0.7**	0.28

* Govt.of India, Press Information Bureau, July 26, 2012.

** Dept.of Agriculture, Govt.of India, Third Advance estimate of production of food grain 2011-12.

Table 34 shows the proportion of different nutrients derived from cereals and millets in ordinary Indian diets.

The most extensively cultivated food grain is rice which is believed to have been first cultivated in India. It forms the staple article of the diet of large numbers in several parts of the country. Wheat is the next major crop produced in this country and has been known from very early times. It is extensively cultivated in Punjab and Uttar Pradesh.

Maize was first cultivated and consumed by only the Red Indians in North America. It was introduced in other countries relatively recently. Today, it is a major crop in India and many people in Punjab, Rajasthan and the tribal people in Gujarat use it as a staple. Wild barley is also consumed in these regions.

Jowar and bajra are the major millets consumed in this country. They are mostly used in Maharashtra, Madhya Pradesh and Gujarat. Kodri or varagu and ragi are cultivated in smaller quantities.

There are other grains such as barley, Italian millet, wild rice, etc., consumed by limited sections of the population.

Wheat and rice are cultivated in fertile lands with a good water supply. The millets are more resistant to drought and are cultivated where the conditions are not favourable for the cultivation of wheat and rice. Maize, although a cereal, resembles millets in its capacity to survive in drought conditions. Other grains such as rye and oats are not cultivated in this country.

The protein content of cereals ranges from 7–12%. But in the amounts taken they contribute the major part of our dietary protein (Table 34). As mentioned in Chapter 2 cereal proteins are lacking in lysine but this can be supplied by including legumes which have a higher protein and lysine content. Many of the legumes are marginally deficient in methionine. Millets such as ragi, kodri, bajra and jowar are better sources of methionine.

Table 34. Proportion of nutrients contributed by cereals and millets in Indian diets.

| Nutrient | % derived from cereals and millets | |
| | Urban Baroda | |
	Lower class	Upper class
Calories	77	34
Protein	77	45
Calcium	36	7
Iron	88	63
Vitamin A	31	16
riboflavin	63	26

The marginal lysine content of cereals and millets may be a problem only in the case of young children because of the increased lysine requirement for growth. As mentioned earlier, supplementation of cereal with legumes or animal foods can take care of this problem.

Rice

Rice is the most extensively cultivated grain not only in India but also in most of South East Asia. The reasons for its popularity are obvious. Cooking of rice is simple as compared to that of other cereals which have to be milled or ground into flour to be made into leavened or unleavened bread. Rice can be just boiled without involving any preparation. It cooks soft and is, therefore, suitable for young children, the toothless aged and convalescents. It has an attractive colour and appearance and a bland flavour and, therefore, blends well with other foods. It gives satiety value because of its bulk without being heavy to the consumer. It lends itself to incorporation in a variety of snacks. Paddy and rice are processed in different ways to yield ready-to-eat or easy to cook foods resembling breakfast cereals.

The harvested grain has a fibrous husk and is called paddy. The husk forms 20–25% of the whole grain and is not edible. The dehusked grain has an outer cover of a brown powdery layer which contains most of the vitamins and minerals in the grain. This powdery layer is intact in hand-pounded unpolished rice.

When rice is dehusked in rice-mills most of this brown layer is generally removed and the grain has a white polished appearance. However, it is possible to produce undermilled rice. Often, hand-pounded rice is polished so that it resembles milled rice.

Polished rice is preferred to hand-pounded or undermilled rice partly because it keeps better and is less susceptible to insect spoilage and partly because people have developed a preference for the taste and appearance of the refined product.

Rice is also prepared after parboiling. The paddy is soaked in water for 2-3 days, boiled or steamed, dried and then dehusked to produce parboiled rice. The grain is slightly coloured and is harder than the original grain. The dehusking can be done by hand or machine. During parboiling, the brown outer layer adheres to the grain and most of the nutrients in it are driven into the interior of the grain. Parboiled rice has a better vitamin and mineral content and a better keeping quality than milled rice.

The nutrient content of parboiled rice as compared to hand pounded and milled rice is shown in **Table 35.**

The process of parboiling was first developed in India and parboiled rice was used by most of the rice-consuming people in this country till a

Table 35. Chemical composition of products derived from paddy*.

	amount per 100 g			
	protein (g)	ash (g)	thiamine (microgram)	riboflavin (microgram)
dehusked rice	6.8	0.12	208	105
parboiled rice	6.8	0.12	200	100
milled rice	6.8	0.10	105	52

* Data obtained in the Biochemistry Department of Baroda University.

couple of decades ago, but unfortunately the consumption of polished rice is becoming increasingly popular and regarded as something of a status symbol. The preference for milled rice is also partly due to the fact that when paddy is soaked for a long time in water, it begins to ferment, resulting in an off-flavour. The difference in colour and appearance is another factor.

A modified method which eliminates both the colour and odour of parboiled rice has been developed by the Central Food Technological Research Institute, Mysore in which instead of soaking the paddy in cold water for 2-3 days at room temperature before boiling, the temperature of the water is increased to 65–67°C and the period of soaking reduced to two to three hours. The increase in temperature as well as the decrease in soaking time help to prevent undesirable fermentation which is responsible for the offensive flavour of some samples of parboiled rice.

During parboiling, the starch in the grain is gelatinized and the grain hardened. Losses during milling are decreased in this process. The yield of parboiled rice from paddy is 5–10% more than that of milled rice.

Parboiling also results in better cooking quality and reduces losses during cooking.

A process similar to parboiling has been developed using modern machinery. The paddy is heated and steam-treated under standard conditions, dried in vacuum and milled. The rice obtained by this method is called converted rice.

Cooking of rice

Rice is generally cooked by boiling in water. During cooking, the starch is gelatinized so that we get discrete grains instead of a lumpy mass. In order to ensure this, the powdery layer is removed by scrubbing and washing several times. This results in further losses of nutrients. The losses are less with parboiled rice as can be seen from the following data*:

Similar losses take place in the case of other nutrients such as riboflavin, nicotinic acid, calcium, iron and phosphorus. Greater losses occur when rice is soaked in excess water and the steeping water discarded after scrubbing. This is done during the preparation of products like idli and dosa.

microgram per 100 g of rice washing.

	thiamine content	Amount lost during		
		1st	2nd	3rd washing
Milled rice	100	22.0	9.0	5.0
Parboiled rice	201	10.0	8.6	2.6

* Swaminathan, M. 1942. The effect of washing and cooking on the Vitamin B1 content of raw and parboiled rice. *Ind, J. Med. Res.* 30, 3.

Further losses occur when rice is cooked in excess water and the surplus water discarded as can be seen from **Table 36**. These losses are more in the case of milled rice.

Old rice and new rice

The cooking quality of rice improves with storage. The starch in rice and other grains consists of amylose and amylopectin which are somewhat different in structure and complexity. The rice is more sticky when cooked if it is richer in amylose. With the aging of rice, the starch granules of rice have a tendency to aggregate and acquire a higher degree of molecular complexity and the proportion of amylose is reduced and that of amylopectin increased, so that the cooking quality of rice is improved. Another change is the slow dehydration as a result of which the outer powdery layer adheres more firmly to the grain with accompanying changes in characteristics. As can be expected losses of nutrients during washing or in cooking water is less in the case of old rice.

Table 36. Change in nutritive value of rice with washing and cooking.[1]

	mg per 100 g raw rice[2]		
	Thiamine	riboflavin	nicotinic acid
Raw rice[3]	1.90 (100)	1.64 (100)	4.20 (100)
Washing	0.27 (13.8)	0.03 (1.8)	0.00 (0)
Washed rice	1.68 (86.2)	1.61 (98.2)	4.20 (100)
Cooked by absorption method	0.87 (44.6)	1.15 (70.2)	4.18 (99.5)
Cooked in surplus water and the conjee discarded	0.49 (25.1)	0.72 (43.9)	2.60 (61.9)
Discarded congee	0.49 (20.5)	0.41 (25.0)	1.52 (36.2)

[1] Data obtained in the Biochemistry Department of Baroda University.
[2] The figures in parentheses are percentages of the amounts in the original rice.
[3] A mixture containing 88 g milled rice and 12 g of a pre-mix fortified with vitamins supplied by the US Agency for International Development, New Delhi.

Generally, more water is needed for cooking old rice than for cooking new rice. One of the problems of cooking newly milled rice is that it tends to cook to a sticky mass. This does not happen in the case of parboiled rice even if it is new.

Old rice increases in length much more than new rice and without disintegration. New rice exhibits greater fragility of cell walls as evidenced by its tendency to burst during cooking. This is consistent with its greater amylose content.

The texture of cooked rice can be improved by heating the rice to a vigorous boil and then allowing it to simmer on slow heat till cooking is completed. The rice should be cooked in just enough water so that all of it is absorbed during cooking. The amount of water needed varies from to 3 cups of water for one cup of rice. When rice is cooked by vigorous boiling throughout, more water and fuel are needed, and the cooked rice tends to be lumpy and to get burnt at bottom and form a dry layer at the top. Contrary to popular belief, cooking by simmering does not take more time than vigorous boiling.

The time required for cooking rice can be reduced appreciably by pre-soaking it in water for an hour or two. The amount of water used for cooking should be reduced to about two cups per cup of raw rice.

The cooking quality of new rice can be improved by roasting it in a pan before cooking so as to result in partial dehydration or by pre-soaking in water or roasting followed by pre-soaking. It can also be improved by first cooking with limited water and then steaming. The addition of a little fat during cooking helps to keep the grains discrete. The addition of a few drops of lemon juice or citric acid improves the colour of the cooked product.

A process has been developed by the Central Food Technological Research Institute, Mysore, for the wet heat conditioning of rice to impart hardness to the grain so that the disintegration of starch granules into cooking water, leading to pastiness, is prevented. The method consists of adding boiling water to fresh rice, heating for 2-3 minutes and then letting it stand for about 2–4 hours during which period the rice is partially parboiled and becomes soft. The rice is then steamed to obtain a product completely free from pastiness.

Although new rice has a poorer cooking quality, it is preferable to old rice for the preparation of certain products such as 'papdi'and 'sev' which are dehydrated macaroni-type products prepared from rice flour. One part of rice flour is cooked with 1.5 to 2 parts of water to form a firm but pliable and smooth dough and the same shaped into balls and pressed in a 'sev' or 'chakli' press (cookie press) so that it comes out in desired shapes. Better results are obtained if the balls are steamed before pressing. This is dried and stored and deep fried in hot fat as needed. The quality of deep fried products prepared from rice flour such as 'chakli' is also improved by using new rice.

The addition of rice flour to products like scotch bread or 'sev' (fried preparation from bengal gram flour) improves the crisp quality of the product and reduces the amount of shortening needed. This may be due to the gelatinization of rice starch during baking or frying.

Other rice products

Paddy lends itself to the preparation of a variety of products which have been popular from the earliest times. Parched paddy, rice flakes, puffed rice and parched rice flakes are prepared from paddy or rice. The preparation of these products will be described elsewhere.

Rice is also used for the preparation of fermented foods such as idli and dosa in South India and dhokla in Gujarat.

Rice has less protein than most other grains but rice protein is of superior quality. It has also less calcium, carotene and magnesium. Polished rice has even less of minerals and vitamins and its exclusive consumption has been associated with beriberi and occasionally with pellagra. These can be prevented by the use of either parboiled rice or under-milled or hand-pounded rice. Beriberi is prevalent in Andhra Pradesh where highly polished rice is consumed and is practically absent in Tamil Nadu and Kerala where parboiled rice is consumed by the majority of people. In Tamil Nadu, the middle and upper classes are switching over to polished rice. The consumption of polished rice is not usually associated with beriberi in the upper classes because of the greater consumption of pulses, milk and other foods.

Fortification of rice

Because of the widespread consumption of milled rice and its association with beriberi, attempts have been made to enrich milled rice with the nutrients lacking in it. However, such fortified rice has a yellow colour which is not acceptable to most people. Further, the rice so fortified is likely to lose some of the nutrients added during washing and cooking. Attempts are also being made to add to milled rice a premix resembling rice and containing concentrated amounts of nutrients. Although the premix is yellow in colour, as only one part of the same is added to 200 parts of rice, the colour and appearance of the resulting products are quite acceptable. But it is possible that some people may carefully pick out the yellow grains before cooking in the belief that they are contaminants unless they are educated about its value. Further, appreciable losses of nutrients occur during cooking (Table 36). The addition of a premix poses problems as small rice mills are scattered all over the country. Popularizing the Use of parboiled rice seems to be a more feasible approach. But fortified rice may prove valuable in school lunch programmes, hostels, hospitals and the like.

Wheat

Next to rice, wheat is the grain most extensively cultivated and consumed. The popularity of wheat is due to the desirable characteristics of chapaties and bread prepared from the same. Wheat contains more protein than other food grains but is deficient in lysine which can be made up by the addition of legumes rich in this amino acid.

Wheat is used mostly in the form of chapaties in this country and in the form of yeast breads in western countries. The unique physico-chemical and rheological properties of wheat dough and its baking quality is due to the protein gluten present in it. Gluten can be separated from the flour by washing off all the starch particles. It plays an important role in the texture of foodstuffs prepared from wheat. When bread dough is kneaded the gluten strands stretch and come into contact with each other and form a net-like structure in which the starch is embedded. This enables the dough to swell. This property is important in the making of breads and accounts for the softer texture of breads prepared from wheat as compared to that from other grains. Chapaties prepared from wheat puff out when they are baked and this quality is not evident in rotis prepared from other grains.

The gluten content of wheat varies from about 9 to 13%. The harder varieties contain more gluten than the softer varieties and are more suitable for bread and chapaties whereas the latter are more suitable for cakes, biscuits and other products prepared from wheat flour such as sakkarpara and nimki. A blend of the two varieties is very suitable for chapaties.

Suji or rava (cream of wheat) and macaroni made from the harder varieties have a better quality. The products tend to become pasty during cooking if prepared from softer varieties.

To get good chapaties, the dough should be kneaded well so as to allow the gluten strands to form. If this is not done, its puffing quality is affected and the edges become cracked. The unpopularity of wheat in South India is mainly because people lack the skills needed for making chapaties and the poor quality of the chapaties prepared makes them unacceptable. The time and labour required for making them seem to be too much for people used to cooking rice by boiling. Preparations such as debra, dhokla and dosa from wheat are likely to be more popular with South Indians as the same are closer to their culinary practice. Their preparation will be described elsewhere.

Wheat Milling

India produces about 80 million tones of wheat. Wheat is mainly consumed in the form of atta,suji and maida. Most of the wheat is milled in small capacity disc mills to produce whole wheat flour consisting of the endosperm the outer layer and bran. Wheat is also milled in capital intensive roller flour mills to produce products such as refined flower or maida used in bakery industry to produce various products. Roller flour milling involves the separation of endosperm, the germ portion and the bran. Apart from maida the roller flour mills also produce resultant atta by combining refined flour with bran in desired proportion. Chakki milled atta has better chapati making quality because of the presence of more damaged starch in it. Starch in the flour is damaged by the heat produced during milling which is more in chakki milling than roller flour milling. Damaged starch is important because enzymes in flour namely alpha and beta amylase work better on damaged starch to produce compounds that converted to simple sugars for feeding yeast during fermentation and to promote brown crust formation during baking. Damaged starch has more water absorption capacity.

Refined flour or maida is used for the making of yeast breads and other wheat products. During the refinement of flour a major part of the vitamins and minerals are lost and protein quality is also affected. In western countries, the lost nutrients are replaced by enriching the flour with the same. In this country, this is not done.

Wheat flour or refined flour which are cheaper than rice-flour can be substituted for the latter in recipes such as chakli after pre-treatment. The flour should be placed over a dry cheese cloth in an idli steamer or colander and heated over steam for about five minutes. This treatment is found to prevent the stretching of gluten strands so as to form a net-like structure. Products prepared from flour treated in this way lose their rubbery texture and become crisp. Pre-treated flour requires less shortening than untreated flour in biscuits, short breads, pastries; etc.

Wheat is also parboiled like paddy before dehusking to yield bulgar wheat. Bulgar wheat and bengal gram similarly treated are the main ingredients in a processed food mixture called laubina used for treating and preventing malnutrition in the Middle East.

Some people advocate the enrichment of flour with lysine and other nutrients. But most of the wheat consumed in rural areas is produced locally and milled into flour at small flour mills and hence this cannot be easily done. Increase in lysine can also be achieved by adding bengal gram flour to the flour used for baking. About one part of the former added to six parts of the latter is found quite acceptable. Bread can also be made from a combination of wheat, bengal gram and groundnut in the ratio 8:1:1. Bread made with fortified flour is sold in large cities such as Bombay but this bread is consumed only by the upper classes whose diet is not likely to be deficient in lysine, calcium or the other nutrients added as they consume plenty of dals as well as milk. Nutritive value of home made products from atta can be increased by altering the recipes of such products. For instance, 'debras' a traditional food of Gujarat made from whole wheat flour, bengal gram and leafy vegetable has high nutritive value in terms of protein quality and vitamins. Rats fed 'debras' were found to gain 12 g per week as compared to 6 g by those fed bread.

Bread production in India has increased 3 times during the past 2 decades. About 3 million tons of bread is produced in India both in the organized and unorganized sections. The reason for increase in bread consumption are many. This include (a) migration of population from rural areas to urban areas (b) both husband and wife going for jobs (c) convenience and affordability of bread.

Since bread is made of refined flour from roller flour mills it can be an excellent vehicle for carrying several nutrients if mixing of these nutrients at desired levels is done during the milling operation. Roller flour mill manufacturers have developed devices for mixing small quantities of nutrients such as lysine, vitamins and minerals to the flour uniformly with minimum additional cost of production.

Bajra, Jowar and Maize

Bajra

Bajra and jowar are referred to as small millet and big millet. They are both widely used in Maharashtra, Gujarat and Madhya Pradesh, mainly for making roti. It is also known as spiked or pearl millet.

Bajra grows on light soil and requires less water and manure for cultivation than other grains. It can be grown twice a year, once in the monsoon and a second time in summer. Another advantage of cultivating bajra is that it is cultivated as a mixed crop with pulses such as red gram, cowpeas, green gram, etc.

Usually bajra does not contain much husk. This is an advantage over rice and wheat from which a considerable amount of nutrients may be removed during the process of dehusking. Bajra protein is relatively richer in lysine, methionine and tryptophan than other grains as it contains a greater proportion of albumin fraction. A much greater variation of 9–18% is found in hybrid strains with an average value of about 14%. A few strains are found to contain as much as 17-18%. Bajra contains 5-6% fat which is of some significance in low fat diets consumed by the poor as 400–500 g of bajra would provide 20–30 g of fat and 10–15 g of linoleic acid.

Bajra is a reasonably good source of thiamine (0.4 mg per 100 g) and riboflavin (0.2–0.3 mg per 100 g) as against average values of 0.10 mg for the latter for most grains. It is also a better source of iron than other grains with the exception of ragi.

Bajra is mostly consumed in the form of roti but can be used in other ways. It can be parched or sprouted and roasted and used in infant feeding. Bajra flour is sometimes cooked in buttermilk with a little salt to make rabdi. Fermented foods can be prepared from a combination of bajra, other grains and legumes.

Jowar and Maize

Jowar is deficient in lysine and has an excess of leucine. The former can be corrected by the addition of legumes. The latter is believed to result in a relative deficiency of isoleucine. Fenugreek is a rich source of both lysine and isoleucine and the addition of fenugreek powder at the 10% level to maize or jowar flour is found to improve their nutritive value to rats.

Debras and spiced rotis made with jowar or maize, bengalgram flour and fenugreek leaves are found to be highly acceptable. Incidentally, in Egypt, fenugreek flour is added at a level of 5–10% to the maize flour used for making bread.

Maize and jowar are consumed mainly in the form of roti and sometimes in the form of rabdi prepared by cooking the flour in just enough water to form a 'mush'. Rabdi is often allowed to ferment overnight.

In South America maize is consumed in the form of 'tortillas' which resemble chapaties in appearance and texture. The traditional method is to soak the maize in lime water, grind into a smooth dough, roll into balls and flatten and cook like chapaties.

Maize is used extensively by certain sections of the population in Gujarat, Rajasthan and the Kangra Valley, mainly in the form of roti.

Yellow maize differs from other cereals in that it has a high carotene content (about 220 i.u. per 100 g) which is highly available. Vitamin A deficiency is reported to be rare in people subsisting on yellow maize.

In studies carried out in the author's laboratory, animals fed yellow maize without any other source of carotene or vitamin A in the diet were found to have a liver vitamin A concentration of 20 micrograms per 100 g as against none in animals fed a diet based on other cereals such as kodri or white maize, which does not have any carotene. At present hybrid strains of white maize are being increasingly cultivated. It would seem desirable to develop high yielding strains of yellow maize.

As mentioned earlier, although maize and jowar have been both implicated in the etiology of pellagra, the disease is rare in this country. This may be because of differences in the form in which maize is consumed. In the preparation of maize grits and degerminated and decorticated maize meal consumed in west, the albumin fractions present in the embryo are lost resulting in lower concentration of amino acids such as tryptophan and lysine. In this country, the whole grain is ground into flour and used. It is interesting to note that no pellagra was found in people consuming maize in the form of tortilla which is also prepared from the whole grain. It was attributed to the soaking of maize in lime water which results in converting some of the bound niacin to the free form but studies carried out by Scrimshaw and Bressani have shown no differences in nutritive value between lime-treated and untreated maize after both are cooked.

Ragi and Kodri

Ragi and kodri are also millets which are cultivated to a lesser extent. The former is used mainly in South India, and the latter, in Gujarat and Madhya Pradesh. They both contain about 6-7% protein. Ragi protein is reported to be a good quality, but kodri is lacking in lysine and produces poor growth when fed alone to rats. However, when one part of a suitable legume, preferably moth bean, peas or bengal gram, is added to 4 parts of kodri, growth is found to be satisfactory. Both ragi and kodri are relatively rich in methionine, which is an amino acid lacking in legumes, groundnut and other cereals, and may prove to be of value when added to combinations of bengalgram+groundnut (e.g. multipurpose flour developed at Central Food Technological Research Institute (CFTRI), Mysore).

Ragi is also found to have a liberal amount of calcium but we do not know how much of this is available as it is also rich in phytate. Ragi has been traditionally used in infant feeding in the south after suitable processing. The grains are steeped in water, allowed to sprout, wet-ground to a smooth paste, tied in a muslin cloth and hung so that the milky fluid from the same drips into a shallow dish kept below. This is dried, ground and used as weaning food. The dried powder is made into a paste and boiled with the addition of water. It can be given with milk and sugar or buttermilk and salt. Alternatively, the sprouted grain can be lightly roasted, ground and used after sieving off the fibrous components. A technology for the production of strained baby food has been developed by CFTRI. This highly nutritious and palatable food based on malted ragi, banana powder a few other ingredients which is affordable to common man.

Ragi flour is mixed with water to form a paste, rolled into balls and steamed. The steamed balls are consumed with curry. This product known as 'ragi ball' is popular in Karnataka.

Kodri is dehusked and cooked as such like rice or ground to flour for making roties. It can be effectively substituted for rice in preparations such as idli, dosa, khichri and pongal.

Use of cereals in infant feeding

Milk is by far the best food for the child just weaned from the breast but in poor families where cereals form the major item in the diet they are the only food available to the child. Among cereals, rice is the most popular one used for infant feeding because it cooks soft and is easily tolerated by children. However, it is low in protein content and is a poor source of minerals and vitamins because of milling and treatment prior to cooking. Both rice and roti are offered with highly spiced dals and broths which the young child just weaned from the breast is unable to tolerate. Other grains such as wheat, bajra, jowar and maize are usually consumed in the form of 'roti' (unleavened bread) which is not suitable as a weaning food. In families where these are the staple the child is subjected to undernutrition. It would seem desirable to process cereals suitably for use in infant feeding. Procedures such as parching, roasting, malting and fermentation are found to be suitable.

Sprouting and roasting

Wheat, chana dal, etc. can be steeped in water for a few hours so as to absorb all the water, dried in the shade so as to get rid of surface moisture and roasted in a hot iron pan. The resulting product appears puffed out like puffed rice and is highly acceptable.

Grains such as wheat, ragi, bajra and jowar can be steeped in water for 12–14 hours and allowed to sprout under moist conditions. When the sprouts become visible, the sprouted seeds can be dried in the shade so as to get rid of surface moisture, roasted lightly so as to develop a characteristic malt flavour, ground and used in the preparation of conjee. In the case of ragi, the coarse fibre can be sieved off.

The sprouting of food grains increases their digestibility and nutritive value. Starch is broken down to simpler starches, dextrin and maltose. Proteins are broken down to polypeptides, peptides and amino acids. Some of the bound iron is converted to a more readily available form. Inorganic phosphate is liberated from phytate. Bound vitamins are converted to the free form. These changes are brought about by enzymes which appear or become active during germination. They help the growing embryo to get its nutrients in a more assimilable form, They also make the cooking of sprouted grains easier.

The vitamins in food grains, riboflavin, nicotinic acid and pyridoxine and phosphorus increase appreciably during sprouting. These increases more than compensate for the small losses involved in roasting.

Parched grains

Parching of grains is an ancient technique in this country. Parched grains and sweets prepared from the same are mentioned in the Ramayana.

Parched grains have high acceptability and are reputed to have high digestibility. Puffed rice is commonly used as a weaning food (mostly given for nibbling). Parched grains or their combinations are eaten as such or in the form of candied products or 'laddus' prepared with jaggery. Not much is consumed in this way because the child has to chew the grains. But parched and roasted grains can be ground into a coarse meal and boiled in water for a few minutes to form a gruel. Puffed rice is particularly suitable for this. Puffed rice obtained from the bazaar can be made crisp by roasting it lightly and then ground into a coarse meal. This can be given with milk or soups or butter-milk. The cereal products can be used along with a similarly processed product from legumes.

Professional methods used for parching in India

Paddy and rice

Paddy is moistened with a little water. It is then put in a frying pan with a long handle containing four times its volume of preheated sand and inserted over an open fire in a specially built oven, the temperature of the sand being about 230–240°C. The grain is rapidly stirred with an iron ladle and thrown over a sieve and the sand sieved off, leaving behind parched paddy which has swollen and burst off the cracked hull during parching. The temperature of the mass immediately after the removal of the sand is between 130–140°C.

Paddy is steeped in warm water the temperature of which is 60–70°C. After steeping overnight during which time the mixture has cooled down to room temperature, the water is drained off. Small amounts of steeped paddy are heated in a shallow pan till the husk begins to crack. This is then transferred to a wooden mortar and pounded rapidly by means of a wooden pestle. The grain is beaten flat and dehusked during pounding. The flattening of the grain is also done by machine. The product is then dried to give flaked rice or 'poha'.

The flaked rice obtained can be parched with pre-heated sand. The flat grain then puffs out and acquires a toasted taste and flavour.

Paddy is boiled in water, dried and dehusked and the dehusked grain parched to give puffed rice.

Other products

Jowar is parched similarly but is subjected to longer pre-treatment. It is washed in warm water and kept tied in a moist cloth overnight and parched the next day.

Grains can be parched at home. They must be first soaked in water. They should then be roasted very rapidly in a hot iron pan containing pre-heated sand. The grain should puff out like popcorn. The sand helps to retain a high temperature and can be sieved off after parching and used again for the next batch. Another method is to pour boiling water over the grains, let stand for about a minute, drain the water quickly, and parch the grains in a hot pan containing pre-heated sand.

The principle of parching is that the moisture in the grain, when subjected suddenly to high heat, comes out as steam with great pressure and results in the puffing out of the grain. This is associated with physical and chemical changes in the grain. The degree of puffing depends on the moisture present in the grain and the speed with which it evaporates.

Puffed breakfast foods prepared from grains as well as milled flours are being increasingly used in the west. Puffed wheat and corn flakes are examples. Streamlined machinery is used for the purpose. The grains or doughs to be puffed are enclosed in a pressure chamber for puffing out and heated at 300° F for 30–40 minutes. The product is subjected to sudden and great aqueous vapour pressure at 175 lbs per square inch for about 3 minutes. The pressure is suddenly released from the retorts causing the grains to 'puff out' because of the rapid fall in pressure. The size of the resulting product is several times the original size. Ready to serve cereal foods are available in the form of flake, shredded, granular, puffed and roasted breakfast foods.

A hybrid strain of corn especially suitable for parching is available. It is wetted and wiped free of surface moisture and parched in a closed pan containing a little fat. Hydrogenated fat is preferred to ghee for this purpose as the latter smokes at a low temperature. This method is not effective when used with ordinary maize which gives a better product with sand-parching.

Parching of grain may result in some destruction of lysine. This can be made up by the addition of bengal gram or other legume after appropriate treatment.

Parched grains can be consumed as such or made into candied balls with jaggery syrup. These can be taken with milk and sugar as breakfast cereal. A mixture of parched grains, bengal gram and roasted groundnut is a handy and wholesome snack for children and others.

The prolonged treatment at high temperatures used in the preparation of commercial breakfast foods results in considerable losses of thiamine and other vitamins as well as lysine. Usually the vitamins are replenished.

The traditional procedures used in this country do not result in more than 5–10% loss of vitamins probably because of the short period of exposure to heat. However, they do seem to affect the availability of lysine.

Role of millets in food security in India

Agriculture scientist Dr. M.S. Swaminathan says "we should enlarge the food basket to include what we call nutria-millets such as jowar, ragi, bajra, madua which have high nutritive value and not just depend on wheat and rice".

Green Revolution was concerned only in areas with irrigation availability. However, in drought prone areas like Orissa, Rajasthan, Madhya Pradesh, Karnataka, Chattisgarh, Maharashtra and Jharkhand more than half of the cropped area goes without irrigation as per the latest available data accessed from "State of Indian Agriculture 2011-12" brought out by Department of Agriculture and Cooperation, Government of India. Almost 35% of India's rural poor reside in these seven states.

Encouraging dry land farming of millets in areas where irrigation is limited is very important in ensuring food and nutrient security in India. Impact of global warming on rainfall and the consequent short fall in the production of grains like wheat and rice is an alarming fact. In eventualities such shortfall in rice and wheat production millets can fill the gap of food and nutrients supply. The limitation in the utilization of millets is the drudgery of their primary processing into utilizable form. Technologies for their processing and production of value added nutritious products are now available with CFTRI, Mysore and University of Agricultural Sciences, Bangalore. However,acceptance of millet based diets by population who are familiar with only wheat and rice is another dimension to this issue. And this is a challenge to nutrition extension workers at the level of the central and state authorities.

Use of fermented foods in infant feeding

Fermentation is another process which can make cereals and pulses more suitable for children in the post weaning period. Fermented foods are also highly acceptable to other groups.

Idli and dosa in South India and dhokla and khaman in Gujarat are some of the fermented foods conventionally used in this country. These are based on either legumes or rice-legume combinations.

The principle used in the preparation of these foods can be applied to combinations of other cereals or millets with legumes. Sprouted legumes can be substituted for dals ordinarily used in fermentation.

Idli

Two parts of rice (three parts of parboiled rice is used) and one part of black gram dal are washed and soaked in water for five to ten hours and ground with water in a stone mortar. The rice is ground coarse and the black gram dal to a very smooth gelatinous paste. The two are mixed together and salt added. The resulting mixture should give a thick batter and more water is added only if necessary. The batter is allowed to ferment overnight at room temperature. The fermented batter appears effervescent with the carbon dioxide produced during fermentation. This batter is poured out with a ladle over moist cheese-cloth in an 'idli' steamer (which resembles an egg poacher) and steamed. Care should be taken not to let out the gas by unnecessary stirring. Otherwise the texture of the product will not be porous.

Khaman

One cup of bengal gram dal is washed and soaked in 1.5 cups of water for five to ten hours, and ground in a stone mortar. The dal is ground coarse and enough salt is added. The resulting mixture should form a thick batter. The batter is kept covered for fermentation overnight at room temperature. This batter is poured out with a ladle in a greased plate and steamed in a suitable pan or steamer. As in the case of idli care should be taken not to let out the gas by unnecessary stirring. The steamed product is cooled, cut into squares and seasoned suitably (e.g. with fried mustard seed, green coriander leaves, grated coconut and hing).

The fermentation of idli and khaman can be simplified by using milled flour. The rice should be coarsely ground and black gram dal finely ground and idli batter prepared from the two. Khaman batter can be prepared from coarsely milled bengal gram dal. Sometimes the microorganisms present in the original grain and responsible for fermentation are partially destroyed during milling. They can be restored by steeping a tablespoonful of the dal used in the preparation in about 2–4 oz of water for about 15 minutes and adding the washing after scrubbing the dal to the batter prepared. The dal used for extracting the washing can be used in other ways or dried and stored. If the grain requires to be washed, the first one or two washings can be discarded and the next washing added to the batter.

In the case of idli a better product is obtained if a batter is first prepared from black gram flour and allowed to ferment for an hour or two before the rice meal (flour) is added.

In all cases, the batter should be thoroughly aerated before keeping for fermentation. This is achieved by beating it with a rotary motion with either the hand or a scoop or eggbeater.

Dosa

Dosa, a traditional food of south Indians, is now a popular food all over India. Dosa batter is similar to idli batter except that the proportion of rice may be increased if desired and the rice ground fine. The batter is fermented as in the case of idli and pan-fried like pancakes. Both idli and dosa are served with chutney, sambhar or chutney powders. They may also be served with jam or honey or molasses. Butter ghee or sesame oil is used as a spread. In South India, it is common practice to use some fenugreek seeds along with black gram dal in the preparation of dosa. This is believed to improve its nutritive value. Studies carried out on rats in the author's laboratory have shown the beneficial effects of such addition. Fenugreek imparts a slightly bitter taste which is masked when the batter becomes sufficiently sour. Also, germinating the seed before grinding it with black gram reduces the bitter taste. Incidentally, germinated fenugreek is consumed as a salad in Egypt and along with onions by the people of Gujarat; the latter believe it to be a cure for debility and fevers. Germination also increases the nutritive value of fenugreek.

Dhokla

Dhokla batter is prepared from coarsely ground rice and dal or a mixture of dals and the fermented batter treated like khaman. Bengal gram, red gram and black gram dals are used in preparing the batter.

Dhokla can also be prepared from combinations of coarsely ground jowar, wheat, kodri or maize with dals such as black gram, moth bean or red gram.

The ingredients of dhokla can be ground in a flour mill and dhokla is a convenient food to prepare on a large scale in school and balwadi feeding programmes. It is highly acceptable to young children as well as school boys and can be given in lieu of a snack or as one-dish meal. Also children do not seem to get tired of it even when it is given daily. In lunch programmes organized by the author's group for school children, dhokla was more acceptable than other foods such as biscuits, debra, poora (dosa) or roti +. dal + greens from the same ingredients. Greens such as fenugreek leaves can be added to the fermented batter to make it an almost complete food.

A convenient steamer for preparing these foods on a large scale is described below:

A circular wooden frame can be made with wooden bars about 2-3 inches wide and 1/2 to 1 inch thick and 2 inches apart nailed together by two or three bars across. The diameter of the frame should be such that it can just fit below the rim of a large aluminium or copper pan to be used as a steamer. Place water in the pan, fit the wooden frame, then place the dishes or plates with the batter to be steamed on the frame and cover with a lid that fits and steam. A couple of bricks placed on the lid will help weigh it down and prevent the steam from coming out.

Fermented batters can also be baked. The batter, prepared thick, should be poured into a greased aluminium pan and baked in an oven at 350°F till done (20–30 minutes). They can also be prepared as steamed breads in closed containers.

Legumes such as peas, field beans and soya beans can also be incorporated in fermented foods. They should be first allowed to sprout and then wet-ground to a coarse or fine paste as desired and a batter prepared from the same and ground cereal. Such sprouting followed by fermentation may be expected to increase the digestibility and nutritive value of the product and break down the trypsin inhibitors present in some legumes.

The process of fermentation can be speeded up, particularly in winter, by adding a little curd and/or keeping the batter in a basin of warm water for 15–30 minutes and then keeping it covered by inverting a larger pan over it.

Fermentation is found to improve the digestibility and nutritive value of foods. The microorganisms involved in fermentation synthesize and secrete enzymes which bring about the partial degradation of starch, protein, etc. and effect the synthesis of vitamins. This is not surprising as both the growing embryo of the plant and microorganisms require nutrients in a readily assimilable form and a generous supply of vitamins.

Chapter 11

Legumes, Oilseeds and Nuts

Leguminous plants belong to the family of Leguminosae. The seeds of leguminous plants are known as legumes or pulses. The latter term appears to have been derived from the latin term 'puis' for pottage.

Legumes have been cultivated from early times. The Ramayana mentions many of the legumes used at present in India. **Table 37** shows the commonly used legumes and the regions where they probably originated.

Table 37. Origin of selected legumes.

Legume	Botanical name	Region where first cultivated	Approximate period when first cultivated
Peas (from Sanskrit pisum)	Pisum sativum	Middle East and India	5000 B.C.
Bengalgram (chick pea)	Cicer ariettinum		
Redgram (pigeon pea)	Cajanus cajan	Middle East and south East Asia.	5000 B.C.
Lentils	Lens culinaris medic		
Black gram	Phaseolus mungo L	India	Prior to 1000 B.C. mentioned in the Ramayana
Green gram	Phaseolus aureus roxb		
Sesame	Sesamum indicum		
cow-pea	Vigna catiang	India and Africa	
Groundnut	Arachis hypogeal	Brazil	Prior to "Inca' Empire
Haricot or kidney bean	Phaseolus vulgaris	Mexico	4000 B.C.
Broad bean	Vicia faba	North Africa	Bronze age
soyabean	Glycine max. merr	China	4000–5000 B.C.

Groundnut and sesame (til) also belong to the family of leguminosae although they are generally referred to as oil seeds because of their use in the extraction of oil.

In this country, bengal gram, red gram, green gram and black gram are the chief legumes cultivated with bengal gram accounting for a major fraction. Other legumes such as moth bean (pronounced mutt), cowpeas, lentils and peas are used on a smaller scale. Field beans and pink beans are used occasionally.

Most of the legumes are used as dehusked and decorticated dals rather than as whole legumes. This is because dals cook better and quicker and lend themselves to incorporation in a greater variety of dishes. They are also more easily digested as the thick outer coating consisting largely of cellulose, is removed during de-husking. They have a better keeping quality and are less susceptible to insect spoilage. But whole legumes have the advantage in that they have a greater vitamin content and they can be sprouted so as to result in further increases in the same.

Dals from peas (split peas) are not available in the market in this country. Apparently, the pulse mills are not interested in dehusking this legume because of its tough coat. It can be easily dehusked and split by common household procedures after steeping it in water for a few hours and drying. Split peas are among the most extensively used legumes in western countries. They can be used as such or in the form of flour in a variety of ways. Whole legumes, like cereals, can be steeped in water for a few hours and allowed to sprout.

As mentioned earlier, the sprouting of food grains results in a number of favourable changes. In the case of legumes, the increase in digestibility and the decrease in cooking time needed are particularly advantageous because dry whole legumes are less easily cooked and digested than whole grain cereals. Further, the Sprouting of legumes is associated with a much greater increase in ascorbic acid.

Legumes such as soya beans and field beans which are not easily digested are well tolerated after sprouting and fermentation. The sprouted legume can be wet-ground and added to cereal flour and a fermented batter prepared from the same for preparations such as dhokla or dosa or idli.

Dry whole legumes have to be pre-soaked in water for cooking and take much longer time than dals to cook. This is partly why they are not consumed often. The time required for cooking can be appreciably shortened by sprouting during which the thick outer coat bursts open and the grain becomes soft, making it easier for the cooking water to penetrate the grain. Dehusking is also easier when the grains are sprouted and dried. Thus sprouting can give us a bonus in terms of increased nutrients and digestibility and decreased cooking time and fuel cost. Even pre-soaking the whole legumes in water for a few hours is found to increase vitamin content to some extent.

The cooking time for dals can be appreciably reduced by pre-soaking them in water for about half an hour. It is also reduced by the addition of a few drops of fat. When the grain to be sprouted is steeped in surplus water, some of the nutrients will be lost in the water discarded. With practice it is possible to use just enough water so that all of it is absorbed.

Usually, the grains are soaked overnight and allowed to sprout for another 24 hours. If they are allowed to remain in water long after maximum swelling has taken place, they acquire a foul odour. The amount of water and time required for maximum swelling will vary with the grain and its quality. Cereal grains such as bajra, jowar and wheat and the softer varieties of whole legumes such as green gram and cowpeas require about half their volume of water for complete swelling. Peas and bengal gram require more, about three-fourths volume. The soaking time required is 6–9 hours in the case of bajra, 9–12 hours in the case of other cereal grains and green gram, 12–15 hours in the case of most legumes but bengal gram requires a longer period (15–18 hours). Sprouting is facilitated by the use of warm water (40–45°C) for pre-soaking, particularly in winter, and in the case of hard grains such as peas and bengal gram. After soaking, the seeds need sufficient warmth and aeration for the sprouts to grow.

The methods commonly used for sprouting and some developed by the author are described below:

1. The soaked grains are tied in a moist muslin cloth or gunny bag, kept on a plate and covered with a large inverted pan so as to keep the temperature even. This is one of the conventional procedures.

2. The soaked grains are placed in moistened earthenware jars, covered with moist cloth. Better results are obtained if the whole is covered with a large inverted pan. Cane-baskets can also be used in the place of earthenware jars.

3. The soaked grains can be placed in a colander fitting over a pan containing some water. The colander is covered with moist cloth whose ends dip into the water in the pan so that it remains moist. A lid is placed loosely over the colander so as to allow aeration. The lid of an idli steamer is very suitable for this purpose. The whole kit can be covered with a large inverted pan in winter.

When cloth is used for sprouting, the sprouts tend to cling to it. The one using a colander is perhaps most convenient for the housewife as it is easy to keep the equipment clean.

Dals

Dals are mostly used in liquid broths such as sambhar and liquid dal.

Bengal gram dal is ground into a flour and used for the preparation of snacks such as 'sev'. It is pre-soaked in water and deep-fried in oil for mixing with chevda.

As mentioned earlier, wet-ground dals are used in fermented foods such as idli, dhokla and khaman. Dals are pre-soaked in water and wet-ground without further addition of water to a coarse texture. The ground material is seasoned and shaped into balls, steamed in an idli steamer or a colander. The steamed balls can be cooled and used as dumplings in soups and gravies. They can also be steamed in an idli steamer or colander as such, or along with chopped vegetables such as onions, cluster beans, cabbage, cauliflower, etc. and seasoned suitably. The resulting product is called 'usal'.

In South India it is common practice to cook dals along with vegetables. The latter are added after the dal is three-fourths cooked and the resulting mixture cooked to completion. As mentioned earlier, vegetables cooked by this method retain larger amounts of vitamin C.

Sambhar is a traditional broth prepared in south India with red gram dal, vegetables, tamarind juice, salt and curry powder. The other ingredients can be added to red gram after it is almost cooked and the whole cooked to completion. Tomato juice or curds and or lemon can be used in lieu of tamarind juice and split peas or sprouted red gram or lentils in place of red gram dal. The taste of the substituted products is preferred by many people.

Sambhar is used along with rice, dosa, idli, upma, bread, etc. Sambhar rice can also be prepared by cooking rice and dal together first and then adding the other ingredients.

It is desirable for people not taking much of milk or animal foods to include more dal in the diet. When dals are consumed in the form of broths, their consumption is limited. The consumption can be increased by incorporating them in chapaties, debras, etc. and using cereal-legume combinations such as 'khichri' and 'pongal'. Khichri is prepared by boiling rice and red gram dal together roughly in the proportion 3:1 or 4:1. Salt, turmeric powder and fat are added towards the end of cooking. Sometimes,dals of green gram and moth bean are used in place of red gram. For the preparation of pongal, 1 cup of green gram dal is roasted lightly in ghee or hydrogenated oil and 2-3 cups of rice and sufficient water added. The mixture is cooked to completion and salt and seasoning added. The seasoning for pongal usually consists of cashew nuts, black pepper, cumin seed, chopped fresh ginger, green chillies and curry leaves. All these ingredients are fried in ghee and added.

Sweet pongal is prepared by omitting the above seasoning and adding jaggery. (1 1/2-2 cups per cup of rice) and ghee after the rice-dal mixture is cooked to a soft consistency. The cooking is continued on very slow heat or over a double boiler till the jaggery blends well with the other ingredients and ghee and seasoning (fried cashew nuts, raisins, cardamom and saffron) added. Burning at the bottom can be prevented by greasing a heavy vessel first, adding jaggery powder and then the cooked rice and dal mixture and heating the whole on simmering heat.

Sprouted legumes can replace dal in many of these preparations such as sambhar rice. Kodri, cracked wheat, cream of wheat and coarsely ground jowar and maize can be substituted for rice.

Dals are also cooked to a soft consistency, the surplus water drained, cooked again with sugar or jaggery and mashed or ground to a smooth paste. The resulting sweet paste can be used as a filling for pastries such as 'puran polis' and sweet puffs. Addition of cardamom, honey, grated, coconut, cream, raisins, milk powder, etc. improves the taste and flavour of the product.

As described earlier, dals can be used after roasting for preparing conjee.

Cooked dals are eminently suitable for incorporation in soups. Split peas, red gram dal, lentils, green gram dal and cowpeas are particularly suitable. Some suggestions regarding their use have been made elsewhere.

The liquid dals used in the daily menu are usually highly spiced and not tolerated by the weaned infant. A portion of the dal can be removed before the spices are added and given to the child. This can be made more acceptable to the child by adding salt, lemon juice and a pinch of cumin powder.

Dals are steeped in water, wet-ground to a thick paste, seasoned and deep-fried like doughnuts to form 'Vadas'. Black gram dal ground fine is used to make a soft vada. A mixture of dals (bengal gram, red gram and black gram) is ground coarse to give 8 crisp product. Split peas and soya bean can replace the dals traditionally used. Chopped onions and cabbage or greens can be added to the dough before frying. Bengal gram flour and finely ground split peas can be used for bhajya (fritters) batters.

Legumes such as bengal gram and peas are also parched to give highly acceptable products. Bengal gram is tied in a moist cloth and kept overnight before it is parched. Peas are soaked in water for 5 minutes, dried partially in the sun for 15 minutes and then parched. Salt and turmeric powder are sometimes added to the steeping water, or the grains smeared with a paste of the same, before they are parched. In Nepal, soyabeans are parched in a similar manner. Parching is found to increase the digestibility and nutritive value of legumes. This may be because of the destruction of trypsin inhibitors and changes in grain structure. As legumes are rich in lysine, some loss of lysine during parching is not a crucial factor. Parched bengal gram has been used successfully in the treatment of protein-calorie malnutrition in children. Parched soya beans can be dehusked and used similarly.

Dals and whole legumes can contribute significantly to the protein content of the diet. In spite of their popularity and the varied ways in which they can be used, their consumption is limited in the poor. It would be desirable to consume at least 50–75 g but the price of dals has been increasing steeply during the last few years, resulting in a decline in their consumption. In rural areas around Baroda pulse consumption was 62 g per capita in 1962, 54 g in 1965, 46 g in 1966 and 25–30 g in 1967. The urban-poor consume 30–35 g or less. Tribal people such as Bhils are found to consume less than 10 g. Although cereal prices have registered similar increases, the poor man looks on cereals as a 'must' and legumes as a frill item in the diet. There is not sufficient awareness of the fact that money spent on cereals can be reduced to some extent by including dals. Even when wheat and bengal gram were available in ration shops at nearly the same prices the poor often let go their rations of the latter. They need to be educated on the fact that they can get better worth for their money by buying 4 kg of wheat and 1 kg of bengal gram instead of 5 kg of the former and that bengal gram flour can be substituted for part of the wheat flour used in making chapaties.

Toxic materials in pulses

Many legumes such as field beans and soya beans have substances which inactivate the enzyme, trypsin, and consequently prevent proteins from being digested. Such legumes are therefore toxic unless these inhibitors are destroyed. Animals fed raw field beans so as to form even one-fifth of the diet are found to die after 6-8 weeks of feeding, According to the nutritionist late Dr. Kamala Sohonie in Bombay, people in scarcity areas of Maharashtra who consumed large quantities of the green legume without cooking were found to suffer from neuromuscular disorders.

Fortunately, trypsin inhibitors are destroyed by heat treatment. Boiling would appear to destroy most of the inhibitors. Soya flour is subjected to dry heat at a relatively high temperature.

Ordinary boiling may not always result in the complete destruction of trypsin inhibitors. It would appear on the basis of preliminary studies carried out in Baroda that the trypsin inhibitors present in sprouted and or fermented soya bean are more readily destroyed during ordinary cooking.

Substances called haemagglutinins are also present in some legumes. They can combine or agglutinise with 'heme' and result in the destruction of haemoglobin. However, they are not generally absorbed. They are mostly destroyed during cooking. Here again, sprouting and or fermentation may help in their speedy destruction.

Flavism is a disease associated with the consumption of certain uncooked legumes such as broad beans. The disease is characterized by haemolytic anaemia, haemoglobinuria (presence of blood in urine) and jaundice.

Cotton seed contains substances called gossypol which is toxic. Techniques have now been developed for its removal.

Guar seed which has a high protein and methionine content is not fit for human consumption because of its tough coat which has a lot of mucilage. It is mainly used as cattle-feed at present. It is the cheapest legume available in the market and has more protein, lysine, methionine, iron and other nutrients than the commonly used legumes. The oil in guar has an unacceptable odour. Both the mucilage and fat in guar are valuable for industry. The former is used for the manufacture of plastics and the latter appears promising for use in the varnish industry.

Lathyrus sativus or kesari dal is a legume cultivated and consumed extensively in Madhya Pradesh. Ordinarily, it is consumed along with wheat or other grains so as to form 25–30% of cereal consumption. The legume is highly resistant to drought and survives when other crops fail. In drought years when the cereal crop fails it is consumed as the staple.

The legume contains a toxic factor ((N-Oxalyl-amino-L-alanine) and lower limb paralysis occurs when it is consumed as the staple for long periods of time. This does not happen when the legume is consumed along with cereals in reasonable quantities. The toxic factor has been isolated from the legume and the same when injected into the blood results in paralysis in young chicks. Studies in the author's laboratory show that the toxic factor is not removed by procedures such as dehusking, boiling, sprouting and fermentation. Studies carried out in the National Institute of Nutrition, Hyderabad show that it can be removed by soaking the legume in water at about 60°C for several hours and discarding the steeping water. However, the difficulty would be in the fuel cost and the feasibility of maintaining this temperature for a long period. Further, the grain is usually ground into flour and used for making chapaties so that the treated legume will have to be dried before milling. The process will be practicable only if some centralised machinery is set up for treating and milling the legume before sale. In many areas agricultural labourers are paid in kind rather than in cash. It appears that many landlords, particularly in a lean year, give the legume in lieu of wages, keeping the wheat for themselves. Legislation would be desirable to prevent this practice. The disease lathyrism is mainly a result of poverty combined with scarce supplies of food grains as the people in these regions are very well aware of the toxicity of the legume.

The toxic factor is found in some strains but not in others. It would be desirable to identify and develop strains which are free from the same. If such preventive measures cannot be taken it would be best to ban the production of the legume altogether.

Kesari dal which is cheaper than other dals is used as an adulterant of dals like toor and masoor and this malpractice has been reported in Maharashtra and few other states.

Aspergillus flavus

Sometimes groundnut is infested with the mold *Aspergillus flavus*, which produces a toxin called aflatoxin. Aflatoxin produces hepatotoxicity. Small amounts of aflatoxin present in contaminated groundnuts and oils can be stored in body fat and exhibit cumulative effects at a later stage. Control of ground cultivation, harvest, drying and storage of seeds are important preventive measures of mold growth. Groundnuts infected with *A. flavus* can be easily identified because of the bluish green colour of the mold. Hand picking and electronic sorting machines are also used to remove the contaminated seeds. There is no danger of toxicity when groundnut is free from mould contamination. Usually the groundnut available in the market in India is free from such contamination. Long distance transport and prolonged storage under unsuitable conditions seem to be responsible for the mould contamination. The toxicity is found only in animals fed groundnut meal as a major item in the diet and has not been reported in man. It must also be pointed out that groundnut meal and groundnut cake are more likely to be infested by molds and the mould is not usually found in whole groundnut consumed by man. It would be wise however, to inspect groundnut for mould contamination before use.

Groundnut flour must be prepared from clean dry groundnut free from shell, foreign materials or defective kernels. The groundnut must be roasted or heat-treated and the red skin removed before it is milled. Flour prepared in this way can be stored for a week or two.

Soya bean

Soya bean is a legume not consumed much in this country although it is popular in Nepal and the Far East. In the United States it is cultivated mainly as a source of oil. Soya bean compares favourably with dals in lysine and vitamin content and has a higher calorie value because of its fat content. It gives reasonable yields per acre. Its nutritive value is compared with that of other legumes in **Table 38.**

The unpopularity of soya bean in this country is due to its beany flavour. In countries such as China and Japan where it is used traditionally, a number of sophisticated techniques have been developed for processing it to various products.

Soya sauce is prepared by a complex process involving several months of fermentation.

Cooked soya beans and steamed rice are incubated with the organism, *Aspergillus oryzae*, and the mixture is fermented to a product with pasty consistency and used in soups and broths. The fermentation takes as long as two weeks.

Tempeh is a product prepared from cooked and skinned soya beans inoculated with a little tempeh from the previous batch (this is similar to adding a little curd to get milk as curd). The mixture is mashed and wrapped in banana leaves and allowed to ferment for 24 hours. The nutritive value of tempeh is found to be superior to that of the unfermented product.

For preparing Natto, a Japanese product, the soya beans are soaked in water, cooked and inoculated with *Bacillus subtilis* or previously prepared Natto. They are then wrapped in barks of pine and are allowed to ferment under warm conditions (40° C) for 20 hours.

It is clear that the above fermentation techniques involving a lot of pre-treatment and prolonged fermentation are much more fussy and time consuming than those used in this country for preparing products such as idli and khaman. As stated earlier, soya beans can be sprouted, wet-ground and added to cereal flour for the preparation of dosa or dhokla after fermentation.

Soya beans can also be parched to give a product resembling parched bengal gram. This is popular in Nepal.

Heat-treated flour prepared from decorticated soyabeans is available in the West. It can be used as a substitute for bengal gram flour in most recipes.

Table 38. Nutritive value of soya bean as compared to other legumes.

	Amount per 100 g							
	Calories	Protein (g)	Fat (g)	Calcium (mg)	Iron (mg)	Carotene (µg)	Thiamine (mg)	Riboflavin (mg)
Grams	340–360	20–24	1–5	70–200	6–10	38–190	0.3–0.5	0.4–0.5
Groundnuts	570	25.3	40.1	90	2.8	37	0.9*	0.30
Soya beans	430	43.2	19.1	240	11.5	420	0.73	0.39

* Roasted ground is reported to contain less than 0.4 mg.

Preparation of soya milk

About 125g of whole soya beans are soaked for 10–16 hours. The hulls are removed by needing the beans and flushing the loose hulls with water. The soaked soya beans are ground with 1 litre of water in a blender. The mixture is sieved in a cheese cloth and soya milk is recovered. The soya milk obtained is boiled and the boiled soya milk can be stored in refrigerator for 3 days. The addition of vitamins and calcium is necessary if the milk is to be used as a substitute for breast or cow milk in infants. Studies all over the world have shown the eminent suitability of soya milk as an infant food. It is particularly used for children who are allergic to cow milk and who have lactose intolerance.

Preparation of Tofu

Tofu is a compressed soya milk curd very popular in South East Asian countries and in the West. It is prepared from soya milk. Soya milk is brought to boiling in a stainless steel vessel. Coagulant solution is then added to the soya milk in hot condition when the curdling of soya protein takes place. Addition of the coagulant is done with stirring till the coagulation is completed as judged by non-coagulation on further addition of coagulant. The curd is allowed to separate and the separated curd is removed from the whey and transferred to a tofu mold lined with cheese cloth. Any container that has many holes can serve as a tofu mold to drain off the residual whey. A lid is placed on the surface of the curd and a weight of 3–5 pounds is placed on the lid for 20 minutes. The resulting block of tofu is placed in a tub of cold water for 1 hour to wash excess diluent if any, left on the tofu. The tofu prepared is stored in refrigerator. Coagulant solution is prepared by dissolving 1 tsp of magnesium chloride or 2 tsp of calcium sulphate in one cup of hot water.

Textured vegetable protein, meat analogues and meat extenders are prepared from soya bean. These products are close to meat in terms of sensory properties and have the potential of substitute for meat.

Soya protein has the highest quality among all the plant proteins. It has all the essential amino acids and the protein quality parameters compares well with animal proteins. Several health benefits are attributed to soya bean because of the presence of Isoflavones. Soya bean contains the isoflavones genestin and daidzin which is recovered along with proteins during the preparation of soya products. Several population studies have shown that consumption of soya bean is associated with reduction of prostrate cancer risk in men and breast cancer among women*. Soya isoflavones have weak

---

* Shu, X.O., Y. Zheng, H. Cai, K. Gu, Z. Chen, W. Zheng and W. Luv. 2009. *Journal of American Medical Association*, **302(22)**:2437–2443.

estrogenic activity and improve several estrogen dependent conditions including premenopausal symptoms (hot flushes) and postmenopausal bone loss. However,these are epidemiological observations in South East countries where soya bean consumption is high.

Idlis prepared from rice and soyabean are well accepted and tolerated by young children including severely malnourished children.

Attempts are also being made to extend the supplies of milk by using a mixture of animal milk and soya milk.

It is unlikely that soya beans as such will become popular in this country, as the grams grown in this country are superior with regard to ease of preparation and digestibility. But it may be possible to popularize products such as heat-treated and ready to use soya flour, soya bean milk and parched soya beans and fermented products prepared from the same. Its superiority with regard to fat, protein, calcium and carotene contents is points in its favour. The Indian Agricultural Research Institute at Delhi is making efforts to popularize the cultivation of soyabean. The tremendous growth of its popularity in other countries during the past 75 years suggests that it may come to be an accepted part of the Indian dietary, if popularized.

Oil seeds

Legumes and other seeds rich in fat and used for the extraction of the oil are called oilseeds. Groundnut, sesame (til) and coconut are the chief sources of cooking oil in this country. Cotton seeds and safflower seeds are also used in some regions. The oils of maize, sunflower seeds, soya beans are used in the U.S.A. and other countries. Palm oil is used in some, African countries.

Sesame or til was probably the first oil seed to be used for the extraction of oil in this country. The Hindi term 'tel' for oil is derived from the Sanskrit word 'tilum' meaning a product from 'tilum' or 'til' (sesame seed). At present, however, the production of groundnut far exceeds that of 'til'.

Groundnut is rich in protein but most of the groundnut produced in this country is used for the extraction of oil and the oil cake is used as cattle feed or manure. The consumption of groundnut as such is much less than 5 g per capita per day.

Groundnut protein lacks in lysine and methionine and its quality can be improved by either adding these amino acids or foods rich in the same. An appropriate combination of groundnut and bengal gram with millet, sesame seed or milk powder should result in a mixture with a favourable amino acid concentration.

In feeding trials with pre-school children conducted in the author's laboratory a combination of sprouted and roasted wheat, water-soaked and roasted bengal gram and roasted and deskinned groundnut have been used for the preparation of conjee for young children. The addition of groundnut helps to improve the fat and protein content of the product and impart a nutty flavour without reducing nutritive value.

About six million tons of groundnut and about 4 million tons of oilcake are produced annually. The latter if utilized for human consumption can contribute about 22 g of oilcake per capita per day providing about 9 g of protein.

The unpopularity of oilcake is due to the fact that it has poor keeping quality and tends to deteriorate very rapidly. If the kernels used for oil extraction are chosen for quality and heat-treated prior to extraction, oilcake of much better quality can be obtained. Also a better product is obtained if the fat is removed by solvent extraction. This method results in a better extraction of oil.

It is necessary to ensure, however, that no solvent residues are left either in oil or the cake as they may be harmful in the long run. The Indian Multipurpose Food (MPF) developed at CFTRI, Mysore is based on a combination of defatted groundnut meal and bengal gram.

Groundnut milk can be prepared from roasted and skinned groundnut. The same should be ground into a smooth paste, water added and the liquid filtered through cloth and boiled. The milk can also be set as curd.

Groundnut can be roasted and ground to form groundnut paste. The same, also called peanut paste, is a popular product available commercially in the west. Groundnut paste or flour can be added to bread, biscuits, chapaties, poories, etc. It may be used in place of shortening in many products such as nimki, sakkarpara, and chakli so as to result in an improved flavour and reduced cost. Roasted and crushed groundnuts can be added to steamed breads, biscuits, cakes, pakoras and the like. Fresh groundnut of good quality can also be used in these preparations and fermented foods such as dosa.

Coconuts give high yield (4000 kg per acre) but their cultivation is confined mainly to the sandy sea-coast of Kerala so that its production is not on a sufficiently large scale. Coconut water is rich in free amino acids, sugars and minerals such as potassium and is easily tolerated by very young children. Coconut milk, which is also used as a weaning food and in cooking, is prepared by grinding grated coconut with water and extracting only the clear liquid by filtering through cheese cloth.

Coconut cake contains a lot of coarse fibre which is not digested, a technique for processing the same so as to make it suitable for human consumption has been developed in the Central Food Technological Research Institute, Mysore.

Fresh coconut oil can be prepared at home by boiling coconut milk till the fat in the emulsion separates out as a top-layer which can be removed by decantation.

The high cost of coconuts is partly because of its value as export commodity. People living outside Kerala and Tamil Nadu consume coconuts only occasionally. Poor people even in the coastal areas of Kerala are seldom able to afford coconut.

Sesame seeds

Like groundnut, this is also a legume containing high protein and fat. The seed is used as such in the preparation of candy and for addition to other foods. The protein lacks lysine but it is rich in methionine. As such, its addition to legumes or cereal-legume combinations may be beneficial.

Sesame seeds can be roasted and candied with jaggery syrup to give a highly acceptable product. They can be roasted and added to cakes, biscuits, snack etc. so as to improve their flavour. Sesame cake has also been used in the manufacture of processed weaning foods.

Poppy seeds

Poppy seeds are used to a minor extent. They share the characteristics of groundnut and sesame seeds with regard to high protein and fat content.

Nuts and other seeds

Nuts such as almonds, pistachio, charoli and cashew nuts are also good sources of protein and calories and are highly popular but their importance in practical nutrition are limited because of their prohibitive cost. Seeds of pumpkin, cucumber and tamarind are roasted and consumed occasionally by limited sections of the population.

Fenugreek

Although this is classed as a spice, it is, in fact, a legume. Egyptian medicine and Ayurveda recommend the use of this legume for many disorders. The seed is rich in lysine, methionine and isoleucine, so that its amino acid composition is complementary to that of grains such as maize and jowar, and also groundnut. The seed is bitter but addition at the level of 5-10% to cereal flour is not found to affect the acceptability of rotis. The bitterness of the seed is due to the alkaloids present in the same. Germination of the seed is found to reduce the bitterness considerably and can be substituted for raw seed in dosa batter. The germinated seed can be used in curries, sambhar, dosa and idli.

Processed foods based on legumes

Because of their high protein content, legumes have been used as milk substitutes for children and many processed foods based on legumes have been developed.

As mentioned earlier, the Indian Multipurpose Food is based on a combination of bengal gram (25 g) and defatted groundnut (75 g) reinforced with vitamin A (3000 i.u.), thiamine (1.3 mg), riboflavin (3 mg) and nicotinic acid (14 mg). Laubina is a product developed in the Middle East and consists of parboiled wheat (68 g), parboiled bengal gram (27 g) and corn oil (2 g), reinforced with citric acid (1 g), vitamin A (5000 i.u.) and vitamin D (500 i.u.). Incaparina is a product developed in South America and consists of jowar (29 g), corn flour (28 g) and gossypol removed cotton seed flour (38 g) reinforced with Torula yeast (3 g), calcium carbonate (1 g) and vitamin A (4500 i.u.).

Other versions of these products such as the infant and weaning foods of CFTRI, Mysore and other combinations of the ingredients in Incaparina and Laubina have also been developed. Oilcakes of coconut and sesame and soya bean flour have also been used. Field trials with these products have shown the value of these products in feeding infants and pre-school children.

Apart from the use of groundnut and soya bean in infant feeding, the milk prepared from them and from nuts such as almonds, charoli, etc. can be mixed with skimmed milk and consumed in place of whole milk by people who wish to cut down the consumption of animal fat. The fats from some of these sources are richer sources of polyunsaturated fatty acids. The nuts should be treated like coconut, groundnut or soya bean for the preparation of milk. Coffee cream based on non-dairy products like soya bean is being increasingly used in western countries.

As mentioned earlier, a combination of wheat, bengal gram and groundnut processed suitably has been used in Baroda in feeding programmes for children. It is found to compare well with the processed foods mentioned above.

The increased cultivation of legumes should be of value not only for human nutrition but also for agriculture and dairy farming. Straws and hays of cereals used as cattle feed are deficient in lysine whereas legume hay is rich in this amino acid and makes a valuable addition to cattle feed. The fodder of cowpeas and the legume itself are found particularly valuable as cattle feed. The cultivation of legumes also increases the nitrogen content of the soil as the roots of most leguminous plants contain nitrogen-fixing bacteria which can convert atmospheric nitrogen into nitrates and nitrites. The nitrogen depleted from the soil by cereal cultivation can, therefore, be replenished by alternating it with legume cultivation. Even in areas where the water supply is not enough to grow the crops to maturity, they can be grown to the stage permitted by water supply and the green fodder ploughed back into the soil to enrich soil nitrogen. It is unfortunate that with the advent of hybrid strains of cereals and millets, legume cultivation has been neglected and the consumption of legumes has actually decreased. The Indian Council of Agricultural Research is currently interested in encouraging legume cultivation and it is hoped that they will succeed in their efforts and will also come out with hybrid strains of legumes with high yields.

Chapter 12

Fats and Sugars

Fats

Fats are necessary for the absorption of fat-soluble vitamins and as sources of essential fatty acids. Their high energy value helps to reduce the bulk of foods. They make diets more satisfying and help to make diets more varied as they can be used in different ways.

Oilseeds, nuts, milk and animal adipose tissue are the chief sources of fat. Man prefers to extract the fat from these sources and use them in a variety of ways. Palm oil and fish oil are also used by some people. Rice bran oil is the preferred oil in Japan and this oil has also been introduced in India.

Cotton seed is a potential source of cooking oil, but most of it is used as cattle feed. The oil-removed seed is found to be better as cattle-feed and the oil extracted could contribute significantly to the availability of edible oils.

In this country, vegetable oils and butter are the chief sources of cooking and table fat. Groundnut, mustard seed, safflower seed, sesame and coconut are used for the extraction of oil. Sources used in other countries include maize, soya bean, sunflower seed, olives and cottonseed and rice bran.

Suet and lard which are fats derived from beef and pork are produced to a minor extent and not sold commercially but they are used for the adulteration of ghee. With the advent of hydrogenated oil adulteration with the same has become more common.

The production of oilseed is of the order of 30 million tons in India during the period 2009-10. The bulk of this is groundnut. Til oil used to be the chief oil used for cooking purposes in many regions but groundnut oil has replaced it in most regions as it is cheaper. Mustard oil is used in Bengal, safflower oil in Maharashtra and coconut oil in Kerala. Although the yield of coconut is very high (2000–4000 kg of kopra per acre) its cultivation is largely limited to the sandy coast of Kerala and other parts of South India. Restricted cultivation as well as its value as an export commodity are responsible for its higher price as compared to groundnut oil.

Hydrogenated oil is produced by saturating the unsaturated fatty acids in vegetable oils by passing hydrogen in the presence of a catalyst. Consequently, its texture and melting point resemble those of ghee. The regular consumption of butter, ghee and hydrogenated oil is limited to the upper classes. Only a small quantity of the butter produced is used as a spread or in baking and most of the butter is converted to ghee. No figures are available for the production of ghee but judging from the figures for the per capita availability of milk (100 g per day) and diet surveys, the average availability cannot be more than 2 g per day. Ninety per cent of 300 families studied in a survey did not consume any ghee except on special occasions. The upper classes consume 10–20 g per day per capita **(Table 39)**.

Even the consumption of vegetable oils is limited to 10–15 g among the rural poor. Tribes such as the Bhils of Gujarat do not buy any oil at all. In rural areas of Tamil Nadu and Kerala the consumption is less than 5–10 g. The low fat content of the diet contributes in part to its low calorie value.

In contrast, the consumption of fats is of the order of 100 g per capita in western countries, a level not reached even by the upper classes in this country. A large proportion of this is animal fat or hydrogenated oil both of which are rich in saturated fatty acids. This, combined with sedentary living and a calorie intake in excess of requirement, is believed to be responsible for the high levels of lipids and cholesterol in blood, and these in turn have been implicated in the etiology of heart diseases.

Hydrogenated fat used in the west is sold mainly in the form of margarine which is used as a butter substitute. The same is blended with skim milk so, as to have a creamy, butter like texture. Oleomargarine is margarine prepared from suet. Because of the role suggested for saturated fatty acids in elevated levels of cholesterol in blood, the shortening used in the preparation of margarine is only partially hydrogenated.

Table 39. Fat consumption in different groups in urban Baroda (1966).

Monthly income Per family (Rs)	Amount(g) consumed per capita per day		
	Butter	Ghee or Hydrogenated oil	Vegetable oil
Less than 150	0	0	15
150–300	0	3	22
300–500	2	7	30
More than 500	3	17	31

The fat consumption per capita is related to the income level as can be seen in table 39. However, today the scenario may be different as more and more people are becoming health and calorie conscious.

Lard is a fat of commercial importance in the West. The quality of lard varies with the composition of the diet fed. The body fat of pigs fed on a high carbohydrate diet contains more saturated fatty acids and the lard obtained from such animals has a greater resemblance to butter. A high carbohydrate diet is, therefore, used for fattening pigs.

Nuts such as cashew nuts, walnuts and almonds are rich in fat but their prohibitive cost puts them beyond the reach of most people in this country.

Different fats are characterized by different physical and chemical characteristics. The melting point of a fat is higher if the fat contains a higher proportion of saturated fatty acids. This accounts for the higher melting points of hydrogenated oil, ghee, and coconut oil. However, melting point is also influenced by the arrangement of fatty acids within the fat. This accounts for the fact that hydrogenated fat which is less saturated than coconut oil has a higher melting point.

The amount of unsaturated fatty acids in a fat can be determined from the amount of iodine it can take up (iodine number) when the same is passed through it under certain conditions.

Refractive index or the deflection of light rays passing through the fat is another measure which varies in different fats.

Saponification number is an index of the amount of alkali required to convert the fatty acids in the fat to soap. The same depends on the number of fatty acid molecules in a given amount of fat and the latter varies in different fats because of differences in the molecular weights of the fatty acids present in them.

These characteristics are used to identify a fat and detect adulteration. Some characteristics of different fats are shown in **table 40. Table 41** gives the amounts of unsaturated and saturated fatty acids in different fats and the proportions between the two. It can be seen from the same that coconut oil, butter and lard contain more of saturated fatty acids whereas the oils of mustard seed, sesame, soya bean, cotton seed, corn, groundnut, safflower seed and sunflower seed contain more of unsaturated fatty acids. Among the nuts, almonds and walnuts are good sources of unsaturated fatty acids whereas cashew nut is a poor source.

Fat is used either as a spread, as in the case of chapaties, bread and rice, or for shallow or deep frying. It is used in the form of an emulsion in products like halwa, mysore paks and cakes and as a shortening agent in pies, biscuits, pastries and crisp snacks such as sakkarpara, sev, chakli, etc. It is also used as such in certain sweets such as laddus or 'magaj' prepared from roasted bengal gram flour.

Table 40. Characteristic of different fats.*

Fat source	Iodine number	Saponification number	Refractive index (15.5 °)	Polyunsaturated fatty acids (P)	Saturated fatty acids (S)	Monounsaturated fatty acids	P/S
Groundnut	93	192	1.472	31	19	50	1.63
Sesame	108	190	1.475	43	14	43	3.07
Safflower seed	133	190	1.474	67	7	26	9.57
Cotton seed	110	194	1.475	47	23	30	2.04
Coconut	9	250	1.440	2	92	6	0.02
Mustard	104	174	1.476	63	5	32	12.60
Butter	32	225	1.447	3	70	27	0.04
Hydrogenated oil	70	179	1.470	--	--	--	--
Soya bean	134	192	1.475	64	18	18	3.56
Corn	120	190	1.476	41	14	45	2.92
Lard	58	200	1.452	10	46	40	0.22
Olive	85	190	1.471	4	11	85	0.36
Almond	97	192	1.473	27	7	66	3.86
Cashew nut	80	184	1.464	8	18	74	0.44
Poppy seed	144	193	1.474	70	0	30	--
Walnut	145	192	1.475	70	8	22	8.75

* Values collected from various source.

When used for deep-frying, the fat left-over after frying is often used again for the purpose. When fats are stored or heated for a prolonged period, certain changes take place in their fatty acid composition. The unsaturated fatty acids present in fats take up oxygen and lose their double bond to become peroxides. They also combine with each other to form 'polymers' which are believed to be toxic.

Apart from the formation of peroxides, the triglycerides may become hydrolysed to free fatty acids which make the fat rancid. The rancidity caused by peroxide formation is referred to as oxidative rancidity and is measured by the amount of potassium iodide oxidized by a given amount of fat. The measure obtained is called peroxide value. The rancidity caused by the formation of free fatty acids is called hydrolytic rancidity and is measured by the amount of the same present.

Varying amounts of natural antioxidants which prevent the oxidation of fatty acids are present in fats. Antioxidants are also added to fats. When the antioxidant is externally added it should be effective at a low concentration and should contribute no objectionable flavour, odour and colour. It should

Table 41. linoleic acid content of different foods and diets*.

| | Values per 100 g edible portion * | | | | | Linoleic acid | |
	calories	Total fat (g)	Saturated fat (S) (g)	PUFA (P) (g)	Linoleic acid (g)	P/S	% of total fat	% of calories provided
Wheat	360	1.4	0.4	0.5	0.1	1.2	11	0.4
Bajra	360	5.7	1.9	2.3	2.3	1.2	42	6.0
Maize	360	3.3	0.7	1.4	1.4	2.0	44	3.6
Rice (milled)	360	0.6	0.3	0.2	≤0.2	0.6	33	≤0.5
Bengalgram	360	3.9	0.5	2.6	2.6	5.2	68	6.5
Blackgram	360	1.1	0.3	0.4	0.4	1.3	37	1.2
Soyabean	430	18.7	2.6	9.7	8.7	3.6	46	19.0
Coconut	660	62.7	57.4	0.9	≤0.9	0.01	≤1.5	≤0.1
Groundnut	550	48.9	12.7	14.0	14.0	1.1	28	23.0
Sesame	560	47.2	6.8	21.5	21.5	3.2	46	34.0
Ghee (buffalo)	900	100	65.8	1.0	1.0	0.01	1.0	1.0
Hydrogenated fat (dalda)	900	100	14.5	-	-	-	-	-
Egg	175	11.8	4.0	2.5	2.5	0.6	21	13
Fish	90	1.2	0.7	0.3	0.3	0.5	25	3
Mutton (muscle)	195	9.6	5.4	0.7	0.7	0.1	7	5
Values per calories**								
Poor diet (Tamil Nadu)		8.3	1.7	2.2	2.2	1.3	27	2
Poor diet (Bhils)		10.0	2.4	4.0	3.0	1.8	29	2.7
Poor diet (Gujarat)		20.0	4.1	6.0	5.3	1.4	27	4.7
Upper class diet (Gujarat)		41.0	12.8	4.4	4.4	0.3	11	4.0

* Rounded figures derived from food tables for calories; other values obtained in the Bio-chemistry Department of Baroda University, Baroda.
** Per capita intake is of the order of 1800 calories among the poor and 2000 calories among the upper class.

be physiologically harmless, readily available and reasonable in cost. Tocopherols are often used as antioxidants.

The presence of moisture in fats speeds up hydrolytic rancidity. Containers made of metals such as zinc and iron speed up rancidity. Cream of tartar is found to prevent it. Rancid fat tends to foam and rise when heated. The frying of tamarind pulp in the fat is believed to prevent this. This may be due to the tartaric acid present in tamarind. Certain herbs such as marjoram are believed to improve the keeping quality of fats.

The peroxide value of a fat increases during use for deep-frying as may be expected and during storage as mentioned earlier. The changes during storage are greater in the case of heated fats. The changes during frying depend on the temperature and period of frying and the type of fat used and are greater in ghee than in groundnut oil. Those during storage depend on exposure to light and air. In studies carried out in the author's laboratory, oil stored in opaque porcelain jars whose lids were sealed with paraffin wax was found to keep better than unsealed porcelain jars suggesting that exposure to air is more crucial than to light.

Different fats smoke at different temperatures and the changes during heating appear to be related to smoking point, being greater in fats such as ghee with a low smoking point. Ghee has a lower smoking point than groundnut or til oil and the latter should be preferably used for foods which require a high frying temperature. For the same reason hydrogenated oil is preferable to ghee.

Different foods require different temperatures for frying. Foods containing milk, sugar, jaggery, cheese or eggs require a lower temperature whereas bhajyas and papads require a high temperature.

When fats are used for deep-frying it is important to control the temperature carefully. It should not be allowed to heat up to a temperature higher than that required for frying. This can be ensured by putting a small piece of the material to be fried and waiting for it to float. The temperature of fat can also be tested by frying a small piece of papad or bread crumb. The papad should puff out at once but not brown. The bread crumb should fry to a golden brown. If the temperature of the fat is too high the food will char outside and remain raw inside. The fat so heated up will have poor keeping quality. If the temperature is too low, the material fried will soak up a lot of fat. If the temperature is just right, a crisp outer layer will be formed which prevents the fat from seeping in and the insides will be uniformly cooked. The secret of good frying is to allow the fat to heat up to the required temperature and not higher and maintain this temperature throughout. The heat should, therefore, be turned down after the first few minutes. If the fat has cooled somewhat during the frying of one batch, it should be allowed to heat up to the required temperature before the next batch is fried. The food fried should 'sizzle' vigorously when put in and be uniformly cooked on both sides and float when taken out.

The keeping quality of heated fat is believed to be improved by frying some potatoes or a piece of tamarind pulp at the end. The oil should be filtered so as to remove the solid particles as the same are believed to speed up rancidity. It should be stored in a closed container. The addition of some fresh oil (1/5 by volume) is believed to improve keeping quality.

Because of the changes which take place during heating, heated fats are poorer sources of unsaturated fatty acids. A diet containing repeatedly heated fats is found to increase blood cholesterol in experimental animals. Further, such fats are not absorbed well. This results in the poor availability of the vitamins which get dissolved in them. In the case of commercially processed fats, antioxidants or substances which prevent the oxidation of fatty acids are added to improve the keeping quality of the same.

The amount of fat absorbed during deep-frying depends on the moisture and fat content of the product fried and the presence of leavening agents. Increased amounts of shortening in the material fried increase the amount of fat absorbed from the frying medium. Leavening agents increase fat absorption by increasing the surface area exposed to the frying medium and the penetrability of the product fried. Sugar, eggs, moisture and low gluten content in the case of wheat flour are believed to have a similar effect.

The use of fat as a shortening agent is because of its ability to bring about a crisp texture of fried or baked products. In wheat products this may be due to the shortening of gluten strands which may make the product rubbery. In other dishes it may contribute to the gelatinization of starch. Butter and ghee are generally preferred as shortening agents, but in some cases (sev, pakora, etc.) groundnut oil is found to be just as good if not better. The amount of shortening needed may be reduced if rice flour is added. This may be because of the gelatinization of starch in rice flours maize flour which is cheaper than rice flour may be substituted for the same. In products prepared with wheat flour, it can also be reduced by steaming part of the flour for a few minutes.

The amount of fat absorbed is also believed to depend on the medium used for frying. Less fat is believed to be absorbed with fats which have a higher smoking point.

Ghee is prepared from butter by heating it till all the moisture evaporates. The heating should be discontinued when the cheesy particles in the same become golden brown. This may be done somewhat earlier as the residual moisture evaporates with the heat of the vessel and the particles slowly turn to a golden brown. Heating the butter beyond this point imparts a burnt odour, results in greater destruction of vitamin A and increases its peroxide value. Under heated ghee on the other hand, develops hydrolytic rancidity because of the moisture present.

In products such as halwa, mysore pak or cake, the fat blends homogeneously with the non-fat components so as to form an emulsion. Beating the cake batter helps the process of emulsification. In the preparation of mysore pak, which is a good example of a product involving emulsification, one part of bengal gram flour and two parts each of sugar and ghee are used. A thick syrup is prepared from sugar which continues to be heated. Small quantities of flour and ghee are added alternatively and the mixture thoroughly blended before each addition so that the ghee is not visible and forms a perfect and smooth blend with the sugar and flour. Towards the end the mixture turns a golden colour and puffs out, showing pores. At this stage it is poured into a greased plate, cut into diamonds or squares after a few minutes and allowed to cool before the slices are removed. Roasting the flour lightly before using it gives a better flavour. Soya bean flour can be used in place of bengal gram flour. The addition of a little cream to the mixture results in a softer product and a more nutty flavour. The preparation of halwas is based on a similar blending of starch, sugar and fat.

Sugar

Sugar is not a dietary essential but ordinarily forms a part of our diet. Most people seem to have a craving for sweet foods. Every festive occasion is celebrated with sweets. The word 'sweet' in everyday language has come to mean lovable or desirable.

Sucrose is sweeter than other sugars. It is possible that a taste for sweets is acquired when bottle milk substituted for breast milk is sweetened so as to resemble the latter in composition. The sucrose added for this purpose is sweeter than lactose present in milk.

Sugar is present in the form of sucrose in sugarcane, sugar beets, etc. As in the case of fat, we prefer to isolate the sugar from these sources and use it in a variety of ways. Palm sugar, honey and maple sugar are used to a limited extent. The most common sugar is cane sugar prepared from sugar cane juice. The refined form of sugar is practically 100% sucrose with all the minerals and vitamins removed during the process of refining. Jaggery and brown sugar are also prepared from cane sugar, but they are not refined to the same degree and as such they contain some amount of minerals, particularly calcium and iron. Unfortunately, white sugar is becoming increasingly popular and is replacing jaggery and molasses.

Molasses is the syrup derived from sugarcane juice and is a byproduct in the manufacture of jaggery and brown sugar. It is highly liked by children and used in families which make jaggery as a cottage industry. Palm-gur is prepared from the sap of the palmyra tree or date palm. It is regarded as an easily digestible food of good nutritive value in Ayurveda and this claim seems justified on the basis of its chemical composition (**Table 42**) and animal experiments. It is found to be a good source of vitamins including vitamin B12 which is believed to be formed by microbial action. The quality

Table 42. Composition of palm gur as compared to that of cane gur[1].

	Amount per 100g in gur from		
	palmyra	date paim	cane[2]
moisture (g)	7.4	9.7	9.0
total sugars(g)	77.2	72.1	87.6
protein (g)	1.5	2.0	1.0
ash(g)	3.3	2.9	1.3
calcium(mg)	195.0	225.0	105.0
riboflavin (mg)	0.38	0.36	0.31
nicotinic acid (mg)	3.30	3.63	2.79

1 Manage, Lata and Kamala Sohonic. 1966. Data abstracted from the following source. *J. Nut. and Diet.* 3, 1,1-5.
2 In contrast refined cane—sugar contains 99.4% sugar, 0.4% moisture and 0.2% of other ingredients.

of palm-gur varies from batch to batch and if techniques can be standardized so as to ensure uniform quality, it can be popularized specially for use with young children before they acquire a taste of refined sugar. Palm trees are resistant to drought whereas cultivation of sugar cane requires the best available land which can be used for the production of rice. Increased production of palm-gur can, therefore, help relieve some of the pressure on land according to many experts.

Honey is another popular sugar derived from flowers and although its popularity is well justified on the basis of its pleasing taste and flavour, its nutritive value has been exaggerated. However, considering the fact that the production of honey does not involve any extra pressure on the land and that the presence of evergreen trees flowering profusely at different times of the year should make bee farming profitable, it is surprising that honey production in this country is practically negligible. The cost of honey is also much higher than in countries such as Australia.

Bee farming can be carried out as a household industry with a small investment and without much man-power. In Australia, as much as 200 kg are obtained from beehive as against 6 kg in this country. Recently, a strain of bees which can manufacture honey from the flowers of alfalfa, which is widely cultivated as cattle feed, has been developed in the United States. Commercially made syrups from corn are also available but their consumption is negligible and is confined to the economically well off.

The sap of the maple tree is used for the preparation of maple syrup and maple sugar in regions such as Canada where the tree is found.

The bulk of the sugar consumed is used in beverages such as tea, coffee and milk. Sugar is also used as such for the preparation of desserts and as a preservative in the preparation of jams, jellies, fruit preserves and cordials. Toffees, chocolates and other popular candies are made almost entirely of sugars.

High Fructose Corn Syrup (HFCS) is a substitute for sugar commonly used in the West for the production of soft drinks. HFCS is manufactured from corn starch. Corn starch is hydrolyzed to glucose and then treated with the enzyme glucose isomerase when glucose is converted to fructose. The resulting product has a composition of 55% fructose and 42% glucose. Higher proportion of fructose in HFCS imparts more sweetness to it. Therefore, it is more economical for beverage manufacturers to use HFCS in place of sugar. It is now reported that consumption of HFCS in beverages may play a role in the epidemic of obesity in the West[*]. Fructose is a highly lipogenic sugar and promote fat synthesis in the body by metabolic process which involve insulin[**]. Incidentally, HFCS industry has not caught up in India due to economic reason and its application in food and beverage industry is doubtful.

Sugar cooking is a task requiring skill. In cakes, biscuits, etc. the sugar has to blend homogeneously with the flour and fat, so as to form a colloidal product which does not crystallize. In products such as laddus, the sugar tends to form crystals on the surface if the syrup is not cooked to the right texture. Preventing crystallization is a major problem in the refrigerator method of preparing ice-creams as crystals tend to form when the milk is frozen without constant agitation. This can be prevented by the addition of whipped cream, beaten eggs, and re-freezing the frozen product after thorough beating and aeration. The addition of a small quantity of custard powder and the use of evaporated or condensed milk also help to prevent crystallization.

Many people such as the Bhils in this country do not buy any sugar at all except once or twice a year for festivals such as Diwali. Sugar consumption among the poor is about 10–20 g per capita per day.

In western countries, sugar consumption is of the order of 100 g per capita per day. This, along with the increased consumption of foods rich in saturated fats, has been believed to contribute to the increase in the incidence or hypercholesterolemia, heart disease, intestinal disorders and diabetes not to mention dental caries. It would be desirable to arrest a similar trend in the affluent sections of this country.

---

[*] Bray, George A., Joy Nelson Samara and M. Popkin Barry. 2004. *Am. J. Clin. Nutr.* **79**:537–43.
[**] Dekker, M.J., Q. Su, C. Baker, A.C. Rutledge and K. Adeli. 2010. *Am. J. Physiol. Endocrinol. Metab*, **299(5)**:E685–94.

Chapter 13

Vegetables and Fruits*

The importance of vegetables and fruits was dramatically brought into focus with the recognition of the role of vitamin C in human nutrition. Barring sprouted legumes, which are not widely consumed, they are the only significant sources of vitamin C in the diet. Salad vegetables and fruits are among the few foods which can be consumed as such without cooking.

Different parts of the plant are consumed as vegetables as shown below:

roots	...	yams, carrots, radish
bulb	...	leeks, onions, garlic
tuber	...	potatoes, sweet potatoes
stem	...	celery, asparagus, banana, amaranth
flowers	...	drumstick, agathi, cauliflower
leaves	...	cabbage, amaranth, colocasia, fenugreek, spinach
pods	...	cow pea, french beans, cluster beans, field beans
immature seeds	...	red gram, peas, bengal gram
immature fruits	...	brinjal, pumpkin, cucumber
mature fruits	...	tomatoes and other fruits

Fruits and vegetables are essentially storage sites where plants store their reserve supplies of nutrients either for themselves or for their progeny. Fruits vary greatly in moisture, carbohydrate, pectin and fibre content and acidity. They also vary greatly with regard to vitamin and mineral content.

---

* Some of the tables in this chapter are partly or fully reproduced from the article 'Horticulture in relation to nutritional requirements' Rajalakshmi, R. and C.V. Ramakrishnan. 1968. PL Fds. *hum. Nuir.* 1:11–14.

The acidity of fruits is derived from different acids such as tartaric acid in grapes and tamarind, citric acid in tomatoes, oranges, and lemons, and malic acid in apple and hydroxycitric acid in Malabar tamarind. These or other acids are responsible for the acidity in fruits such as raw wood apple and different kinds of berries. The acids in fruits are formed from intermediates of carbohydrate metabolism which accumulate in the raw fruit. As the fruits become mature, the activities of enzymes capable of converting these organic acids to sugars increase, resulting in increased sugar content. The sweetness of fruits is mainly due to the presence of sucrose, fructose and glucose, different fruits containing different proportions of the same.

An increased cultivation and consumption of vegetables and fruits is certainly desirable for several reasons. They make for a pleasing variety in the meals. They require less land per capita and their production can give more nutrients per acre than other foods as can be seen from **Table 43.**

Starchy vegetables

Vegetables can help correct the basic deficiencies in our diet of calories, calcium, iron, carotene and riboflavin. The cultivation of bananas and roots and tubers can help increase our calorie supplies as they give high yields per acre. Leafy vegetables can contribute significant amounts of vitamins and minerals.

In the cultivation of vegetables and fruits as energy sources the yield per acre and nutrient content must be taken into account. Bananas are popular but they have a low protein content. But they have the advantage that they are highly relished and can be eaten as such and are easily digested and tolerated even by children. As such, they form a welcome addition to the diet. Roots and tubers are also good sources of calories. Tapioca, yams, potatoes, sweet potatoes and colocasia roots are used as substantial sources of calories in different parts of the world. Upto 200 g of roots and tubers can be consumed in dayas this will provide only about 10% of total calories. Tapioca gives high yields but its consumption must be along with that of cereals, pulses and oil seeds as they have a low protein content and their exclusive consumption results in protein malnutrition. The same applies to sweet potatoes. Potatoes seem to be the most suitable as they have high energy value and also contain appreciable amounts of essential nutrients. They form a staple for the poor in Ireland and their prolonged consumption is not attended with any adverse effects. Thus if the cultivation of roots and tubers is considered for meeting part of our calorie requirements potatoes would be a suitable crop. However, elephant yams and wild yams which are grown in this country not only give a higher yield per acre but also have a greater content of calcium, carotene and riboflavin as will be seen from the following data:

Table 43. Relative efficiency of vegetable foods and animal foods as suppliers of nutrients from an acre of land.

Foodstuffs	Gross yield per acre (kg)	Calories x 10⁵	Protein (kg)	Approximate amount available per acre (a) Protein (kg)	Iron (g)	Carotene Vitamin A (i.u x 10⁵)	Riboflavin (g)
Cereals	350	12.0	35	0.10	21.0	3.5	0.35
Pulses	250	8.6	60	0.20	20.0	2.5	1.00
Oilseeds	300	16.5	78	0.15	4.8	1.8	0.90
Milk	360	2.9	11	0.76	0.7	3.6	0.36
Animal foods	20	0.4	4	0.05	0.4	0.1	0.06
Leafy vegetables	5000–10000	24–48	200–400	12.5–25.0	750–1500	3500–7000	5–10
Root vegetables	5000–10000	50–100	100–200	1.0–2.0	30–60	50–100	1–2
Other vegetables	2500–5000	10–20	50–100	1–2	50–100	75–150	1.5–3.0
Fruits	10000–20000	50–100	80–160	3–6	120–240	50–100	2–4
Sugar	2000	80	---	---	---	---	---

* Calculated from figures for yield and average nutrient composition of different food groups derived from values given in food tables for commonly consumed foods.

	Per 100 g edible portion						
	Calorie	Protein (g)	Calcium (mg)	Iron (mg)	Carotene ((i.u)	Ribo-flavin (mg)	Yield per acre (kg)
Potatoes	97	1.6	10	0.7	40	0.01	5000–10000
Elephant yam	79	1.2	50	0.6	434	0.07	10000–20000
Wild yam	110	2.5	20	1.0	943	0.47	10000–20000

Elephant yams are a hardy crop. Trials in this laboratory have shown that elephant yams and other root vegetables can be readily incorporated in cereal and legume dishes such as debra, stuffed paratha, dosas, cutlets, steamed dumplings, etc. and can thus be used in feeding programmes organized for children. The recipes can be formulated in such a way that protein calories form at least 10% of total calories and the cost works out to less than 50 paise for 1000 Calories. It should be mentioned here that the cost worked out is based on the prices of food commodities prevailed when the data was collected. However, the cost can be extrapolated to the present prices. On the basis of the present prices of food commodities

Table 44. Cost and composition of recipes based on cereal-legume-vegetable combinations.

	Cereal (g)	Pulse (g)	Root vegetable (g)	Leafy vegetable (g)	Other vegetables (g)	Oil (g)	Calories*	Protein Calories (g) %
Debra	75	25	100	50	---	5–10	515–560	12.4–13.5
Stuffed Parathas}	75	25	100	50	---	5–10	515–560	12.4–13.5
Dhokla	75	25	100	50	---	5–10	515–560	12.4–13.5
Poora (dosa)	75	25	100	50	---	5–10	515–560	12.4–13.6
Khichri	75	25	100	50	50	5–10	545–580	12.4–13.6
Sambhar rice	75	25	100	50	50	5–10	545–580	12.7–13.6
Dumplings		50	100	---	---	5–10	317–362	15.5–17.6
Macaroni	25	25	50	---	---	5–10	297–342	10.3–11.6

* Cost per 1000 k calories 55–60 paise (1 Rupee =100 paise).

the cost may work out to Rupees 10–15. A few selected recipes conforming to these criteria are shown in **Table 44.**

In recent times elephant yam has elicited lot of interest among nutritionist working in the field of dietary supplements and alternate medicine*.

Elephant yam is an ideal food for satiety without adding much to calorie intake. The polysaccharide glucomannan composed of glucose and mannose present in elephant yam is a soluble fibre which is not digested. It will increase several times its volume after absorbing water. This leads to sensation of fullness after consumption of elephant yam. It acts as a prebiotic supporting the growth of useful bacteria called probiotic like *lactobacillus bifedus* in the gut. The dried powder of elephant yam is available in the health food market of western countries with the name 'Konjac'.

Tapioca is widely consumed in Kerala usually along with parboiled rice and fish. But when the latter two are reduced, especially in the case of children, protein malnutrition is the result. Wheat which contains more protein is not accepted by the people in this State. Studies in the author's laboratory have shown that dishes commonly prepared in Kerala can be made with a mixture of tapioca, bengal gram and wheat so as to provide

Table 45. Recipes based on cereal – legume – vegetable combinations.

Food stuff	Outline of procedure
Debra	Make a dough with cereal plus pulse flour, finely chopped leaf greens, cooked and mashed potatoes, shape into balls, roll out and bake like chapaties.
Stuffed parathas	Cook and mash the root vegetable and add chopped and cooked leaf greens. Shape into balls and use as stuffing for chapaties. Make the dough with the cereal-pulse mixture.
Dhokla	Let ferment batter of coarsely ground cereal-pulse mixture. Add boiled and mashed rootvegetable and chopped leaf greens. Steam in greased plates for 20 minutes, cool, cut into pieces and season.
Poora (dosa)	Prepare a batter as above but somewhat thinner. Shallow fry like dosas (pancakes).
Khichri	Cook the cereal, pulse and vegetable together.
Sambar rice	Dehusked dal or sprouted pulse may be used. In the case of grains other than kodri and rice, 'cracked'grain may be used. Cook the cereal-pulse mixture. When it is almost cooked add the vegetables, tamarind juice, salt, spices etc, and cook again to 'sambhar' rice consistency.
Dumplings	Add boiled and mashed vegetable to bengal-gram flour. Add salt and seasoning and shape into balls. Steam, garnish and serve (can also be used in soups and broths).
Macaroni (cereals may be omitted)	Boil and mash the vegetable and add tapioca flour or pulse flour cooked in simmering water so as to form a dough. Knead, roll into balls, steam, press through a 'sev'press, season and serve. This combination can also be used for 'puttu', a common tapioca preparation in Kerala.

* Chua, M., T.C. Baldwin, Y.J. Hocking and K. Chan. 2010. *J. Ethnopharmacol.* **128(2):**268–78.

more than 10% protein calories. These dishes have been subjected to sensory evaluation using subjects from Kerala. Their recipes have been included **in Table 45**. Although products like tapioca macaroni have been developed by the Central Food Technological Research Institute, Mysore, education of the house wife in the preparation of such dishes will meet the twin objectives of improving the protein intake and increasing the acceptability of wheat in Kerala. A similar consumption of root vegetables in other parts can relieve to some extent the demand on cereals.

Studies with rats have shown that the addition of yam to a wheat-bengal gram mixture in the amounts suggested does not affect the protein quality of the diet.

Leafy vegetables

As mentioned earlier, leafy vegetables are excellent sources of carotene. In diets based on plant foods they are almost the only good sources of calcium, iron and riboflavin. In studies carried out on rats the addition of leafy vegetables to a mixture of cereal or millet+legume is found to result in an improved nutritional status. In other animal studies such addition is found to promote bone calcification. In our field centre, children fed a wheat, bengal gram dhokla with leafy vegetables were found to have a better skeletal development and vitamin A status than those given ordinary dhokla. Many of the fruit vegetables are good sources of riboflavin and vitamin C. In the choice of vegetables for increased cultivation and consumption, some attention must be paid to their composition with regard to carotene, oxalic acid, calcium, iron and vitamin C.

Among the leafy vegetables, fenugreek leaves seem to be excellent as their amino acid composition is favourable, the carotene in the same is well utilized and they are rich in iron and do not contain much of oxalic acid. They can be chopped and added to fermented batters of dhokla, dosa, etc. or cooked with green gram or with potatoes and onions. In these forms they are well-accepted although they are a little bitter in taste. Some jaggery can be added if necessary. In our rural centre in Gujarat young children are found to prefer dhokla with fenugreek leaves to many other foods.

Other leafy vegetables low in oxalic acid are cabbage, coriander leaves, mint, and safflower leaves. The oxalate content of many other leafy vegetables is not available.

Fruits and salad vegetables can be consumed as such and form a welcome addition to foods. Vegetables and fruits of low calorie value have an important place in the diets of persons such as obese people and diabetics who have to restrict their calorie intake. Even in normal individuals, the consumption of vegetables and fruits helps move the bowels regularly and prevent constipation.

It is not realized that a liberal consumption of vegetables can reduce the need for other foodstuffs and relieve the demand on cereals. About 250–300 g of vegetables and fruits can be consumed in a meal in the form of 50–100 g of roots and tubers, 50g each of leafy vegetables and other vegetables, and 100 g of fruits. In fact, in households including such liberal amounts of fruits and vegetables, there is less demand on cereals and pulses. Thus they should have a sparing effect on food grains which require more land for cultivation. We need only to visualise the appearance of the following menus in order to realize how much more attractive and appetizing a meal with liberal amounts of vegetables and fruits can be:

Menu including vegetables and fruits	The routine menu
tomato juice	chapaties
or pumpkin soup	dal
chapaties	potato or
dal	other vegetable
mashed spinach	curd
baked or cooked potatoes	
cauliflower with peas	
salad or carrots and cucumber	
serving of fruit curd	

Although it would seem that fruits and vegetables have to be taken in greater bulk in order to provide the nutrients present in other foods they compare well with other foods as sources of different nutrients if their moisture content is taken into account as their dry weight is only about 1/5 of fresh weight **(Table 46)**.

About 2-3% of the cultivated land used for the production of grains, oilseeds, etc. should be used for vegetable and fruit cultivation. Much less is actually cultivated. In Baroda District in Gujarat for instance, less than 1% of agricultural land is used for vegetable and fruit production. This results in a deficient supply in relation to demand. This in turn, results in high prices in spite of their high yields. Reasons for their lack of popularity with the farmer are the high losses prior to and after harvesting. Losses due to insects, birds, rats and monkeys are heavy. A man who grows vegetables has to find a ready market or perish whereas the cultivator of grains can afford to hoard and sell at higher prices. Facilities for storage, quick transportation and marketing and for refrigeration and canning will improve this state of affairs. Commercial dehydration and canning of vegetables at source is also likely to be useful.

Even at the prevailing high prices of vegetables they compare favourably with animal foods with regard to nutrients which can be derived

Table 46. Different foodstuffs as sources of selected nutrients.

Foodstuff	Moisture Content %	Approximate amount (g) giving					
		100 Calories	10 g protein	100 mg calcium	3 mg iron	1000 i.u vitamin A or carotene	1 mg riboflavin
Cereals	10	30	100	330	50	1000	1000
Pulses	10	30	40	125	40	1000	250
Oilseeds	5	20	40	200	200	600	330
Milk	84	125	330	50	1500	1000	1000
Animal food	75	70	40	700	150	3300	330
Egg	72	60	75	170	150	50	555
Leafy vegetables	90	200	250	40	20	15	1000
Starchy root vegetables	80	100	500	500	500	1000	5000
Other vegetables	80	250	500	250	150	330	1700
Fruits	85	b. 100				d. 100	
			1250	330			5000
		a. 200				c. 2000	

a and b – fruits low and high in carbohydrate.
c and d – fruits poor and rich in carotene.

from a rupee's worth of foodstuffs as can be seen from **Table 47.** Though the figures given in the first column of this table will be different today the pattern is expected to be the same. The time involved in preparing vegetables inhibits many people from consuming them regularly. Most poor people are accustomed to one dish meals. Such one dish meals have been worked out using cereal-legume-vegetable-leaf green combinations which have been described earlier (Table 45) and they need to be popularized.

The use of vegetables and fruits

Vegetables and fruits can be consumed in a variety of forms such as soups, juices, salads, etc.

Soups

Soups make an appetizing addition to meals and are very suitable for infants and the convalescent. They do not ordinarily form part of the Indian dietary,

Table 47. Nutrients provided by a rupee's worth of different foods*.

Foodstuff	Approximate amount (g) in rupee's worth	Nutrient present in rupee's worth foodstuff					
		Calories	Protein (g)	Calcium (mg)	Iron (mg)	Carotene or vitamin A (µg)	Ribo-flavin (mg)
cereals (wheat)	600	2100	72	180	36	210	0.60
pulses	280	1000	72	240	28	180	1.20
oilseeds (ground nut)	200	1100	50	100	3.2	72	0.60
milk (buffalo)+	500	300	15	1000	1.0	150	0.50
animal food (mutton)	250	485	50	30	5.0	23	0.68
egg (hen)	75	125	10	45	1.5	350+270	0.13
leafy vegetables (amaranth, fenugreek, spinach)	2500	1250	100	6250	375.0	105000	2.50
Root vegetables	1500	1500	30	300	9.0	900	0.30
Other vegetables	2000	800	40	800	40.0	3600	1.20
Fruits (bananas)	1000	1000	8	300	12.0	300	0.20

+   milk containing 3% fat, 3% protein and 5-6% carbohydrate.

but preparation of soup is not as difficult as might seem to the housewife. Some simple suggestions for soups are given **in Table 48.**

Fresh buttermilk which is not too sour or coconut milk can replace milkin the recipe given. Fried or toasted bread crumbs or bits of fried papad can be added at the time of serving. Whole green legumes or roasted cowpeas can be cooked and added.

If soups with a fine consistency are desired they can be sieved through a colander or blended in a mixer.

Juices

Fruit juices can be prepared from fruits such as water-melon, rock-melon, chani bor, jamun, phalsa and tomatoes. In the case of tomatoes, add boiling water and keep covered for a few minutes (this is called blanching). Peel off- the skin after immersing them in cold water, if necessary, churn with an egg-beater, wooden churn or electric beater to a homogenous

Table 48. **Suggestions for making soups.**

Vegetables	Other ingredients	Procedure	seasoning
Pumpkin, carrots, potatoes	Milk and/ or green gram dal	Cook and mash vegetable, add milk and bring to a boil roast dal, cook soft and churn and add to soup	Salt. Black pepper, cumin seeds, curry leaves fried in ghee
Tomatoes	Flour, milk, onions	Fry finely chopped onions in a little fat and add blanched and pureed tomatoes and bring to a boil, roast a little flour add milk, mix well and add gradually to the tomatoes, add salt and seasoning.	Fried cumin seeds
Tomatoes and a mixture of other vegetables such as cabbage, cauliflower, beans etc	Onions	Fry onions, add water , and cut the vegetables, cook soft, mash and add tomato puree or juice in soup, bring to a boil and season.	Salt, cumin powder, an extract prepared from mint, basil, curry leaves, coriander, ginger, lemon leaves etc.
Tomatoes, lemon	Redgram dal	Cook dal soft, churn well, add blanched and churned tomatoes and boil for a few minutes.	Celery salt, ajma powder, salt, cumin, coriander or curry powder, lemon juice, coriander leaves, ginger.

liquid and chill with salt and lemon juice added. If desired, add suitable seasoning such as cumin, mint, coriander or ajma. A little sugar may also be added. The tomatoes can also be homogenized as such without blanching if an electric mixer is available. The same can be used for homogenizing a juice from other salad vegetables such as grated carrots, cabbage, etc. Juicy mangoes can be pre-treated like tomatoes and the juice expressed. Such treatment makes the extraction of juice easier. Rock-melon and water-melon can be freed from skin and seed and cut into pieces and homogenized.

Chani bor, phalsa, jamun, etc. can be boiled in water for about 5 minutes under cover, allowed to keep for 10–15 minutes, churned, filtered and sugar and lemon juice added and the juice chilled. Juices prepared from these berries have an attractive colour and flavour.

These juices can also be used as a base for fruit punch. A fruit punch is essentially a combination of lemon or orange juice, other fruit juice, sugar syrup and tea to which aerated water is added at the time of serving. Suitable spices such as cardamom can be added.

Vegetables

Tomatoes, cucumber, carrots, onions, green mangoes, tender coconut, capsicum, lettuce, cauliflower, radish, etc. can be used in different combinations to make salads. Lemon juice, salt, oil, mustard seed (in vagary), chopped ginger, coriander leaves, cut pieces of coconut etc. make desirable additions. Curd can also be used along with or in place of lemon juice. A sweet-sour salad can be prepared from grated carrots by adding lemon juice, sugar, honey and fruits such as pineapple, banana, dates and raisins. They are highly popular with children. Boiled beets, potatoes etc. can also be added. The salad vegetables can be sliced (e.g. tomatoes and cucumber) or cut into sticks (e.g. carrots) and served as such.

Fruit salad

As mentioned earlier, fruit should be sliced into a bowl containing lemon juice and sugar. Papaya flavoured in this way is highly acceptable to people who do not like the fruit as such. A mixture of fruits can make an attractive fruit salad. The cores and seeds should be removed in apples and pears before they are cut. If seeded grapes are used, they should be cut into halves with a sharp knife and the seeds scooped out before they are added.
Green bananas, pumpkin, potatoes etc. can be boiled and served as a salad with curd, salt or sugar and seasoning added. Ripe bananas can be added to a mixture of curd, milk, honey, jaggery and cream or ghee. Black raisins, cashew nuts, cardamoms, walnuts, dates, etc. can also be added.

Baked dishes

Potatoes, sweet potatoes etc. may be baked with their skins. Sweet potatoes can also be boiled, skinned, mashed, brown sugar and butter or ghee added and baked. The same may be topped with a layer of nuts, sesame seed, raisins, coconut, etc. and flavoured with cardamom.

Chutneys

Mint, corianders and curry leaves, onions, tomatoes etc. can be ground into a paste and seasoned to make a chutney. Additions of tamarind pulp, grated coconut, chana dal roasted in ghee, etc. may be made before grinding. Chutneys can also be made from vegetables after pan-frying or cooking. Onions, green tomatoes, egg plant, ridge gourd, pumpkin, galka, elephant yam and raw wood apple can be prepared by this method. Tamarind pulp, salt, hing, chillies and jaggery may be added before grinding. Vaghar and lemon juice (in place of tamarind pulp) may be added after grinding. The vegetables may also be prepared in the following ways:

Method	Procedure	Example
Sauteed	heat oil in a pan, turn in the vegetable and cook with a sprinkling of water under cover snake gourd	cauliflower, potatoes, ladies fingers, snake gourd
Cooked with Dal	cook green gram or red gram to three-fourths consistency, add the vegetable and cook to completion	fenugreek, field beans, onions, cabbage.
Cooked with coconut paste	cook vegetables and add coconut paste and suitable seasoning	'Aviyal' vegetables, cauliflower, cabbage, greens, tomatoes
R o a s t e d whole	roast and peel the vegetable, mash and season suitably.	sweet potatoes, green bananas, bringals
cooked with t a m a r i n d juice	cook the vegetable, mash in the case of greens,add tamarind juice,salt, a little jaggery and seasoning; roasted and powdered sesame or fenugreek or curry powder can be added depending on the flavour desired	p u m p k i n , l a d i e s fingers, amaranth, spinach,bringal, drumstick, carrots
cooked with m a s h e d tomato juice	tomato juice to be substituted for tamarind juice. Fried onions or coconut paste may be added.	roasted and egg plant, a mixture of cauliflower, onions, potatoes, peas and drumstick.
cooked with butter milk	use butter milk in place of tamarind juice	m a s h e d s p i n a c h , amaranth, potatoes
s t e a m e d with ground dal	pre-soak dal in water,grind into a coarse paste, add the chopped vegetables, season, steam and turn into a pan containing heated oil and cook for 5–10 minutes.	banana flowers, onions, cluster beans, cabbage, colocasia leaves rolled as rollypollies with dal paste
cooked with jaggery	cook, mash and cook again with jaggery. In the case of wood apples mash the pulp and add to jaggery syrup.	p u m p k i n , s w e e t potatoes, carrots, wood apple
Cooked in Jaggery syrup	steam an cook in jaggery syrup.	Cut pieces of raw mangoes, green tomato
Pastries and Breads	the vegetables may be boiled together and used as filling in pies and pastries(samosas) Or in yeast breads.They may be mashed and added to debras.	p e a s , o n i o n s , cauliflower, potatoes, cabbage, carrots etc.
Casseroles	the cooked vegetables can be topped with a layer of cheese and coconut and baked.	potatoes, cauliflower

Method	Procedure	Example
Halwas	cook in water or milk or over steam, mash, add ghee and sugar and continue to cook to a halwa consistency.	pumpkin, bottle gourd carrots, sweet potatoes.
Preserves	cook grated and steamed carrots or cooked pumpkin in sugar or jaggery syrup to a jam type consistency and store. Lemon juice, raisins and spices may be added. Remove surplus juice from blanched Tomatoes and cook with sugar.	carrots, pumpkin, green tomatoes, ripe tomatoes

Vegetables are also used in vadas, bhajyas (vegetable fritters), cutlets, dumplings, etc.

In spite of the varied ways in which vegetables can be used, most housewives tend to cook them in stereotyped ways with a lot of spice so that many children have to be coaxed into consuming them.

The distinctive flavour of different vegetables is lost by prolonged cooking and excessive seasoning, both of which should be avoided. Children should be encouraged to consume plain boiled or baked vegetables or those cooked with nutritious foods such as dals, coconut paste, tomatoes and curd.

Chapter 14

Foods of Animal Origin

Milk, eggs, poultry, sea foods and meats are the main foods of animal origin. As stated earlier, animal foods are rich in methionine and are the only sources of vitamin B12.

Milk

Milk is the most widely consumed of these foods. Even people who are opposed to taking animal foods obtained by killing, because of either family tradition or personal conviction, do not object to milk, as the same is obtained without killing the animals. However, people such as the vegans in Britain do not include even milk in their diet.

Since early times, man has tamed many mammals and used the surplus milk produced as food. Cows, buffaloes, goats, sheep, camels and donkeys are all used as milk animals. Yaks are used for milking purposes in mountain regions. In this country, cow milk and buffalo milk are the most important from the commercial standpoint. Reliable estimates of the amount of goat milk are not available as most of the milk produced is consumed by the family. It can be used with benefit for those who are either allergic to cow milk or are unable to tolerate it. It is also used in the manufacture of special varieties of cheese. Camel milk and donkey milk are used in desert regions. The latter is also advocated for medicinal purposes.

Animal milk because of its being the food for the mammalian infant is nearly complete food for man. It is a source of protein and fat soluble vitamins and the best source of calcium. It is easily digested and tolerated and is very useful in the feeding of infants and convalescents. However, milk obtained from animals is lacking in iron and vitamin C. As milk is a food intended by nature for the infant of the species and most of the mammals can synthesize vitamin C it is not surprising that milk obtained from animals is deficient in the same. In contrast, human milk contains a generous amount of vitamin C, a fact which is consistent with the need of the human infant for this vitamin.

For the newborn infant who is born with a surplus store of iron, a deficiency in milk of iron is of no consequence. But when milk is continued as the sole food after the first six months, the child tends to develop iron deficiency anaemia.

The per capita availability of milk in this country is of the order of 280 g per day as on the year 2010. About one-third of the milk produced is consumed in urban areas which contain about 20% of the population. About 5–10% of the urban population consumes more than 400 g of milk per capita per day. Restaurants in urban areas use up a good proportion of milk for the production of tea and coffee. There are many families which hardly consume any milk.

Milk is the only source of animal protein in vegetarian diets. Generally, the production of animal protein involves extra pressure on the land as about 10 g of protein have to be fed to the animal in order to derive 1 g of protein as food from the animal. In the case of dairy animals, however, about 3 kg of plant proteins are converted to 1 kg of milk protein. Further, the dairy animal is able to utilize foods such as hay and grass which are not edible for man and needs only a small supplement of foods which are edible for man. Even these are mostly in the form of oil-cake, cotton seed, cluster beans, etc. which are not used in our diets at present. The dairy animal, therefore, does a very valuable service to man by converting non-edible food to edible food of the highest quality and provides in addition valuable manure in the form of dung and urine. In spite of the low yields obtained at present milk compares in cost and nutritive value with other foods of animal origin such as eggs and meat.

Milk is used mainly as such or in the form of curd and butter milk and beverages. It is also used for the preparation of ice-cream, milk chocolates, malted beverages and milk sweets such as khoa, peda, gulabjamun, rasgollas, sandesh and cheese.

Curd is the major product obtained from milk in this country. Milk is fermented by certain bacteria which convert the lactose in milk to lactic acid which is responsible for the sour taste of curd. These bacteria are introduced into milk by the addition of a little curd from the previously prepared batch. For these bacteria to multiply rapidly, the milk should be neither too hot nor too cold. The curd gets too sour in summer and does not set readily in winter because of variations in environmental temperature. These variations can be avoided by setting curd under standard conditions. The milk should be warm (35-40°) when set (the right temperature can usually be achieved by boiling about one-third to half of the milk to be set as curd and adding it to the remainder. A standard quantity of curd should be added to the milk (about one-half teaspoon per cup, or less, if the curd is too sour) and the container kept insulated in winter by inverting a large pan over it. Under these conditions the curd should set in about 5 hours.

The preparation of curd is an ancient process. The difference in the flavour of curds is believed to be due to those in the microorganisms involved in the fermentation. The presence of Torula yeast is found to impart a cheesy flavour. The curd or yogurt prepared in Bulgaria is fermented with *Lactobacillus bulgaricus.*

The preparation of curd is a way of preserving milk. The growth of acid-forming bacteria prevents the growth of other microorganisms which cause milk to spoil. Many pathogenic microorganisms including those causing amoebic dysentery do not multiply in curd.

Although there is no difference between curd and milk with regard to nutritive value, some people who are unable to tolerate milk, especially infants, are able to tolerate it in the form of curd. In conditions such as diarrhoea and dysentery, curd is preferable to milk. Preparations such as 'eledona' used in the treatment of dysentery in young children are based on buttermilk powder. Curd prepared at home after boiling the milk and diluted to buttermilk with boiled water is equally suitable and much cheaper.

Buttermilk is obtained by adding water to curd and churning it or as a byproduct in the process of preparing butter.

Butter making is an ancient process and involves the separation of butter from milk in which it is present as an emulsion. This separation is achieved by centrifugation, as in churning, so that the lighter fat layer floats to the top. Either whole milk or cream can be used for the preparation of butter. In households cream is separated as a top-scum or malai which forms when milk is heated and allowed to cool with exposure to air. For a good separation of malai, the milk should be heated till it foams up and then cooled with exposure to air by covering it with a colander or a sieve in place of a lid. The milk should not be disturbed before the malai has set. Milk needed for immediate purposes can be boiled separately so that the remaining milk can be left undisturbed. The milk can be cooled for 3-4 hours (after first cooling to room temperature) in a refrigerator or in a basin of cold water for better separation. The malai can be removed and set as curd and the same pooled every two or three days and churned for butter. The addition of some fresh malai or milk over the top layer will prevent it from going too sour or getting mouldy. Alternatively, it can be stored in the refrigerator after it has set.

The fermentation of cream before churning brings about its acidification and the easy separation of butter. It also imparts a desirable flavour and aroma to the butter. Butter is also prepared from unfermented cream in creameries. In this case, the microorganisms are added to the butter to bring about the required flavour.

When butter is prepared from fermented cream the liquid left is buttermilk with a pleasant taste and flavour. Both are poor when cream is allowed to ripen spontaneously without the addition of curd. The agitation caused by churning exerts an effect similar to centrifugation and brings about the de-emulsification of fat and causes the fat globules to accumulate and form a solid mass at the top. When this layer is largely free from moisture it is removed, squeezed gently to remove liquid and stored in a cool place. Its keeping qualities are better if it is formed into a firm ball and floated in cold water so that non-fat substances are washed off. Standard colours and salt are added to butter for table use.

The churning of butter is easier in winter if warm water (40°C) is added to the fermented cream initially and cold water added after a layer of butter forms at the top.

Many people find a double egg beater more convenient than the traditional churn. An electric mixer can speed up the process. The buttermilk obtained during the preparation of butter can be used as such or in soups, khadi (buttermilk sauce), rabdi prepared from flour etc.

In this country, as skim milk is not available the removal of malai yields not only fresh butter and ghee but partially skimmed milk for those who want to cut down fat consumption. It is possible to remove, in the form of malai, more than 25% of the fat in milk by cooling to room temperature after boiling, and more than 50%, by cooling in refrigerator. The milk should be loosely covered (eg., with a colander) for this purpose.

As mentioned earlier, ghee is prepared from butter by removing all the moisture. The other non-fat components separate out as cheesy particles. To get ghee with good flavour as well as keeping quality the butter should be heated till all the moisture evaporates. The heat should be turned down towards the end and overheating should be avoided. When it is prepared just right the cheesy particles which separate out are golden brown in colour. The ghee can be strained off and the residue can be added to many dishes to add a pleasant taste and flavour. When ghee is cooled to room temperature, it becomes partly solid, the solid portion having a typical granular structure.

Various forms of milk such as homogenized milk, evaporated milk, and non-fat dry milk are now available in the west. Homogenized milk is obtained by subjecting milk to a temperature of 57–60 C at 1000–5000 lb pressure through a very small orifice and in this process a reduction in the size of fat globules takes place and the milk does not easily form a top scum. With the reduction in size, the number of fat globules increases and there is a corresponding increase in total surface area which increases the adsorption of proteins and phospholipids resulting in a high degree of emulsification.

Because of the larger surface area of the fat globules, homogenized milk increases the thickness of certain products and coagulates more easily. The cooking quality of homogenized milk therefore differs from that of non-homogenized milk when used in puddings etc.

Evaporated milk

The evaporation of milk is accomplished by removing a considerable amount of water from whole milk. After the removal of 60% of the water the product is homogenized and sterilized in sealed cans. The cooked flavour characteristic of evaporated milk is not usually detected in cooked food and improves the flavour of certain foods such as those made with cocoa and chocolate.

Condensed milk

Condensed milk is milk which has been concentrated from full cream milk by removal of its water with or without addition of sugar. The removal of water is achieved at a relatively lower temperature by bringing down the boiling point (which is about 100° at atmospheric pressure) to 55–63° by reducing the pressure. The total milk solids are not less than 28% and milk fat not less than 9.5%.

Toned milk

Milk sold as 'toned' milk in this country is milk with reduced fat content, the reduction being brought about by either partial skimming or by addition of skim milk. Skim milk and fat are also skillfully blended so as to give 'reconstituted' milk.

Dry milk

Dry milk is milk from which most of the water has been removed leaving a fine creamy white powder. It is prepared from whole milk or skim milk, the latter giving a product with better keeping qualities. Non-fat dry milk (skim milk powder) can be used with or without fat to replace fluid milk in a recipe or to enrich the product. It can be either reconstituted or used in dry form. Milk prepared from skim-milk powder forms good curd. In the west, milk powder which readily mixes with water is available but the milk powder available in this country has to be treated carefully as it tends to form lumps otherwise. A thick homogeneous paste should be prepared from one cup of milk powder and cold water. Then about four cups of simmering water should be added and the milk churned well and strained through a tea-strainer or colander. If the powder has become lumpy, it should be crushed with a rolling pin and sieved before being used.

Pasteurization of milk

Pasteurization of milk is very essential because milk is an excellent culture medium for the growth of bacteria. It can be done by holding milk at 62°C for 30 minutes or flash-heating of milk at 72°C for 15 seconds. Thus pasteurization is simply a process for the destruction of pathogenic or other heat labile species of bacteria. Because of the short period of heat and immediate cooling, losses of nutrients are not significant.

In India surplus milk is used for the preparation of 'rabdi' and khova. Rabdi is made from whole milk which is boiled down to thick consistency and sweetened. Khova is whole milk concentrated in an open pan till a granular solid mass with a low moisture content is obtained. Khova is an ingredient of several Indian sweets, however, these products are sold at a high price. Sandesh is prepared from the cheese separating from whey. The separated cheese is kneaded with powdered sugar and pressed into desired shapes to make 'sandesh'. The kneaded cheese is shaped into balls and steeped in sugar syrup for a few hours to form rasagollas.

Khova is mixed with powdered sugar, kneaded well and shaped into desired shapes to form 'peda'. Nuts such as pistachio are sometimes sprinkled on top and the product coloured and flavoured with cardamoms.

Khova is mixed with a little flour, curd and baking soda, kneaded well, rolled into balls, deep-fried in ghee or hydrogenated oil at a low temperature and the fried balls put in thin sugar syrup to form gulabjamuns. Saffron and rose-water may be added to the syrup. Hundred grams of the same can be mixed with 20-30 g of maida (plain flour), 20–25 ml of curd and a pinch of baking soda. Milk and baking powder can be substituted for curd and baking soda.

The preparation of khova needed for making gulabjamuns is a time consuming process. Khova obtained from the bazaar is often of poor quality. Gulabjamuns can also be prepared from milk powder. As khova contains about 33% fat and 17% moisture a product resembling khova can be prepared by kneading together 6 parts by volume of skim milk powder, 1 parts of ghee or hydrogenated oil, (or 7-8 parts of whole milk powder and a little ghee) 2 parts of curd. 1 part of maida (plain flour) and baking soda or baking powder (1/2 teaspoon for 3 cups of milk powder). The dough is shaped into balls, deep-fried and put in sugar syrup prepared from 8 parts of sugar and 12 parts of water.

Skim milk powder can also be used in the preparation of ice-cream. One cup of skim milk powder should be thoroughly blended with one cup of previously chilled milk, sweetened, and frozen. The frozen milk should be beaten up, the desired flavouring added and the mixture frozen again.

Cheese is prepared by allowing milk to ferment so as to result in a slight souring of the same. This is achieved by adding the appropriate microorganisms. The soured milk is heated when the milk protein separates out. This is freed of surplus moisture and used as cottage cheese. It is further fermented to form different varieties of cheese by adding different microorganisms under different conditions.

Cottage cheese can be prepared at home by adding lemon juice to boiling milk or by boiling milk which has been allowed to sour at low temperatures (for instance, in the lower shelves of the refrigerator). Souring of milk at a low temperature prevents the multiplication of pathogenic organisms.

Cheese is also prepared from milk by the addition of rennin, an enzyme present in the digestive system of the calf. Some plant enzymes and microorganisms are also able to bring about a similar change. The liquid which remains after the separation of cheese is called whey. It contains valuable, minerals and vitamins. When cheese is prepared at home, whey can be used for preparing butter milk or khadi or in soups. Commercially, whey is evaporated to form whey solids which are used as cattle feed. They should prove a valuable supplement to the diet of the poor in developing countries.

Malai can be used in place of cream or milk and butter in cakes biscuits etc. It can be mixed with milk and churned with an egg-beater till it blends with the milk to make coffee cream.

Basundhi is prepared by heating milk for a prolonged period at a low heat so that some cheesy particles are formed. It is then sweetened, seasoned and served as a dessert.

Milk, curd, buttermilk, milk powder, butter and ghee have versatile uses. Milk and milk products are easy to use, highly relished and well-tolerated by groups such as infants and convalescents. It is not surprising that a prosperous land has been conceived of as one flowing with milk and honey.

Meat

The most common meats in this country are those of goat and chicken. Beef, lamb and pork are used to a minor extent. Among the tribal people many other varieties of meat are consumed but these are not commercially available. These are mostly meat of 'game' animals. Indian cuisine is famous for its chicken curry and 'tandoori' chicken.

Meat is a good source of protein and has the advantage that it has a relatively low carbohydrate content which makes it useful in the formulation of high protein, low carbohydrate diets. The fat content of meat varies considerably. In this country meat is used mostly in the form of curry, kabab or pulavs and occasionally roasted as such.

Contrary to popular opinion a large percentage of people in this country (more than 70%) are not vegetarians by either conviction or family tradition. In practice, however, most of them are obliged to live on vegetarian diets because of economic necessity. In most states, the consumption of animal foods including meat, fish and eggs is less than 5 g per day. It is somewhat greater, in areas where fish are available as for instance, West Bengal Kerala, Karnataka and Tamil Nadu. The poor consumption of meat is because of the fact that breeding of animals for meat production involves more pressure on the land. As stated earlier, about 10 g of protein have to be fed to animals to get 1 g of protein in the form of meat. Also, there are strong prejudices against pig meat which is the most easily produced kind of meat.

The cooking of meat makes it tender and easy to chew and allows the digestive juice a more rapid access to the protein. In addition to muscle cells, meat contains some fibrous connective tissue. This fibrous tissue is not as easily digested as muscle protein and makes the meat tough. That is why the meat of older animals which contains more fibrous tissue is not as tender as that of younger animals. When fresh flesh of slaughtered animal is hung for some time, certain postmortem changes acids develop due to enzyme action and they help to soften the meat tissue. Thus, animal flesh is converted to meat due to these changes.

Meat forms a very favourable medium for the growth of pathogenic microorganisms and as such involves the problem of transportation and storage, particularly in the hot and humid conditions prevailing in this country. It may also be a source of infections if the animals are not carefully inspected before and after slaughter. This perhaps accounts for the fact that some groups of people will not eat meat slaughtered by others.

As stated earlier, the carbohydrate content of meat, fish etc. is negligible which makes it useful in the formulation of low carbohydrate, high protein diets. It was, therefore, fashionable to include liberal amounts of meat in diets planned for diabetics. But with a recognition of the association between diabetes and heart diseases and of the capacity of animal protein and fat to promote cholesterol formation, fish and poultry are considered preferable to meat in such, diets.

Many other varieties of animal foods have formed part of man's diet. The Ramayana mentions the meats of peacocks, deer, buffalo, pigs, etc. and describes a method of roasting the whole animal complete with skin and hair over an open fire. Apparently the animal was held with a long fork and turned over the fire, very much in the manner of 'barbecues' which are popular in the west.

In most countries the upper classes consume more flesh foods. In this country vegetarianism is more common among the upper classes. In fact, communities which want to climb up to social ladder used to give up meat. Even among the Bhils, who love flesh foods, a person who gives up meat acquires some prestige. Most of the non-vegetarian communities abstain from meat during religious festivals. Consequently, in the case of meat, we do not find the kind of relation between income level and amount consumed found in the case of other foods. In Baroda, families with an income of more than Rs. 500 per month consume about 5–10 g of animal foods per capita per day mostly in the form of eggs, whereas those with an income of Rs. 150–500 per month consume an equal amount in the form of fish, chicken and meat. The poorest group with a monthly income of less than Rs. 150 per month hardly consume any meat.

Eggs

Eggs of hens, ducks and other species of birds have formed part of the diet of man. The traditional prejudice against eggs as a food of animal origin is disappearing. This is mainly because eggs produced by large farms are unfertilized eggs. In other words, the hens are not allowed to mate and the eggs produced are consequently not fertilized and contain no embryo. As the consumption of such eggs does not involve killing an embryo, more and more vegetarians are coming to include eggs in their diet. This is responsible for the greater consumption of eggs by upper classes a large percentage of which is traditionally vegetarian. However, the cost of eggs is well beyond the reach of most people and their production requires more land than that of milk; Eggs are now sought to be produced from a certain species of ducks which feed on grass and, therefore, involve less pressure on land.

Eggs which are a complete food for the embryo are naturally rich in essential nutrients. An average hen's egg available in the market weighs 30–40 g and contains about 4-5 g each of protein and fat. Egg proteins are of high biological, value. But egg is not as good a source of calcium as milk. Eggs can be easily boiled or otherwise cooked to form a variety of dishes: They also lend themselves to incorporation in a variety of dishes such as cakes, puddings, pan-cakes, ice-creams, etc.

Fish

Fish is a major article of diet in communities living on river basins and along the sea coast. Fish proteins have high biological value, and like meat, fish contains only a small amount of carbohydrate.

Oysters and crabs are also consumed, generally by the poor classes. The small varieties of fish are salted and dried. Dried fish is quite popular among the poor. In regions such as Bengal and Kerala where the diets are predominantly based on rice, fish are a very valuable addition to the dietary. Further, in contrast to animal food, the production of which entails a greater pressure on the land, sea foods relieve the pressure on land. The fishing techniques used in this country are primitive. It is believed that the production of fish can be enormously increased by using modern techniques. Collaboration with other countries such as Japan and Scandinavian nations is now being sought to achieve the same.

Recently a technological process has been developed by which small fish are converted to fish flour. Fish flour, prepared from whole fish is considered to be a very nutritious food. Also, it does away with the major problem of preservation during transportation. The use of fish flour has been enthusiastically advocated by some people. However, fish flour is not acceptable in chapatis etc. because of its off-odour and colour but acceptable when added to soups, curry, etc. which are highly spiced and disguise its flavour. While fish flour may be a welcome addition to foods that can alleviate malnutrition, the more so because it does not involve more pressure on land, its relative nutritive value as compared to vegetable foods appears to have been overestimated. In animal experiments carried out in the author's laboratory, the addition of either fish flour or legumes to cereals is found to bring about an equal improvement in nutritive value.

Apart from the seas and the rivers, the reservoirs and tanks used for storing water can be used for the development of fisheries.

There are over 1800 varieties of fish in the Indian waters. They include small fish which are consumed whole and big fish weighing as much as half a ton.

Some experts fear that if we resort to indiscriminate fishing with a view for immediate gain forgetting the needs of long-term survival and multiplication of species, we may annihilate them in a few decades. It would seem necessary to shift the site of fishing operations from region to region, so that each region is left undisturbed for some time and to avoid fishing during the breeding season. The development of good transport, storage and distribution facilities is essential if fishing is to be a popular and successful industry.

Other sea foods such as crabs, oysters and lobsters are also popular. Whales and sharks are also caught occasionally.

By-products such as fish manure and fish oil are obtained from the fishing industry. The oil obtained from the liver of cod fish and sharks is a rich source of vitamin A.

Chapter 15

Miscellaneous Foods and Drinks

Many other foods and drinks not mentioned earlier are also included in our diet whether or not they contribute to the nutritive value of the diet. They are discussed here regardless of their nutritive value because they form part of the diet.

Beverages

Coffee, tea and cocoa are the chief beverages.

Coffee

Coffee is believed to have derived its name from kaffa, a city in South West Ethiopia where it was perhaps first cultivated. Others trace the word to kahve, the name for it in Arabia. Coffee was first cultivated in Arabia and Ethiopia where it grew as a weed. According to one legend, a goat herd in Arabia is believed to have noticed the stimulatory effect of the weed on goats grazing on the same and coffee was subsequently developed as a beverage.

The cultivation of coffee spread from the Middle East to the East Indies and south and south East Asia in the late 17th and early 18th centuries. It was introduced in the New World by a young French naval officer who brought a coffee plant with great difficulty (During the last days of his voyage he was short of drinking water and had to share it with the coffee plant) and cultivated it in Martinigue, an island in the West Indies. From there coffee cultivation spread to the Americas. Today coffee is most extensively cultivated in Brazil and to a smaller extent in other tropical countries including the Middle East, East Indies and India. In this country coffee was introduced by the European planters about 200 years ago as a commercial crop. Its consumption became popular less than hundred years ago and it was confined to south India in the beginning and is now spreading to other regions.

The coffee cherries are picked when ripe, washed and spread out on cement floors to dry. The dried beans are run through farring and hulling machines to remove the hull, dried pulp and parchment. Alternatively, the cherries are first crushed so as to squeeze out the bean and the pulp surrounding the beans allowed to ferment in large tanks for 24hours. This makes it easy to remove the pulp and the beans are washed thoroughly and spread out to dry in the sun for 2-3 weeks. Alternatively, they are dried in perforated drums through which hot air is passed.

Preparation of coffee powder involves the roasting of the coffee seeds to a temperature of about 200–250°C by which the moisture is driven off, sugars are practically caramelized, and the fat, amino acids, alkaloids and other constituents are changed to certain aromatic compounds which give coffee its characteristic flavour. Coffee is rich in trigonelline which is partially converted to nicotinic acid during roasting. (A similar conversion takes place in fenugreek which is another food rich in trigonelline). Two varieties of coffee seeds are used, namely coffee Arabica and coffee Robusta. The latter is more expensive and has a delicate flavour. The former gives a strong extraction. A blend of the two in the ratio of 1:2 is found to be a good combination. Differences in flavour are partly due to strain differences and partly due to conditions of cultivation. The coffee plant is cultivated at altitudes varying from 1500–6000 feet, the finer varieties being cultivated at higher altitudes.

The important constituents of coffee are caffeine, sugars, cellulose, protein and small quantities of fat and essential oils.

Coffee is often roasted and ground at home and used for making the beverage. A small quantity should be roasted at a time so that the beans can puff out well. The temperature should be high initially and lowered when the seeds begin to crackle. If the temperature is high in the latter stages, some of the volatile substances which are responsible for the typical aroma of good coffee are lost. The roasted beans should have puffed out well and should be capable of easily being crushed with the hand and the insides should be uniformly brown. If the roasting is not done well, the seeds are deep brown outside and green inside. The colour of the properly roasted seed varies with the strain of seeds used. Over-roasting turns the seeds black and the resulting coffee is very bitter and lacks a good flavour. The roasted seeds and the ground powder lose their flavour if stored for more than a week. They should be stored in clean dry, airtight containers, preferably made of glass.

The ground coffee is used in different ways. It is boiled in water and the powder allowed to settle down and the clear extract decanted off or filtered. This method is used with percolators. Alternatively, the ground coffee is placed in dripper or a filter and boiling water poured over it gently. In the 'filter', a perforated lid is placed over the powder so that the water seeps through the coffee powder and drips down into the bottom container as a clear coffee extract or decoction. The decoction obtained by this method is quite strong and can be diluted to the required strength with either hot milk or hot water. It has a good flavour which is lost if it is heated again. A good cup of coffee can be prepared by adding coffee to 1/2 cup of very hot milk till the right colour is seen. More hot water, if necessary, should be added to make up the volume to one cup.

A coffee dripper can be improvised with a funnel and flask or other container into which it can fit. A filter paper should be placed into the funnel in the form of a cone and the coffee powder placed in the same. Boiling water poured over the powder will drip down into the flask below. The coffee should be ground coarse for boiling and fine for use in filter. For the preparation of 'espresso' coffee, boiling water with steam is passed through a layer of coffee under pressure so that a strong extract is obtained almost immediately.

Instant coffee, now very popular, is prepared by drying prepared coffee under certain conditions. Because of its flavour, coffee is used in cakes, ice-creams, etc.

Cold coffee can be prepared by mixing previously chilled milk with strong coffee and sugar and diluting it to the required strength by adding ice-cubes.

Coffee is consumed mainly for its stimulatory effect. The caffeine in coffee acts on the nervous system so as to result in a temporary stimulation followed by depression. The stimulatory action of coffee on the central nervous system also results in other effects such as excessive secretion of hydrochloric acid in the stomach. Coffee from which most of the caffeine is removed is also available in the west. This is believed to be done by soaking the coffee in a benzene derivative. Strains of coffee plants which yield beans with a low caffeine content have also been developed. Decaffeinated coffee is taken for its aroma rather than its stimulating effect.

Green coffee refers to coffee produced from coffee beans that have not been roasted. It is ground and brewed like normal coffee. Green coffee has very little taste. Joe Vinson et al* have reported significant correlation between green coffee and weight loss. Weight loss is attributed to the

* Vinson, Joe, Mysore V. Nagendran, V. Burnham and R. Bryan. 2012. Jan. 1, Diabetes, Metabolic Syndrome and obesity.

polyphenol chlorogenic acid present in green coffee which is thought to reduce the absorption of glucose and lower the hyperglycemic peak. However, these results need further confirmation.

Tea

Tea is a beverage prepared from dried leaves of the plant, Thea, used from very ancient times in China. It was also known as 'cha' in Canton. (According to one tradition, Bodhidharma, a Buddhist priest in China was annoyed with himself for having gone to sleep during meditation, chopped off his eye lids and threw them on the soil. Tea plants grew in the place where the eyelids were thrown, presumably to help in preventing sleep during future meditations.) In this country, people living near the north-east border areas appear to have known the use of tea from early times. However, it did not spread to other regions till it was introduced by foreign planters in the 19th century. Tea drinking became popular first in north India and is now becoming popular in south India also.

Tea leaves used for beverages are of various species of Thea, the common being *Thea sinesis, Thea bohea, Thea viridis and Thea assamica*. The tender leaves of the tea plants are plucked, spread out in bamboo trays and withered, and rolled out so as to be partially crushed and allowed to ferment for 0.5 to 4.5 hrs. The fermented leaves are dried and packed. For the preparation of green tea, the leaves are steamed, rolled and dried. The steaming helps to preserve the green colour by inactivating the enzymes.

The U.S. used to be a major consumer of tea till the famous Boston tea party after which coffee became more popular.

Tea is valued for its flavour which is a combination of taste, aroma and texture. The chief constituents of tea related to flavour are caffeine and tannins, flavonoids (polyphenols), theanine and volatile oil. Dry tea has more caffeine (3%) content than coffee. However, more coffee is used to prepare a cup of coffee than a cup of tea and hence caffeine consumption is more when a cup of coffee is taken than when a cup of tea is taken. The main polyphenol in tea is catechin. In black tea the catechins are dimerized to theaflavin and oligomerized to thearubigins. Green tea has more flavonoids than black tea as some of the flavonoids must have undergone oxidation during processing.

Teas, especially green tea has become very popular as a health drink. The health benefits of teas are attributed to the flavonoids, especially the catechins present in it. The French have lower incidence of heart disease and the reason is attributed to red wine which contain the polyphenol resveratrol that limits the negative effects of fatty diet. In a study in 1997 at the University of Kansas, epigallocatechin gallate (EGCG) a tea polyphenol is twice as powerful as resveratrol which may explain why the rate of heart disease among Japanese men is quite low and Japanese are known for their tea drinking habit. Green tea is now known for its calorie burning property as reported from Geneva, Switzerland*. Green tea has thermogenic property that promote fat oxidation.

Preparing tea by boiling the leaves in water results in a high tannin content and loss of some of its flavour. To get the typical aroma of tea, boiling water should be poured over the tea leaves and the same kept under cover. The water used should have just begun to boil and not have been boiling for a long time. The tea should be strained off after 3–5 minutes. Soft water makes a better tea.

Most people take tea with milk and sugar. It is claimed that tea with a better flavour is obtained when tea is added to milk than vice versa. Some people take it as such or with lemon juice. In summer strong tea can be mixed with lemon juice and, sugar, chilled and served with ice so that it gets diluted to the required strength. Fresh or dried rose-petals, peels of cardamom and green lemon grass can be used along with tea leaves to get a drink with a pleasing combination of flavours.

Cocoa

Cocoa is the seed of the cocoa or cocoa tree, *Theobroma cocoa*, cultivated first in south America by the Mayas and Aztecs (Incidentally, Theobroma, in greek, means the food of the gods). It was introduced in Spain in the 16th century. The cocoa seeds (or nibs) are roasted in their shells so as to develop a pleasant flavour. The shells arc then removed and the nibs ground to a fine powder.

Cocoa contains theobromine and caffeine, both of which are stimulants. The cocoa beans are rich in fat and saturated fatty acids. Unsweetened or baking chocolate is prepared by grinding the nibs to a fine paste, moulding them into slabs and drying. For the preparation of cocoa powder, used for making beverages part of the fat is removed. The fat obtained, namely, cocoa butter, and the product is treated with alkali in order to neutralize the acid and make it more soluble. The fat butter is used for the manufacture of chocolates, candies, cosmetics and pharmaceuticals. It is also used such as cream for the skin. Cocoa powder is used for flavouring in milk based foods such as ovaltine, proteinules, etc., and for the preparation of chocolates, biscuits, cakes, ice-cream etc.

To develop the full flavour of cocoa, boiling water or milk should be added to the cocoa powder. The flavour can be improved by allowing it

---

* Dulloo A.G., C. Duret, D. Rohrer, L. Girardier, M. Fathi, P. Chandre and J. Vandermander. 1999. *Am. J. Cli. Nutr.* **70(6)**:1040–5.

to simmer for a few minutes. Mocha is a drink prepared by mixing coffee and cocoa. It has an interesting flavour and is used in cakes, ice-creams, etc.

Miscellaneous foods and drinks

Aerated drinks

Aerated waters and beverages contain carbon dioxide incorporated under pressure. The bubbling waters of certain springs were believed to be beneficial for health. Priestley was the first to artificially produce aerated water to simulate spring water. This was soon followed by large scale production of aerated water or soda in Switzerland and U.K. In America a Philadelphia physician believed in the beneficial effects of aerated water and persuaded Speakman to produce it on large scale for the use of his patients. Speakman improved on the idea and produced aerated beverages using fruit juice and sugar. Later, organic acids such as citric, tartaric and malic acids, artificial sweetening agents such as saccharine and artificial fruit flavours came to replace fruit juice and sugar either partly or fully. Extracts of roots (eg: ginger) and herbs also came to be used in place of fruit and sugar. Minerals found in spring waters also came to be added for table water as well as aerated water. The minerals usually added are sodium carbonate, magnesium chloride, calcium chloride, sodium chloride and sodium sulphate. To produce a foaming beverage saponin bodies, liquorice extracts or certain gums are used.

Aerated waters may contain 1 to 4 parts by volume of carbon dioxide depending on the temperature used during incorporation. The carbon dioxide needed is readily obtained as a byproduct during fermentation or when limestone is converted to quick lime.

Fruit juices, if used, have to be freed of albuminous and pectinous matter which is why acids and flavours have largely replaced fruit juices. Only the best sugar which does not form 'scum' when made into a syrup is used.

The cost of aerated beverages is out of all proportion to the cost of the raw ingredients. Lemonades and squashes can be prepared at a much cheaper cost at home.

Lemon squash can be prepared at home from lemon juice or citric acid and lemon flavour and sugar. A 'bubbling' drink can be prepared by adding a pinch of soda at the time of serving to fresh or bottled fruit drinks.

The cost of the beverages and drinks described above (coffee, tea, coca-cola, etc.) is out of all proportion to nutritive value. Yet they are making steady inroads into the poor man's budget. Poor and middle class families may spend 15–25% of their total food budget on tea and coffee. The large scale diversion of milk for tea and coffee during the past few decades has resulted in a somewhat greater consumption of milk by adults and less by children. Some thirty years ago it used to be common practice for a poor family to buy about 200 g of milk and give it to the youngest child whereas now the same amount of milk is used for making about 4 cups of tea with the child getting about half a cup.

Spices, condiments and herbs

Spices form a 'must' in the diet of most people in this country. For several centuries, India was known as the land of spices which found their way to Europe through the Middle East. It is well known that the search for new routes to India following the interruption of the spice trade through the Middle East led to the discovery not only of North America but also South America, Australia, South Africa and the Arctic Ocean by people trying to reach India by travelling in different directions. Many spices such as pepper popularly known as natives of the East Indies were probably first cultivated in India as they are mentioned from very ancient times.

Turmeric, chillies, mustard, coriander, cumin, fenugreek and black pepper are the most common spices used. The less commonly used ones include cinnamon, ginger, nutmeg, omum (ajwain) and variyali.

Pepper is commercially one of the most important of spices. The berries are dried in the sun. White pepper is prepared by soaking black pepper in water after rubbing off the skin. Fresh green pepper is used in areas where it is cultivated for preparing pickles. Pepper is so well known for its pungency that chillies and pimento came to be called red pepper and Jamaica pepper because of their pungency although botanically, they have no resemblance to pepper. The whole seeds are fried in hot fat till they 'crackle' and added to preparations such as 'Pongal'. This makes them less pungent and imparts a characteristic flavour.

The mint family includes marjoram, sage and thyme which are also used as flavouring agents. The leaves are dried and powdered. Their aromatic flavour is due to the oil secreted by the oil glands present in the skin and stem.

Tamarind pulp is used as a source of acid, particularly in South India. The extraction of juice from tamarind pulp is easier if the pulp is steeped in boiling water for half an hour, churned well with an egg-beater and passed through a colander. A second extraction can be prepared similarly. Sweetened tamarind juice is used as a drink in Latin America. It is used in curries, chutneys and sauces in this country. Dry garcinia fruit *Garcinia indica* (kokum) is used in Maharashtra and *Garcinia cambogia* (Malabar tamarind) is used in Kerala and mango and amla powder in parts such as Gujarat. These contain ascorbic acid and some other vitamins and minerals.

Lemons and tomatoes when in season can substitute for these in many preparations. It is also handy to have a supply of edible grades of citric acid and tartaric acid which can be substituted partly or fully for these traditional sources.

Most spices are rich in minerals, particularly iron, but this may not be of any significance from the point of view of nutrition. The amount consumed varies from 10–25 g per day per capita. Spices are certainly expensive but any suggestion to the effect that the money on spices should be otherwise spent is not likely to be accepted in this country.

The popularity of spices is due to their stimulating effect on appetite. They increase the secretion of gastric juice. They also mask any unpleasant flavours in foods which is why meat is always highly spiced in this country. When used discretely they can enhance the flavour of foods but the tendency is to dress all vegetables with heavy doses of the same spice mixture so that the distinct taste of different vegetables is not perceived. Spices and condiments vary in their irritating and stimulating characteristics. Those such as turmeric, fenugreek, coriander, cumin, caraway seeds, hing, garlic and saffron contribute interesting flavours without being irritant. All spice cinnamon and nutmeg are only very slightly irritating but the strongest ones are chillies, black peppers and mustard.

Raw mustard is very irritating and contains a cyanogen which is destroyed when the seeds are crackled in fat (the seeds are put in hot fat and allowed to "crackle"). They should be taken off the heat as soon as the noise begins to subside and transferred to another vessel to retain their full flavour. Cumin and ajwain can be similarly treated. In this country, the common variety used is black mustard or *Brassica nigra*. White mustard or *Brassica alba* is used in the West. Powdered mustard is a powerful emetic. Table mustard is prepared by mixing the powdered seeds with vinegar and other spices. A good salad dressing can be prepared from roasted and powdered mustard seed, lemon juice, salt and sesame oil.

People who are prone to gastric acidity or ulcers or intestinal inflammation should avoid the more irritating spices. Spices such as coriander, cumin and fenugreek can be taken in relatively larger amounts as they are practically non-irritant. They are rich, in certain nutrients. In Ayurveda these spices are claimed to have a medicinal effect. The claim made for fenugreek as a cure for anaemia has been vindicated in studies carried out in rats in the author's laboratory. Blood haemoglobin in rats given fenugreek as the only source of iron was found to compare with that in rats given standard iron salts.

Fresh coriander leaves are used in chutneys and as a dressing and flavouring agent (like parsley) for salads, vegetables, curries, etc. They can be cultivated all round the year.

The botanical name for fenugreek, *Trigonella foenum graecum* (Greek fodder) owes its origin to the fact that it was grown as fodder in Greece. This was also the case in India. Fenugreek leaves, although bitter are a popular vegetable.

Turmeric and ginger are the tuberous rhizomes of erect perennial herbs. They resemble the cannas plant in appearance. Ginger is reputed to stimulate digestion and relieve "gas". But it can be strongly irritating. Dried ginger is prepared from the fresh rhizomes gathered young. Ginger tea or a pinch of ginger can be added to fruit punches and the like.

Turmeric is widely used as a spice both as a colouring and flavouring agent. It is popularly believed to be anti-inflammatory. Pharmaceutical doses of the same are found to have an action comparable to anti-allergic or antihistamine drugs. Turmeric is also found to reduce blood cholesterol levels. It can be added to boiling milk. An extract prepared from turmeric by boiling crushed bits of fresh or dry turmeric in water can be consumed as such and also used for saline gargles to relieve and prevent sore throats. Fresh turmeric is used along with lemon and mango ginger for preparing a salad type pickle.

Curry powder is prepared from a mixture of spices. The South Indian "Sambhar" powder contains chiefly, coriander, fenugreek, cumin, mustard, black, pepper, red chillies, turmeric and hing which are roasted and powdered. A less pungent powder can be prepared at home by grinding after roasting 5 parts each of coriander, and Bengal gram dal, one part of fenugreek and smaller quantities of cumin, mustard, pepper, etc. Roasted and powdered dals especially those of red gram and black gram are also used. The curry powder sold in the market can be 'diluted' by mixing it with coriander and cumin. A pinch of cumin powder can be used for flavouring tomato juice, soups etc.

The North Indian spice mixture includes in addition cloves, cinnamon, nutmeg, variyali, etc. The flavour of cardamoms, cloves, etc. is due to the essential oils present in them.

The high consumption of irritant spices such as pepper, cloves and chillies combined with diets low in fat and protein was thought to be responsible for the wide incidence of peptic ulcers in this country. But it has been now proved by Nobel Laureate Barry Marshall (2005), that ulcers in the gastrointestinal tract is produced by the bacterium *Helicobacter pyroli*. Consumption of spices only aggravate the symptoms of ulcers already produced by *H.pyroli* Incidentally, the yogic system recommends a diet free from irritant spices.

Dry garlic is a popular condiment whose consumption is reported to promote the intestinal synthesis of vitamins. Hing or asafoetida is a gum resin obtained by drying the 'milk' of certain plants growing in Iran and Afghanistan.

Saffron, a bright yellow flavouring and colouring material consists of the dried stigmas of the common yellow Crocus (*Crocus sativus*). Kashmir is traditionally famous for its saffron crop. It is also cultivated in Asia Minor and Spain.

Sweet pepper has the flavour of chillies without being pungent. It is dried and powdered and sold as paprika in the west. It can be used to give the rich red colour of chillies and a mildly pungent flavour to pickles, curries, etc. especially by those who find chillies too pungent and irritating. It is not readily available in the Indian market, but when it is available as a green vegetable it can be ripened, dried and stored.

Substances such as variyali, dhaniya dal, etc. are often consumed after a meal particularly in Gujarat.

Herbs such as curry leaves, coriander leaves, and parsley are also popularly used. The leaves of the basil (Ram tulsi) and the lemon tree can be used similarly to give interesting flavours. A tea prepared from these leaves can be added to soups and curries to give them an interesting flavour.

A tea prepared from fresh or dried rose petals can be used in fruit punches, 'kheer', etc. or in lieu of rose-water in sweet dishes. Rose-petals (dry or fresh) added to tea leaves enhance the flavour of tea. Gulukhand is a delicacy made from rose petals and honey and is believed to have tonic properties.

In South India the tender leaves of citrus trees are pounded to a coarse meal with salt, a little oil, chillies and hing and stored to be used as chutney powder.

The aromatic leaves of the common mint plant are ground into a paste along with salt, tamarind, tomatoes or mangoes, chillies and other materials (onions, coconut, etc.) to make chutneys. Mint leaves can be used for flavouring soups and sauces.

Most of these leaves can be dried, powdered and stored. Lemon and orange peels can be treated similarly. Fresh orange peel can also be used for preparing appetizing chutneys and sauces. They can be steamed, cut into pieces and cooked in sugar syrup to make candied product which can be used as such or in cakes, biscuits, etc. Cut pieces of orange peel can be put in vaghar and cooked till they become tender. Green chillies, fresh ginger, curry leaves, etc. may be added along with the peel. Tamarind juice, hing, a little salt and jaggery are added and the mixture allowed to boil to make a very appetizing sauce. Lemon peel can be similarly pancooked, ground to a paste with salt, chillies and hing and seasoned with a little lemon juice to make chutney.

In South India a variety of berries such as sundaikai and mana-thakkalikkai are dried and stored. They can be steamed, soaked in sour curd or butter milk and salt for 24 hrs dried and the dried berries fried in fat as needed. They are reputed to have medicinal properties.

Neem flowers can be used similarly. They lose most of their bitterness when processed in this way.

Phytonutrients in the diet

Apart from major food principles carbohydrate, proteins,fats, vitamins and minerals with established functions of energy source, tissue building, coenzymic functions and various body processes large number of food items we consume contains invaluable compounds in them. These substances are known as phytonutrients or plant derived chemical substances. Inclusion of such plant foods which contains phytonutrients in the diet is important since the potential benefits of these plant based food items in terms of health promotion and disease prevention are enormous.

Changes in life style and dietary pattern have resulted in illness like coronary artery disease, diabetes,stroke,cancers etc. in higher frequency today than ever before. Epidemiological studies have suggested that inclusion of certain food constituents in the diets of certain sections of population have lead to decreased prevalence of certain illness in such population. Consequently, new interest has arisen in the health giving properties of certain chemicals in food items like, herbs, spices,vegetables and fruits.

In the previous sections references have been made of these substances and their mode of action in terms of health promotion. The aim of this section is to consolidate all of them and add new insight into this aspect of nutrition. Attempts are also made to include a comprehensive account of the bioactive principles in the commonly consumed plant materials used as food and their mode of action at molecular level in the human body.

The phytonutrients identified in herbs, spices,fruits and vegetables have antimutagenic, free radical scavenging,antiallergic and immunity boosting functions and these properties attribute to disease prevention and health promotion. Phytonutrients are now referred to as 'nutraceuticals'. Nutraceuticals prevent diseases from occurring where as pharamaceuticals cure diseases.

The following are the class of compounds occurring in plant foods and their abundant sources:

1. Antioxidants

These are compounds that have the ability to scavenge and neutralize free radicals formed in the cells as a result of various metabolic processes, environmental factors such as pollution, sunlight, smoking and alcohol consumption. Super oxides formed in the body are molecules with free radical structure and they are highly reactive. They can react with highly sensitive macromolecular structures in the cells the most vulnerable being the DNA of the cell which undergo oxidative stress. Under oxidative stress the purine bases which constitute the DNA structure undergo certain chemical changes and this leads to lesions in the DNA at specific points. It is now known that more than 30 different base lesions occur when DNA is exposed to free radicals*. Normally, body has the capacity to repair most of these damages. However, some of the damages are stable and excessive generation of free radicals under various conditions mentioned above will bring about DNA damage. It is in this respect the role of a variety of Antioxidants present in various constituents of the food such as herbs, spices, fruits vegetables is vital in terms of protecting the DNA damage. The antioxidants can react with the free radicals as soon as they are formed so DNA is protected from attack by free radicals.

The consequence of DNA damage on the health and normal functioning of the body is a subject of study all over the world. The most important outcome of such studies is that DNA damage can alter the ability of the affected genes to transcribe resulting in either synthesis of a defective protein or an uncontrolled protein synthesis. The ultimate effect of these molecular events that take place in the cell is the development of various types of cancers, diseases of the cardiovascular system and the brain.

Having discussed the importance of antioxidants in foods in terms of health promotion and disease prevention it is pertinent to examine some of the commonly consumed plant foods and the antioxidant principles in them. Antioxidants are ubiquitous in nature. However, the plant materials included in the diet should be free from substances that are toxic to human body. It is imperative that as the human civilization has evolved these plant materials that contain toxic principles might have been eliminated from the diet. The best known antioxidants in foods and their distribution are as follows:

Beta carotene : Fruits and vegetables, carrots, spinach, oregano, papaya, mango

Lycopene : Tomatoes, grape fruit, watermelon

Resveratrol : blue grapes

Anthocyanin : Mulberries, apples, pomegranate, bringal

Ascorbic acid : Amla (Indian gooseberry), and most of the fruits

---

* Isao Kuraoka et al. 2001. *J. Biol. Chem.*, 276, (No. 52), pp. 49283–49288.

2. Phytosterols

Phytosterols are compounds similar is structure to cholesterol. Because of the structural similarity with cholesterol they interfere with the absorption of dietary cholesterol thereby reduce the serum cholesterol level.

3. Natural acids

The fruits consumed as a dietary item contains organic acids that are synthesized by the fruit during its development. Each fruit is characterized by the prevalence of certain organic acid. For example, citric acid in citrus fruit, malic acid in apples, tartaric acid and so on. Fruits have great importance as a necessary constituent of the diet not only because of presence of vitamins like vitamin C, minerals and soluble fibre but also due to organic acids and phenolic acids. There is a recent trend to promote vinegars prepared from the fruits as phytonutrient for preventing various ailments. The fruit juices are fermented to fruit wines by yeast and further to vinegar by selective bacteria. Historically vinegars have found use as an acidulant and preservative in foods. Apart from these uses vinegars of fruits are also used as health promoting items in the diet. The fermented products of fruits contain several organic acids including phenolic acids of the source material, and acetic acid and ascorbic acid at certain concentrations. Apple cider vinegar prepared by the fermentation procedure mentioned above has become popular in the West as a health food and has been recommended for management of hypertension. Vinegar consumption is associated with diminished post-prandial glucose response following a high glycemic load meal.

4. Non-digestible carbohydrates

Several plant foods contain carbohydrate that are not digested by the digestive enzymes of the gastrointestinal tract. These macromolecules are broadly classified as dietary fibre. Dietary fibre is composed of soluble and insoluble fibre. Insoluble fibre such as cellulose and hemicellulose are widely distributed in plant foods. Soluble fibres are pectin, inulin, mucilages, glucomannan and glactomannan. Pectin is widely present in most of the fruits. Inulin is a polysaccharide made up of fructose units present in agave (generally not used as a food in India). Glucomannan is present in elephant yam about which mention has already been made elsewhere. Soluble fibres are more important from the health point. These carbohydrates regulate bowel movement and promote the growth of useful bacteria in the gastrointestinal tract (G.I tract) and keep the G.I tract in healthy condition. It is now known that many of the ailments originate from G.I tract which acts as a detoxifying system for harmful substances generated in the body.

5. Enzymes

Some of the fruits grown in India contain enzymes which aid the digestion of proteins in the diet. Papain in papaya and bromelain in pineapple are proteolytic enzymes.

6. Papaya and Jack fruit

These two fruits deserve special mention in this section because of many reasons. They are the most widely available and cheap fruits in many parts of India. Papaya is easily cultivated in kitchen gardens and jack fruit is a large tree yielding a large quantity of fruits every year. They contain most of the vitamins, minerals, isoflavones, saponines, and carotenoids such as lutein, cryptoxanthine and beta carotene.

7. Bioactive compounds in spices and herbs

It is now known that role of spices extends beyond flavouring and seasoning. Some of the spices and herbs contain compounds that are bioactive and health promoting.

Piperine is the pungent principle while volatile oil is the flavour principle in black pepper. Piperine has bioenhancer activity. It increases the bioavailability of several nutrients, drugs and xenobiotics. The intestinal absorption of nutrients such as vitamin C,vitamin A, Vitamin B6,and beta carotene is increased in presence of piperine*.

Turmeric is used in foods as a flavourant and as a colourant. The flavour of turmeric is due to the volatile oil and the yellow colour is due to the pigment curcumin. Curcumin is a phenolic compound which is now used as a natural food colour in many manufactured food products.

There has been an enormous volume of literature on the biological properties and health benefits of curcumin in terms of prevention and cure of several ailments**. Recent studies at Jonssen Comprehensive Cancer Centre, University University of California has shown in pilot study using human subjects that curcumin suppresses a cell signaling pathway involved in the head and neck cancer. The human saliva contains proinflamatory cytokines that promote cancer growth the expression of which is suppressed by curcumin.

Wound healing properties of turmeric is known for ages in India. The biological properties of curcumin is due to its anti-inflammatory effect. Curcumin inhibits the enzyme cycloxygenase 2 (COX 2), the enzyme

---

* Atal, N. and K.L. Bedi. 2010. *J. Ayurveda. Integr. Medicine.*
** Jayaprakasha, G.K., L.J. Rao and K.K. Sakariah. 2005. *Trends Food Sc.Tech.* **16**:533.

involved in the formation of prostaglandin from linoleic acid. Prostaglandin is implicated in the inflammatory process in the body such as joints, wounds etc.

The molecular mechanism as to how curcumin suppresses cancer growth in animal models and human subjects has been a subject of research in several laboratory all over the world. There is a consensus among authors that down regulation by curcumin of a protein called nuclear factor kappa B (nF kappa B) which promote cancer growth is the mode of action of curcumin and that is the reason why turmeric consumption is beneficial for human health.

University of California at Los Angeles Veteran Affairs study reports that "India dietary staple as potential Alzheimer's weapon". Curcumin inhibits the accumulation of destructive beta amyloid plaque in the brain causing Alzheimer's Disease. Alzheimer's Disease in India is the lowest in the world and turmeric which is widely used in this country is attributed to this.

Garcinia indica (kokum) and *Garcinia indica* (Malabar tamarind) are fruits grown in Kerala,Coorg,Konkan coast and Maharashtra. They are used as a food acidulants and flavouring in several culinary preparations and they go well with meat and fish. Though they are fruits, they are not consumed as table items used as ingredients in many preparations and hence discussed in this section.

The acid present in both the fruits is (-)hydroxycitric acid(HCA).The chemistry and biological property of HCA has been comprehensively reviewed by Jena *et al**. HCA inhibits the enzyme ATP: citrate lyase a key enzyme in the biosynthetic pathway of conversion of carbohydrate to fat in mammalian system. In the earlier chapters it has been discussed that the excess carbohydrates after meeting the energy needs of the body is converted to fat and stored in the body as adipose tissue leading to obesity. This process is inhibited in the presence of HCA thereby preventing the development of obesity.

Carcinia cambogia extracts and formulations containing this extract is available as commercial product in the nutraceutical market.

Garlic is a must in several of Indian culinary preparations and those in many other parts of the world. Garlic contains the sulphur compound Allicin. Garlic increases the high density lipoproteins in the blood and keep the arteries and heart healthy.

---

* Jena, B.S., G.K. Jayaprakasha, R.P. Singh and K.K. Sakariah. 2002. **50(1):**10–22.

Chapter 16

Effects of Cooking on the Digestibility and Nutritive Value of Foods

Man took a major step towards civilization when he learnt how to light a fire and use it for cooking foods and for keeping himself warm. Except for nuts, fruits and salad vegetables, most of the foods we eat are cooked. Wheat is consumed in the form of bread, biscuits, cakes, chapatis, upma, sakkarpara, breakfast cereals, macaroni, pancakes, buns, dough-nuts, etc. Such, a large variety of foods differing in taste, texture and flavour is possible because of different methods of cooking. Cooking not only improves the taste of foods by bringing out new flavours, but also improves their digestibility and rids them of harmful bacteria.

The starch granules in foods are often surrounded by a tough cellulose wall. Mastication in the mouth is incapable of disrupting this wall and the digestive juice cannot completely break it. When foods are cooked the starch swells and breaks the cell wall and thus becomes more accessible to the digestive juices. Cooking destroys substances such as avidin in eggs and trypsin inhibitors certain legumes which interfere with the utilization of nutrients in foods.

'Wet' methods of cooking such as boiling, simmering, stewing and steaming involve cooking in the presence of liberal amounts of moisture. The temperature of boiling water remains steady so that in these methods, a uniform temperature is maintained and the food gets uniformly cooked. It is not surprising, that boiling is the most common method used for cooking. When foods are cooked by boiling, the food should be brought to a vigorous boil first and the heat then turned down as violent boiling throughout tends to break up the food. Further the temperature of the water cannot be increased any further after it begins to boil and continued vigorous boiling only results in excessive evaporation of water and waste of fuel and foods like rice are likely to get burnt at the bottom and form a dry crust at the top. When charcoal stoves are used for cooking it will be a good plan to use two, one burning vigorously to bring things to a boil and the other to continue to cook them on slow heat. Three to four pieces of glowing charcoal will be quite enough for the latter. Boiled foods are not considered tasty by some people but this is often because the water used for cooking is discarded. If just enough water is used for cooking discarding of excess water is not necessary. Boiled foods retain their natural taste and flavour and can be made palatable and attractive by simple seasoning. Simmering and stewing are essentially variations of the method of boiling.

Vegetables have to be cooked on high heat first and then on moderate heat if they are to retain an attractive colour. Vegetables such as brinjal will harden and fail to cook to a soft texture if they are cooked on slow heat to begin with. The addition of a little acid can prevent the discolouration of brinjals, remove the soapy quality of ladies fingers, and remove the alkalinity and bitterness of vegetables such as elephant yams and bitter gourd. Lemon juice, sour buttermilk or tamarind juice maybe added as the source of acid. Vinegar or citric acid may also be used.

Steaming or cooking with steam can be direct as when the food is placed over a perforated plate or dish as in an 'idli' steamer or indirect as when the food is placed in a closed container and then cooked with steam. The loss of nutrients with the latter procedure is practically negligible. In direct steaming, there is no leaching out of minerals but some of the vitamins may get oxidized. The loss of vitamins may be as much as in boiling.

However, both direct and indirect steaming are very convenient procedures and have several advantages. Steamed foods such as idli, khaman, and dhokla are very popular. A variety of interesting puddings, steamed breads and savoury dishes can be prepared using the indirect method which is also an excellent method for heating leftovers. Left over rice can be loosened into separate grains and steamed over a colander so as to result in excellent texture and appearance.

Cooking under pressure

The principle of cooking under pressure has long been known but it is only recently that convenient and practical cookers have come within the reach of the housewife. The food is placed in containers and the latter placed in the cooker which contains a little water. When the cooker is heated, the water boils and the pressure of the steam generated speeds up the cooking.

There are appropriate devices for the escape of steam when the pressure of steam inside exceeds the safety limit. Safety cookers need relatively less fuel and time. Where the different foods have to be seasoned differently as in Indian cooking, pressure cookers are not as convenient as they seem. But they are very handy for making marmalades and cooking whole legumes on a large scale. In most families dal is cooked as a routine. A steamer can be improvised by fitting with a colander the pan in which the dal is cooked. Vegetables can be placed in the colander and covered with a heavy lid. By the time the dal is cooked it is possible to cook 2 or 3 vegetables over the colander one after the other so that they can be cooked without extra time or fuel. The cooking time for dal is also shortened by this procedure. This simple kit if properly assembled is much easier to manipulate than a pressure cooker.

Dry methods of cooking

It is likely that the first cooking attempted by man was roasting the food over open fire. This method is still used for chapatis, papads, corn,sweet potatoes, green bananas, brinjals, etc. The food has to be turned around so that it is uniformly cooked on all sides. This requires some skill and a careful control of the heat-source.

Baking in a closed oven is essentially a modification of this process with the advantage that a more uniform temperature can be maintained and there is no need to turn the food constantly. Baking with, a little fat is sometimes referred to as roasting. Baking is relatively recent in this country. Many foods such as chakli which are deep fried can be baked with a little extra fat added to the dough. This does away with the problem of leftover fat. For instance, the dough used for chakli, sev, etc. can be baked as savoury cookies after suitable modification of the recipe. Fermented batters (they should be thick) can be baked as breads.

An oven is not generally a part of kitchen equipment in Indian homes. A 'dutch oven' is essentially an insulated metal box with a hole at the bottom so that when placed over heat source, the air inside can get heated up. The box is usually fitted with a glass door at the front and can be used over gas or kerosene or charcoal stove.

An oven may also be improvised with a large aluminium pan and lid. A small inverted pan with a flat bottom can be placed at the centre of the large pan and the material to be baked placed on this so that it does not touch the sides of the container. Alternatively, the stand sold for use in 'dhokla' steamers can be used. The pan is placed on the stove and covered with a lid over which glowing charcoal is placed. This helps to maintain a uniform temperature. The material to be baked should be inserted only after the pan gets hot enough. The temperature of the oven (pan) can be judged by the time taken for a piece of paper to brown. Baking requires more fuel than other methods of cooking. But pies, cakes, pastries, etc. can be made at a smaller cost at home once the technique is acquired. Also, unlike deep-frying, baking does not require continuous attention.

Parching is essentially a method of cooking by dry heat in a semi-open oven.

Leavening agent

When cakes and breads are baked, they rise due to the leavening action of carbon dioxide present in them. In yeast bread the same is produced during the fermentation of sugars to alcohol by yeast. In cakes either baking soda or baking powder is added which result in the evolution of carbon dioxide. The same comes out with pressure when the foods are heated causing the foods to swell. Steam has a similar action. As mentioned earlier, steam coming out at great speed is responsible for the puffing out of cereals during parching. If the cereals are very dry they will not parch which is why they are usually moistened before parching

Baking soda or potassium bicarbonate gives out carbon dioxide when heated to become sodium carbonate or potassium carbonate which gives an alkaline reaction. This may result in an unacceptable taste and also result in the destruction of vitamins. In baking powder the baking soda is combined with other substances such as citric acid and tartaric acid which can neutralize the alkalinity. Baking soda is, however, cheaper and more readily available. Its alkalinity can be neutralized by substituting butter milk or sour cream for milk or cream in the recipe. One gram of baking soda can be used in place of 2-3 g of baking powder suggested in the recipe.

Frying

As mentioned earlier, foods are also cooked by shallow and deep frying. In shallow frying, a small quantity of oil is used. This can be further reduced by just greasing the 'tava' (grid iron) and allowing the product to cook on moderate, heat (pan-frying or broiling). Dosas, pan-cakes etc. are prepared by shallow frying.

To make crisp dosas, the batter should be somewhat thin. The tava should be hot to begin with (the temperature can be tested by sprinkling a little water over the same—it should dry up almost immediately) and the batter poured or spread as a thin layer of uniform thickness. The heat should then be turned down and the dosa allowed to crisp slowly on both sides.

Cheese-toast (grilled cheese sandwiches) can be prepared like dosas. Place a layer of grated cheese between two slices of bread toast or pan-fry the same using butter or ghee so that both sides are cooked to a golden brown. The lid of an idli steamer can be used to cover the toast during cooking. It can also be used while preparing dosa if a softer texture is desired and to shorten cooking time in winter. The tava used for dosas should preferably be thick and flat and not concave like the ones used for making chapatis.

If an oven is not available, biscuits can be baked on a hot flat tava maintained on slow heat by covering them and turning them on both sides.

Deep-frying and the changes with which it is associated have been described earlier. Deep-frying of 'papadis' is actually similar to parching. They are dehydrated foods with small amount of residual moisture. When they are put in hot fat the pressure of the steam generated causes them to puff out. If the fat is not hot enough, the pressure generated is not enough to make them puff out well.

Cooking is associated with both beneficial and adverse effects on nutritive value. As mentioned earlier starchy foods are better digested after cooking. The biological value of proteins is generally increased by wet methods of cooking.

The protein value of pulses increases when subjected to heat, because of the destruction of trypsin inhibitors. Some lysine is lost with dry heat but this is not a crucial consideration in pulses which are rich in lysine. In cereals, on the other hand, dry methods of cooking result in a decreased protein value because of the loss of available lysine in which they are already deficient. Dry heating of foods like baking of foods rich in lysine and glucose leads to non-enzymatic browning reaction. This is called Maillard reaction in which the free amino group of lysine residues of protein reacts with the aldehyde group of glucose which produces a brown colour. This brown colour is desirable in some foods such as bread and biscuits the golden brown on the crust of these products is due to non-enzymatic browning which is a desirable attribute. However, in foods where lysine content is vital for nutritional quality this reaction leads to making lysine unavailable to the body.

As mentioned earlier, fats deteriorate in nutritive value when subjected to prolonged heat combined with exposure to air. The changes in fat quality may be expected to be less with baking and negligible when used in steamed breads, puddings, etc.

There is no significant loss of minerals during cooking unless the water used for cooking is discarded. This can be prevented by cooking foods in just sufficient water. Some losses occur when food grains and vegetables are washed before cooking. The former should be rinsed lightly and the latter should be washed before they are cut. Scrubbing the vegetables well before they are cut will also help remove the pesticides which are often sprayed on vegetables. If grains are pre-soaked in water some losses may occur in the surplus water discarded. The amount of water used for pre-soaking should, therefore, be carefully adjusted.

Considerable amounts of carotene and vitamin A are lost during cooking specially in shallow and deep frying. The losses may vary from 30–50%. Sun-drying also results in substantial losses.

Thiamine and riboflavin are lost during both wet and dry methods of cooking. The losses are more in the former case and more with increased exposure to air and in the presence of an alkali. They are less in an acid medium and during deep-frying since fat forms a protective layer. As mentioned earlier, although total nicotinic acid may decrease or show no change, the amount of free nicotinic acid in foods increases during cooking. The losses, if any, are not considerable.

Vitamin C is readily destroyed by heat. As mentioned earlier these can be minimized by proper methods of cooking. The losses are less with deep frying.

As stated earlier, sprouting and fermentation can bring about increases in the vitamin content of foods and these increases more than compensate for losses during subsequent treatment such as roasting. When sprouting is followed by fermentation there are further increases in vitamin content. Some additional data on changes in vitamin content during sprouting and fermentation are presented in **Table 49**.

Several factors influence the nutritional content of foods and the level of losses. The effect of processing on the nutrient content will depend on the sensitivity of nutrients to various conditions during processing such as heat, oxygen,pH and light. The nutrient retention may vary with a combination of conditions such as characteristic of the food being processed and the concentration of the nutrient. For example, the sensitivity of vitamin C to heat varies with pH. **Table 50** shows how some nutrients are affected by conditions of processing.

Repeated use of oils for frying

In frying the oil is usually heated to 170 to 220 degree centigrade. When heated to this temperature in presence of air oil undergoes chemical changes such as hydrolysis, oxidation and polymerization. The amount of degradation products increases with duration of heating. The toxicity of degradation products present health concerns. Some of these products are carcinogenic.

Thermal oxidation forms volatile and non-volatile decomposition products. The latter present the most risk to health. Diet high in lipid

Table 49. Increase in vitamin content during sprouting and fermentation*.

| | % increase in | | | | | | | | | Ascorbic acid[5] (mg per 100 g) | | |
| | thiamine | | | riboflavin | | | nicotinic acid | | | | | |
	S[2]	F[3]	S&F[4]	S	F	S&F	S	F	S&F	S	F	S&F
Wheat	44	17	50	42	60	81	44	60	80	10	7	26
Maize	10	10	15	47	50	100	47	50	100	10	6	---
Black gram	15	8	15	48	50	90	52	50	90	60	40	85
Month bean	15	9	20	65	95	115	96	110	163	90	70	135
Green gram	33	11	33	56	70	96	48	77	96	80	65	106
Bengal gram	18	15	22	52	60	100	45	52	93	60	---	86
Lentils	15	6	21	45	60	100	45	60	100	17	12	43
Soya bean	20	16	22	49	61	85	54	86	92	---	---	---

* Values obtained in the Biochemistry Department of Baroda University.
2 S, soaked in water for 6–12 hours and allowed to sprout under warm moist conditions for 24 hours.
3 F, batter prepared with coarsely ground grain, water and salt and allowed to ferment for 10–15 hours.
4 S&F, sprouted, wet ground with coarsely ground with salt to from a batter and fermented.
5 the raw grain contains negligible amounts.

Table 50. Stability of nutrients under various processing conditions.

Nutrient	Effect of processing
Fat	oxidation
Protein	Denaturation and improves digestibility
Amino acid	Lysine availability reduced
Vitamin C	Decrease during drying, oxidation takes place. Less destruction in acidic conditions.
Vitamin B1	Destroyed by high temperature especially in Neutral and alkaline conditions
Vitamin B2	Sensitive to light. Fairly heat stable
Niacin	Stable to heat and light
Vitamin B6	Heat stable
Vitamin B12	Heat stable
Carotene	Destroyed by heat. Oxidized by light
Vitamin A	Heat stable
Vitamin E	Oxidizes

oxidation and polymerization products (found in used frying oils) are associated with cellular alterations and reduced endothelial functions. Endothelial function is the normal biochemical process carried out by the cells that line the inner surface of blood vessel including arteries and veins as well as internal lining of heart and lymphatics. A diet high in products formed from repeatedly fried oil has been shown to induce glucose intolerance in rats.

It has been a practice in the market to mix the filtered used oil to fresh oil and sell at reduced rate. There is a word of caution that filtration though removes the suspended particles in the used oil will not remove the toxic degradation products present in the repeatedly used oil. Two things one has to look for in buying oils are (1) clear golden yellow colour and good smell. (2) Brown edges and dark colour are bad.

It is a healthy practice to adopt shallow frying as against deep fat frying wherever possible in order to minimize the use of repeatedly used oils. Where deep fat frying is unavoidable as in the case of certain preparation recycling of oil should be done with caution and this comes with experience.

Chapter 17

Food Microbiology and Hygiene

Our knowledge of foods would be incomplete without some understanding of the role microorganisms can play in the production and spoilage of foods.

Microorganisms are so called (micro means minute) because they are not visible to the naked eye and can only be seen with a lens which can magnify their size several times. Microscopes used ordinarily for the purpose have the power to enlarge their size 1000–1200 times.

Yeast, mould and bacteria resemble plant cells whereas protozoa resemble animal cells. Viruses are also classified as microorganisms but they lie at the border between living and nonliving matter. They multiply like living cells but can only do so in plant or animal tissue which is called host tissue. In contrast, bacteria, yeast and molds can be grown in sugar solution with some added nutrients. Although an individual mold cell is not visible to the naked eye, we can often see the moldy growth on foods.

Fortunately for man, most microorganisms are either beneficial or harmless. A few, however, cause foods to spoil and others cause diseases when they enter the human body. The different microorganisms can be distinguished by their shape, appearance and the way in which they cluster together etc. For instance, some microorganisms can use sucrose whereas others cannot. They also differ in the products they form during growth. Some strains of *Aspergillus niger* produce citric acid, whereas others do not. Some microorganisms produce a particular vitamin whereas others may remove the same from the medium as they require it for growth. Microorganisms also differ with regard to the conditions which produce maximum growth. Some may grow best at a temperature of 37°C whereas others may do so at a temperature of 30°C. Their appearance as seen under the microscope also varies. It is possible to study the various characteristics of the microorganisms found in any material and identify them on the basis of these characteristics.

A pure culture of a microorganism (i.e. a colony consisting of cells of only one particular microorganism) is obtained in order to study its characteristics. This is done by adding water to a small sample of the material containing the organism and cultivating it in a nutrient medium. The colony formed is again diluted with water and a small sample treated similarly. This process is repeated several times till examination under the microscope shows only one kind of organism in a drop of the sample. Then, the microorganisms so separated are allowed to grow to large numbers to form a pure culture.

Most microorganisms require air, moisture and an optimum temperature for survival and growth. A temperature of 30° to 40°C is usually favourable for their growth. At high temperatures, they die. At low temperatures, as in freezing, they remain inactive but become active again when exposed to favourable temperatures. In other words, we can kill microorganisms by sterilization at high temperature but we can only inactivate them by freezing. Foods preserved by freezing should, therefore, be free from initial contamination.

Microorganisms in fermented foods

Curd

Some microorganisms are capable of converting lactose in milk to lactic acid. This also brings about other chemical changes as well as changes in texture and flavour. The chief change is the separation and acidification of casein from milk. Conditions required for the formation of good curd have been described earlier (Chapter 13).

Bread

Leavened breads made from fermented dough are becoming increasingly popular in this country. In most breads, the fermentation is brought about by yeast. The cells act on the sugar present in the dough and produce alcohol and carbon dioxide. The carbon dioxide formed causes the dough to 'rise'. When the fermented dough is baked, the alcohol evaporates and the bread gets its typical porous texture. Other chemical changes also take place during fermentation.

Commercially dried yeast is available which gives live cells on mixing with water. But if it is stored too long the cells lose their activity. Professional bakers mix a portion of the fermented dough with the fresh dough just as we incubate milk with a little curd. This is possible if baking is done frequently. However, fresh yeast has to be used at least every few days. Yeast cultures can also be maintained in a medium of potato starch. Other microorganisms such as *Streptococcus lactis* are also used in making certain varieties of breads. Yeast is also used in the preparation of doughnuts and some varieties of cakes. If a little yeast is added to a batter prepared from milk or buttermilk with a mixture of flours such as rice flour, maida, corn flour, etc. and allowed to ferment, the fermented batter makes good 'dosas' (Pan cakes) with the characteristic formation of pores. Sterilized yeast, used as a food supplement, is rich in 'B' vitamins.

Ordinarily, plant foods lack vitamin B12. But small quantities of the same may be found in some foods because of the synthesis of the vitamin by the microorganisms present in them. Recently it has been reported that even rain water contains some vitamin B12 believed to be produced by the microorganisms present in the dust particles in air.

Most plant foods such as cereals and legumes contain microorganisms. Species of lactic acid bacteria are found in most of them which is why batters prepared from the same ferment without the addition of any culture.

The fermentation of idli batter is associated with an increase in batter volume and acidity because of the production of CO_2 and lactic acid. These changes enhance the taste and texture of the steamed product and are brought about primarily by the bacteria *Leuconostoc mesenteroids* which is a dominant organism in fermented idli batter. Other organisms playing a role in fermentation are *L. delbruckii* and *L. fermenti*. They bring about increases in vitamins and inorganic phosphate and the partial breakdown of proteins and starch. Similar changes occur in the fermentation of khaman batter. Many of the microorganisms present in fermented batters are found in the food grains.

Commercial uses of microorganisms

Microorganisms are also exploited for the production of valuable substances such as citric acid, proteases, lipases, amylases and vitamins. They are also used in the conversion of starch to simpler carbohydrates such as dextrin and maltose and for the production of protein hydrolysates from proteins. Before the use of microbial fermentation substances such as citric acid were very expensive and in limited supply. Their importance in the production of antibiotics such as penicillin is well known. Most of the antibiotics used to treat infections are manufactured commercially by fermentation process using specific microorganisms.

Intestinal microflora

Normal intestine contains many microorganisms which make their appearance soon after a baby is born. *Lactobacillus bifedus* (bifidobacterium) is one of them. It helps the environment in the G.I tract at a higher level of acidity. Pathogenic organisms which cause various diseases can grow only in an environment that is less acidic. Therefore, *L.bifedus* do not allow pathogens to grow under normal conditions.

Microorganisms play a valuable role in nutrition. They break down the undigested material to simpler substances and help in the formation of feces. They also play an important role in digestion and in the synthesis of several vitamins particularly of B vitamins and vitamin K. Because of intestinal synthesis, some individuals do not show deficiency symptoms even when the diet is lacking in some of the vitamins. The use of antibiotics and sulfa drugs has the effect of suppressing this synthesis. Poor people on marginally adequate diets often develop deficiency symptoms following treatment with these drugs.

Pathogenic microorganisms and parasites

Some microorganisms bring about favourable changes in foods but other microorganisms cause foods to spoil and make them unfit for human consumption. The substances secreted by them are toxic to the human body. Foods must, therefore, be protected from the action of harmful microorganisms. Techniques used for the same will be described in the next chapter.

Pathogenic microorganisms are those which cause disease when they are present in any part of the human body. Those in the intestine compete with the body for valuable nutrients, interfere with absorption, and cause intestinal inflammation. They lodge themselves in tissues such as the liver, kidney, lung, bone, mucous membrane, joints and blood and affect the body in a number of ways. They may erode the tissue where they have lodged themselves causing a lesion and inflammation. They also produce substances which are toxic to the body.

Diseases such as enteritis, typhoid, paratyphoid, dysentery, and cholera are caused by microorganisms which spread through food and water and lodge themselves in the intestine. Tuberculosis may also spread through milk or food although it spreads mainly by the respiratory route. *Salmonella enteritidis* in animal foods causes a disease similar to typhoid. *Clostridium Botulinum*, present sometimes in non-acid canned foods, can result in a deadly disease. Various types of molds present in foods result in food poisoning.

The pathogenic microorganisms are usually derived from food, water, air, or through direct physical contact. It is necessary to take precautions to prevent the spread of harmful microorganisms through these media.

Pathogenic organisms may spread from a diseased person to others if the utensils used by him are not cleaned well. Utensils used for eating and drinking should, therefore, be sterilised before they are used again. A simple practice may be to allow them to dry in the sun for a few hours. In rural areas, a mud platform can be used for the purpose. Utensils and personal effects used by a person suffering from active infection should be kept apart, sterilised after use where possible and not used by others.

Milk

Milk animals can be carriers of diseases such as tuberculosis. The udder of the cow, the hands of the milker and the milking pail used must be cleaned thoroughly before milking as milk is very good medium for the growth of microorganisms and may become a vehicle for the transmission of organisms of diphtheria, streptococcal infections, typhoid, paratyphoid, cholera, dysentery and scarlet fever. Contamination during transit is likely if the container is not covered with an air tight lid. Also, the milk must be held in refrigerated rooms till it is transported and distributed. Cold storage during transportation is desirable. Fortunately, the practice of boiling milk is universal in this country but sometimes the milk is just heated, and not quite brought to boiling point. Another undesirable practice in homes is transferring the raw milk from one container to another for boiling and putting back the boiled milk in the original container without washing it so that the residual milk present in the original container provides an inoculum for the organism present. Pasteurized milk is milk which is held at a temperature of 62°C for about 30 minutes. If a higher temperature is used, then heating is done for a shorter period. Milk can be pasteurized in a tank and then transferred to hot sterile bottles or the holding done after the milk is transferred to the bottles and sealed. The latter procedure is to be preferred as there is no danger of contamination after treatment. The pasteurized milk is cooled and kept in cold storage till distribution. When milk is obtained front retailers in the open market it often collects a lot of dust in transit. It is necessary to filter such milk before boiling.

Milk sweets kept in warm and unhygienic conditions serve as fertile media for the multiplication of pathogenic microorganisms resulting in several cases of food poisoning. Moist sweets such as 'srikhand' may be agent for spreading typhoid and dysentery. It is unwise to buy such sweets except from places of established standards.

Catering institutions

Pathogenic organisms also spread through persons concernedwith preparation of foods. If they handle food without washing their hands with disinfectant after using the toilet and if they happen to be carriers of diseases such as typhoid and dysentery, they spread the infection to others. Cooks and helpers working in catering institutions should be particularly instructed to observe certain rules of hygiene. They should clip their nails short and keep their hands and nails clean. They should be examined and treated for the presence of intestinal parasites periodically. They should use a spoon or a scoop to mix food as far as, possible. They should not scratch their body, smoke, cough or sneeze during cooking. It would be desirable to use a clean cap and apron. Foods should be subjected to minimum handling with the hand after they are cooked.

Care of utensils

Another source of contamination is through the contamination of kitchen utensils with microorganisms present in unclean soil, While 'clean' soil is a good cleansing agent, soil frequently trodden over by men and animals is likely to be major source of infection. Economic conditions being what they are we shall be hardly justified in asking poor people to use hot water and soap.

Where soil is used for cleaning, it is necessary to collect it from clean and unpopulated place. Clean soil can be kept in a flower pot, dealwood box or kerosene tin which can be used for growing a plant such as tulsi. Powdered charcoal, bricks and ash are safer cleansing materials in the absence of modem soaps and detergents.

In school lunch programmes carried out under author's direction each child washes his own vessel, dips it in a large pan in which water is kept simmering and keeps it on a mud platform so as to allow it to drain and dry with exposure to strong sunlight. At least this practice can be followed in institutions.

Care should be taken to clean drinking glasses and dinner plates thoroughly after use in institutions which have to cater to many individuals some of whom may be carriers of infection consciously or unconsciously.

In most institutions washed dishes are wiped with a dirty cloth. They should be allowed to drain and become dry without wiping. Otherwise separate clean dish towels must be used for the purpose. They must be washed daily and dried in the sun.

In many homes cooking is done on raised platforms which are not trampled upon. This is safer than cooking on the floor. But the cloth used for mopping the floor is also used for the platform. This should be avoided.

Drinking water

Drinking water in most villages is fetched from some open and unprotected water source such as river or lake. The operation of the oxygen cycle would cleanse river water ordinarily, but when this is polluted by indiscriminate practices, purification by the ways of nature is no longer adequate. The problem is aggravated by the draining of sewage water and industrial waste into the river. People should be educated in the wise use of water sources. The scriptural injunctions in this country which declare it to be a sin (crime) to perform ablutions or spit at or near water source perhaps deserve respect. Where the water source is a river, the minimum that can be done is to prohibit at least the upstream area from being used for washing clothes, cleaning utensils, etc. Where the water source is a lake, only transportation of the water should be allowed and no cleaning and washing should be done at site. This is strictly enforced in some villages in Tamil Nadu where a guard is posted day and night to prevent violations of this rule. Where the water source is a well, the sides should be cemented for a depth of at least 10–20 feet so that no dirty water from the surrounding area seeps through. The immediate vicinity must be cemented and the well provided with a boundary wall. Where the water is drawn by a pulley it is also necessary that a bucket or pot must be reserved exclusively for this purpose and that they are not used for cleaning utensils, washing clothes, etc.

Since many pathogenic microorganisms spread through drinking water, the best thing to do in the absence of a protected water supply is to boil the water used for drinking. However, boiled water is not liked by many and in poor families the cost of fuel is also a problem.

Drinking water can be filtered by having two earthenware pots fitted one over the other. The bottom of the upper one should consist of a layer of clean sand and charcoal so that water filters from this into the lower one. Such pots can be provided at low cost by the Panchayats.

Storage in copper pots is believed to have an inhibitory effect on the growth of pathogenic organisms.

In many families, the cleanliness of the drinking water is taken care of, but the people are generally casual about the water used in cooking. While this is not so harmful for foods that are boiled, only drinking water should be used for the preparation of buttermilk, chutneys and the like.

Intestinal parasites

Apart from microorganisms, intestinal parasites such as hook worm, tape worm and round worm also cause great harm by interfering with proper absorption of food. Vegetables and fruits are often contaminated with these parasites because of their presence in the soil in areas where modern sanitary facilities are not available. Animals help to spread the infection. Hook worm eggs cannot hatch and grow outside animal body. It is important to realize that hookworms and other parasites spread through fruits, vegetables, greens and other foods which have been lying on contaminated ground. The worms are present in the excreta of affected individuals and when excreted they lay eggs on the soil if the excreta are not sanitarily disposed off. Thus they spread through soil or water contaminated with feces containing the parasites.

When walking barefoot on contaminated soil, eggs of hook worm can enter the blood stream through the skin. They too attach themselves to vegetables etc. but they cannot hatch and thrive outside the body of the host (man or animal). Hook worm disease can, therefore, be entirely prevented by sanitary disposal of feces and reduced by wearing shoes.

If care is taken to ensure that food consumed is free from these eggs the spread of disease can be avoided. All vegetables and fruits should be thoroughly scrubbed and washed with clean water before cutting. In areas affected with epidemics such as cholera it is desirable to soak them in a solution of potassium permanganate or salt. This particularly applies to green chillies, ginger, coriander, salad vegetables and fruits which are consumed as such without cooking during an epidemic.

Disposal of night soil

Fields and vegetable gardens should not be considered as public lavatories. The best solution is to provide amenities for the hygienic disposal of night soil by the construction of bore latrines of the type used in army camps. These can be constructed at a relatively low cost and the Government or Municipality will benefit in the long run by subsidizing their construction. The minimum that should be done is to cover the feces with sand so that flies do not spread infection. Spread of infection through animals,flies, cockroaches, ants, rats and birds help spread infection. Their access to food should be prevented and they should be exterminated periodically.

The common housefly is a major carrier of diseases but seems a difficult pest to control even in western countries. However, care can at least be taken to prevent flies from coming into contact with sources of contamination or with food. Garbage and waste matter must be collected under cover and burnt or buried. Where they are used to form compost they must be covered with soil. Food must not be allowed to rot on the ground. Drainage water must not be allowed to stagnate. A good practice is to have trees such as coconut palms or banana trees which will absorb all the drainage water and give in return valuable food.

Personal hygiene

Often children play in the garden with bare feet and washing soiled hands and feet with clean water before meals should be enforced. Similarly, 'orthodox' Injunctions against entering the house after an outing without washing feet and hands can be invoked.

In the warmer regions of India as the southern states, even the poor man is accustomed to daily bath where water facilities permit. All the same, the importance of daily bath and change of cloth and desirability of drying cloth in the sun should be emphasized. At present soap may be beyond the reach of poor people. In this connection, leaves such as leaves are reputed to have antiseptic properties. In studies carried out in author's laboratory a boiled extract of neem leaves is found to inhibit the growth of pathogenic organisms such as *E.coli*. Since neem leaves are to be had for the picking, it would be desirable to popularize the use of neem extract and neem leaf powder as a cleansing agent.

Incidentally, in ayurvedic preparations neem leaves are used to for the treatment of intestinal disorders. Traditionally, water boiled with neem leaves has been used for bathing by women after child birth.

The simple measures suggested above should be possible for implementation in rural areas if the municipal,public health and social agencies operating at village level make concerted effort (1) to educate the villager on mode of communication of disease and the need for personal and public hygiene (2) to enforce these measures to the extent possible and 3) to provide basic amenities needed at low cost.

Microorganisms involved in food and water borne diseases

In the foregoing discussions the various sources by which food and water can be contaminated by disease causing microorganisms and parasites enter food and water. The precautions that need to be taken at household and community level in terms of hygiene and sanitation have also been dealt with. It is now pertinent to discuss in detail the food and water borne illnesses and the causative organisms involved in these illnesses. A summary of the microorganism involved in various food and water borne diseases, the sources and symptoms of diseases is given in **table 51.**

Exotoxins

In addition to disease caused by direct bacterial or viral infection some food born illness are caused by exotoxins which are excreted by the cells as the bacterium grows in food. Foods containing exotoxins can produce illness

Table 51. Food and Water Borne Diseases and Causative Organisms.

Bacteria	Where found	Transmission	Symptoms
Campylobacter Jejuni	Intestinal tract of animals, birds, raw Milk, untreated water Sewage sludge	contaminated water	Fever, muscle pain diarrhea, 2–5 days after eating
Clostridium botulinum	Widely distributed in nature. Grows only in absence of air Improperly canned Foods.	Bacteria produce toxin that causes illness.	Toxin affects nervous system Symptoms Appear 18 to 36 hours but can appear after 4 hours. Difficulty in speaking, breathing.
Clostridium perfringens	Soil, dust, sewage intestinal tract. Grows in the absence of air.	Outbreak result From food left for long period At room temperature.	Diarrhea, gas pain May appear 8 hrs after eating.
Escherichia Coli 0157:H7	Intestinal tract of some mammals, raw milk Unchlorinated water	Contaminated water, raw milk, unpasteurized cramp, nausea.	Diarrhea, abdominal Begin 2 to 5 days After eating.
Lysteria Monocytogenes	Intestinal tract of humans, milk, soil, Leaf vegetables.	Ready to eat foods, such as hot dogs, Luncheon meat, Sausage deli-style Meat and poultry	fever, head ache, stomach upset, diarrhea.
Salmonella typhimurium	Intestinal tract of humans and feces.	water contaminated With feces of affected persons.	produces Typhoid. Fever, Stomach upset nausea. Appear 8 to 72 hours.
Shigella	Human intestinal tract. result from salads handled by workers with poor hygiene.	fecal contaminated water. Most outbreaks blood, mucus, fever. with poor personal After ingestion.	Disease referred to as shigellosis Diarrhea containg occurs 12 hours
Staphylococus aureus	human skin, infected cuts, pimples, nose	Person-to-person through food handling. multiply rapidly at room Temperature to produce toxin thatcause illness.	severe nausea, abdominal cramps, vomiting. Occur 1 to 6 hours of ingestion.
Vibrio cholerae	intestinal tract of humans	Drinking water and food contaminated with feces of affected persons.	produces cholera
Hepatitis A virus	Human liver	Food and water produces contaminated with feces of affected persons.	jaundice

even after the microbes that produced these toxins have been killed. Keeping non-acid cooked food such as meat, fish and poultry at room temperature in dusty atmosphere at public places poses risk to the microbial safety of such foods.

Dust particles are carriers of microorganism and if toxin producing bacteria like *Staphylococus aureus* gets entry into foods mentioned above can multiply fast at room temperature producing toxins that are dangerous to health

E. coli is normally present in the gastrointestinal tract of human being. Only certain strains like 0157:H7 is pathogenic the rest are not pathogenic. Presence of *E.coli* in food and water is an indication of fecal contamination and if *E.coli* is detected in food and water detailed examination of the same for other pathogenic organisms needs to be done to ensure microbial safety of water and foods.

Chapter 18

Food Preservation

Some foods such as fruits are available in some seasons and not in others. Other foods are more abundantly available in some seasons than in others. For instance, with buffaloes, milk supply is more plentiful in winter than in summer. Many crops are harvested only once a year. Civilized man tends follow a similar dietary pattern throughout the year and faces the problem of making foods produced in a particular season available throughout the year.

Causative factors of food deterioration:

1. Rodents and pests

Food grains such as wheat, rice,legumes are susceptible to rodent and pest attack. Not only there is a loss of food grains due to rodent and pest attack but also spoilage due to contamination by excreta in the infested grain. The nutritive value of the infested grain has been found to be inferior to the uninfested grain in terms of protein quality as the endosperm of the grain is eaten away by the rodents and pest. It has been a great concern of the government of India to reduce the wastage of food grains due to rodents and pests and concerted efforts are being made to reduce the wastage due to this factor. Pest proofing of gunny bags,design and construction of godowns that are safe from rodents and insects and fumigation of stored grain with appropriate fumigants are the strategies adopted to ward of deterioration of food grains due to rodents and pests.

2. Microbial

Molds, yeast and bacteria of various strains attack the raw food grains, fruits, vegetables and animal foods and cause deterioraton of foods and make them unfit for human consumption. Post-harvest operations of food grains is the determining factor of growth of microorganisms on the fresh agricultural produce. Drying the harvested food grains need to be dried at safe moisture level in order to prevent the growth of molds during storage.

The safe moisture level varies in different food grains between 10–12%. Storing the harvested food grains after drying to safe moisture level is also important to prevent deterioration due to germination of the grains.

During the season there is a glut of fruits and vegetables and due to the temperate climate prevailing in India they are attacked by microorganisms and also deteriorate by biological process by the action of various enzymes in the tissues of fruits and vegetables. Deterioration of fruits and vegetables by microbial and enzymatic activity can be prevented or minimized by storing them in cold storage. It is known that vegetables that are freshly harvested from the field have what is known as field heat. The temperature of the freshly harvested vegetable is favourable for the activity of enzymes involved in the loss of freshness of farm produce. Pre-cooling of fruits and vegetables at farm level removes the field heat and this helps in deterioration of quality while transporatation to the market place or cold storages located in distant places. Where refrigerator or cold room facilities are not available at farm level the procedure of Evaporative Cooling can be applied for pre-cooling at farm level. The details of this procedure can be obtained at CFTRI, Mysore.

Principles of food preservation

Food preservation revolves around 4 major parameters namely moisture, temperature, pH and oxygen. Food can be preserved by controlling these parameters.

Water activity

Water is necessary for the activity of enzymes and for microbial growth. Certain minimum level of water is necessary in the food for microorganism to grow on the food. The term 'water activity' refers to the available water content of the food for microbial growth. Water activity (aw) refers to the ratio of vapour pressure of water in food to the vapour pressure of pure water. Water activity depends on the nature of the food material and varies in different foods. Water activity of selected examples is given below:-

Substance	aw
Distilled water	1.00
Tap water	0.99
Milk	0.97
Saturated NaCl	0.75
Fruit juice	0.97
Honey	0.60
Dried fruit	0.60

Microorganisms do not grow at water activity less than 0.90

The two main methods used in reducing water activity of foods are:

1. Dehydration

Dehydration is the process of removing water from the food to the desired moisture level so that the water activity is kept at the cut off level for microbial growth.

a) Sun drying is the traditional method of dehydration wherein solar heat is used for removing water from the food material.

b) Mechanical drying by using various types of driers such as tray driers, tunnel driers, fluidized bed dryers, vacuum shelf dryers, roller drying, spray drying and freeze drying. The selection of the dehydration method depends on a number of factors. Spray drying, drum drying and roller drying are applicable to liquid foods such as milk and fruit juice. Accelerated freeze drying is another type of drying wherein the material is dried in frozen condition under vacuum. This is capital intensive and hence applicable to high valued products.

c) Osmotic dehydration: The water in the food material has the osmotic pressure of a plant or animal cell. If the material is immersed in a solution of higher osmotic pressure the water from the material will flow out to the surrounding solution due to the difference in osmotic pressure. The water in the material is thus removed till a stage wherein the osmotic pressure in both the compartments are the same. At this stage more solute is added to the solution to increase the osmotic pressure of the solution. This will enable more water from the material to diffuse out to the solution. This process is repeated till the food material has lost water content to the desired level. Solutes most often used in osmotic dehydration are sodium chloride and sugar.

2) Pickling

Pickling also known as brining is the process of preserving food by anaerobic fermentation in brine (a solution of salt in water) to produce lactic acid, or marinating and storing in acid solution usually vinegar (acetic acid at 0.1% level). The resulting solution is called pickle. Edible oil is used as pickle medium with vinegar. If the food contains sufficient moisture pickling brine may be produced by simply adding dry salt. For example, sauerkraut and Korean kimchi are produced by salting the vegetable to draw out water and natural fermentation by lactic bacteria to produce required acidity. The principle of pickling is that at pH 4.5 and below bacteria do not grow and salt is an extra hurdle for bacteria to grow.

3) Food preservation by thermal processing

Addition of heat to foods kills the microorganisms present in the same. The destruction of microorganism depends on factors such as thermal death time of the organism, the type of food, the pH of the food and the composition of the medium in which the food is immersed. The following are the practical application of preservation by thermal processing:

a) Sterilization

In this method the food is heated at a particular temperature for a specified period of time which kills the bacterial cells and their spores so that the food has achieved what is known as commercial sterility. The heating is done in the container in which the sterile product is packed. Usually cans made up of stainless steel coated with tin and glass containers are used for packing the food. Process of food preservation by thermal processing using metal cans for packing is called canning. In this method the cans are filled with the food material in appropriate size and topped with liquid such as brine or syrup. The filled cans are exposed to steam or hot water. This causes air in the head space to be driven out. The cans are then sealed with lid in an automatic machine air tight or hermetic. The sealed cans are then transferred to a retort and sterilized at 120 degree centigrade for a specified period. During sterilization heat from the cans is transferred to the brine or syrup and then to the food material by convection. The sterilized cans are then cooled gradually.

The vital point in successful canning operation is the time temperature relationship. The time taken for convection of heat to the coldest point in the food piece that is being canned is to be determined. This data has to be obtained to fix the processing time for successful canning of various food products. Under-processing leads to the survival of spores of the toxin producing *Clostridium botulinum* and the spores will germinate and grow during storage of the cans. Consumption of products from such cans leads to botulism which can be fatal if not attended to immediately. This is especially important in canning of low acid foods such as meat and fish. However, this problem is not as severe in acid foods such as most of the fruits because low pH is not conducive for sporulation and growth of bacteria. Over-processing of foods can lead to loss of texture, flavour and nutrition quality of foods. The method for calculation of processing time for canning of various foods at commercial scale is described by Ranganna*.

Canning of food can be done at home scale or at cottage level without a commercial caning line. Metal cans of various sizes are available from

---

* Ranganna, S. 1977. In Manual of Analysis of Fruit and Vegetable Products, Tata McGraw-Hill Publishing Company Limited, New Delhi.

the can manufacturers. Cans are available in the flattened form with open ends. The process of making the cans cylindrical is called reforming. The ends can be sealed with the lid and this process is called seaming. Both reforming and seaming can be done with hand operated reformers and seamers. Community canning centres located in various districts of India impart training in canning of fruit and vegetables at cottage level.

Where facilities such as can reformer and can seamer are not available canning can be done at homes using glass jars which can withstand pressure and which are sealable. A protocol for home scale canning using glass bottles is given in Appendix 1.

b) Pasteurization

It is the process by which vegetative cells (viable cells) of bacteria are killed by heat treatment. Heat treatment is not severe enough to kill the spores which will survive in pasteurization. This process is applicable to liquid foods such as milk and fruit juices. Pasteurization is done by two methods, namely heating the food at 63 degree centigrade for not less than 30 minutes and heating at 72 degree centigrade for not less than 16 seconds. Pasteurized food has to be stored under refrigerated conditions as storing at room temperature will enable the spores to germinate and spoil the food. Storage life of pasteurized milk is 10–20 days depending on the temperature of the refrigerator.

c) Aseptic packaging of foods

In this process both the food and packaging container are separately sterilized. The sterilized food is filled into the sterilized packaging container in aseptic condition and sealed. This process is most convenient for liquid foods such as fruit juices, fruit pulps etc. The fruit juices in tetrapack available in the market are aseptically processed and packed. Aseptically processed and packed foods are superior to conventionally canned products in terms of flavour and nutrient content.

3. Freezing preservation of foods

Where as in thermal processing heat is added to the food in freezing heat is removed from the food. Preserving food by freezing is one of the easiest and least time consuming. The disadvantage is the initial investment which is high. In this method the food retain its natural colour, flavour and texture. In this process the bacteria are not destroyed but the growth is only temporarily stopped as long as the food remains in frozen condition. Growth can take place when the food is taken out of the freezer and kept at room temperature for certain length of time. The frozen food undergo thawing at room temperature and the bacterial growth takes place.

The enzymes of the raw food continue to be active even after harvest and bring about changes in texture, flavour and colour in foods. Plant foods like vegetables undergo browning due to the enzyme polyphenol oxidase. Freezing slows down the activity of these enzymes but does not destroy these enzymes. Therefore, it is a normal practice to blanch the vegetables before freezing either by steam or by boiling water till the enzymes are inactivated. Blanching also kills the bacteria present on the surface of the material. Steam blanching is superior to water blanching as leaching of nutrients to the surrounding water is not involved in the former.

Rancidity development is a concern in preservation of food that contain fats such as meat, fish and poultry. Oxidation of fat leads to development of rancidity and off flavour. Such foods should be wrapped air tight before freezing to avoid air contact.

While freezing water contained in the food become ice. When water becomes ice it expands and the ice crystals formed cause cell walls of the food to rupture. As a result the product will be much softer when it thaws. These textural changes are most noticeable in fruits and vegetables that have higher water content. Such foods are not suitable for freezing. Textural changes due to freezing are not apparent in products that are cooked before eating because cooking also soften cell walls. Textural changes are not noticeable in high starch vegetables such as peas, corn and beans.

Rate of freezing is an important factor that determines the texture of frozen foods. Quick freezing brings about less textural changes than slow freezing. Moisture loss or ice crystal evaporation from surface area of the product produces freezer burn. Freezer burn appear as fuzzy, grayish white spot on the surface. Freezer burn is not harmful but causes off-flavours. Wrapping the food in moisture proof container prevents freeze burns in frozen foods. Covering fruit with syrup and cooked meat in gravy or sauce can help to prevent freeze burn.

Two types are freezers are generally used in commercial practice namely plate freezer and blast freezer. Plate freezing is done for products such as pastries, fish fillets, beef patties as well as irregular shaped vegetables that are packed in brick-shaped container. The food is firmly pressed between metal plates that are cooled to sub-freezing temperature by internally circulating refrigerant. The temperature of freezing preservation of food is normally less than -17degree centigrade. Blast freezing is a method of cooling food quickly to a low temperature that is safe from bacterial growth. Bacteria multiply fast between 8 and 68 degree centigrade. By reducing temperature of cooked food from 70 degree centigrade to 3 degree centigrade or below the food is rendered safe for later consumption. This method of preserving food is commonly used in food catering and in preparation of 'instant food' as it ensures safety and quality of foods product.

Blast freezers operate with blowers which force chilled air over the food in the freezer to cool it rapidly. Blast freezers tend to consume lot of energy and most commonly seen in industrial and commercial applications.

A third method of freezing preservation of food is individual quick freezing (IQF) which is fairly recent origin. By this method virtually all the properties of most foodstuff can be preserved. The important feature of this method is ultra-rapid freezing to a very low temperature (-30 to -40 degree centigrade). Fruits and vegetables frozen by IQF can be stored in the fresh condition for more than one year.

In IQF each piece of food is frozen individually using the technique of fluidization resulting in freezing of fruits, vegetables,fish etc. only in 10 to 12 minutes which otherwise would take 3 to 4 hours in blast freezer. This result in better texture, no lump or block formation and the product with free flowing properties. One does not have to thaw out the entire packet but only the required portion and the remaining can be kept undisturbed.

4. Cold sterilization using hydrogen peroxide, ethylene oxide and ionizing radiation

These methods are not applicable in all food commodities and processed foods as per Indian laws. Ethylene oxide is used to reduce the bacterial count in spices like black pepper exported from India to countries where the use ethylene oxide is permitted. Ionizing radiation is used mainly for prevention of sprout formation in potatoes.

5. Chemical preservation of foods

There are several chemical agents which do not allow microorganism to grow if added to foods. These agents have been tested for their safety to human health by national and international agencies have laid down specifications for their use in foods. The specifications include the foods in which a particular chemical can be added as a preservative and their maximum permissible levels in foods. The following chemical preservatives are being used in India for preserving various food items:

Sorbic acid	: soft drinks, chapatis and cheese
Benzoic acid	: soft drinks
Sulphur dioxide	: fruit juices, dehydrated fruit and vegetables.
Potassium nitrate	: curing of meat
Butylated hydroxy toluene (BHT) and Butylated hydroxyl anisole (BHA)	: as antioxidant to prevent rancidity

The specifications with regard to use of these chemicals in foods have been laid down by regulatory agencies and reference to these aspect is made in the next chapter.

Often vegetables and fruits are preserved by completely submerging them in brine (salt water) or by adding salt. Amla, citrus fruits, mangoes and vegetables are preserved by this method. The presence of salt at a high concentration prevents the water from being available for bacterial growth. This is because when the concentration of salt in the water is higher than that in the bacterial cells, water cannot be absorbed by the cellular membrane. Rather, the flow will be in the opposite direction and the cells will be depleted of their water content and shrink. This would account for shrinking of tender mangoes when preserved in brine.

The same principle is employed in using concentrated sugar syrups for preserving.

Use of acid

When the medium in which the food is preserved is strongly acidic, most organisms cannot survive. The use of vinegar for the preservation of pickled vegetables, tomato sauce, ketchup etc; ensures such an acid medium.

Use of oil and spices

Spices such as chillies, fenugreek and pepper are used in the preparation of pickles. They not only improve the flavour of foods but are also believed to create an environment unfavourable for the growth of bacteria.

Similarly when oil is used in pickles a top layer of oil is formed which prevents the microorganisms in the air from coming into contact with the food. Coating fruits such as lemons with a thin layer of oil can keep them fresh for a longer time. In Gujarat it is common practice to coat dals of green gram and red gram with castor oil, a procedure also used sometimes for other grains such as wheat and rice.

The application of the techniques described above to selected foods is described in Appendix I.

The life of perishable foods can often be prolonged and their wastage avoided by easy household procedures applying the above principles. Some suggestions are made below:

Moist foods

The life of perishable left-over foods such as sambhar, rice, vegetables etc. can be prolonged to some extent by simple procedures which are described below. The use of such techniques will cut down the frequent waste of foods specially when there are large quantities of left overs after a party or a feast.

Liquids such as dal, sambhar, rasam and khadi

Heat the liquid in an open container. Bring to a boil and continue to boil for a few minutes. Clean the lid, sterilize separately by heating over an open flame and clamp down over the pan and let simmer for 5–10 minutes, so that the container becomes almost free from air inside. Remove from the stove and keep in a cool place. Do not open the container till before use. Metal 'Dabbas' with lids are most suitable for this purpose. The life of liquid foods can be prolonged by this method by as much as 24 hours. Milk can also be preserved by this method for a longer period.

Vegetables and cooked pulses

When these are left over, they can be preserved for the next day by adding tamarind juice, salt and chilli powder. The mixture should be brought to a boil and simmered under cover for about 10 minutes and stored as described above.

Rice

Loosen the rice grains and pour boiled water over the same so that the rice grains are completely submerged and are at least 2′ below surface level. Rice can be stored by this method for 24–48 hours. The steeping water can be drained off and the rice eaten with curd and pickles. The steeping water tastes like fermented barley and makes a good and nourishing drink either by itself or with the addition of salt, buttermilk, curry leaves, mint leaves, etc. This is a common method of storing rice in Tamil Nadu where such treatment is believed to improve the nutritive value of rice. Fermented rice with curd used to be a common breakfast for children and labourers in Madras. Alternatively, loosen the grains, put them in a colander, steam in a closed container and keep closed till use. The shelf-life of rice can be extended by an additional 12 hours by this procedure.

Chapatis

If chapatis are left, they can be toasted on slow heat till they become crisp and stored in a tight container. They can be served with butter or ghee or crushed and served with milk and sugar as a breakfast cereal.

Curd and buttermilk

Add lime water to the curd or buttermilk to prevent rapid souring and keep covered with a moist cloth in a cool place.

Fresh fruits and vegetables

Bananas and other delicate fruits can be kept on wire or cane baskets. Sometimes they are hung from the ceiling in a cool, well-ventilated place. It is better if the fruits are kept separated and do not touch each other. Lemons can be coated with oil.

Waxing of fruits also prevents exposure to air. The fruits are coated with a thin layer of molten paraffin wax or dipped into the same quickly and taken out.

Green leafy vegetables should be wrapped in moist muslin cloth and kept in a cool place. Cabbage, cauliflower and other similar vegetables can be wrapped in two or three folds of old newspaper and stored.

A home-made 'refrigerator'

In summer when milk spoils quickly, curd sours and vegetables dry, a 'refrigerator' can be improvised using one or other of the following procedures:

Use wide-mouthed earthenware pots. Keep them in moist sand or a basin of water. Cover with a moist cloth whose ends dip into the basin or moisten it from time to time. Use one pot for vegetables, fruits, etc. and another for milk, curd, etc. The foods stored in this way will keep fresh for a longer period.

Alternatively, use a cupboard with wire-doors and sides for storage. Cover the safe on three sides with moist jute cloth whose ends dip in pans containing water. Sprinkle water periodically if the cloth dries up.

Chapter 19

Food Safety and Standards

The palatability and nutritive value of the foods we eat is also affected by their quality. Foods of excellent nutritive value to begin with may become unfit for human consumption during storage or handling. Insect-infested grains, rancid fats and contaminated milk and sweets are examples. "How safe are the foods we eat and the water we drink" is a major concern of government authorities all over the world and international organizations under the United Nations Organization. In India The prevention of Food Adulteration Act (PFA) was passed in 1956 and the standard and specifications for various commodities of foods as applicable to this country and the processed foods under various categories were formulated and enforced. The Codex Alimentarius Commission established by the FAO and WHO of the United Nations Organization in 1963 set out standards and specifications which covers all foods whether processed, semi processed or raw with more emphasis on foods that are marketed directly to the consumers.

Food industry is a major industry with a very large turnover in most of the countries. In this country, except among the very rich, the money spent on food accounts for a large share of the budget. In a sample survey in Baroda 80% of income was found to be spent on food in the low income group, 55% in the middle income group, and 40% in the high income group. Food supplies are dwindling in relation to population in the case of pulses, oils, milk, meat and eggs. At the same time the demand for foods other than food grains is increasing with industrialization. In the case of spices, tea and coffee, because of export possibilities, the home market is sometimes strained. Thus in the case of both foods which are in short supply and foods which are abundantly produced, there is a real or artificial gap between supply and demand. When this happens, there is a great temptation for shop keepers for either adulterating the food sold or selling food of inferior quality. Any food article is considered to be adulterated if its nature and quality are not up to the standards which it professes or which do not conform to the specifications laid down under the FSSAI guidelines.

The quality of foods is affected in various ways as indicated below:-

Addition of extraneous matter

For example, food grains often contain a lot of extraneous matter and grains of sand as make-weights. Addition of water to milk to increase the volume is another instance.

Mixing inferior quality materials with superior ones

Mixing infested grains with those of better quality or used tea leaves with fresh tea would come in this category.

The use of prohibited dyes and preservatives

This type of adulteration is found very commonly in the case of cheaper varieties of sweets and in the colouring of spices such as chilli powder and turmeric powder.

Extraction of valuable ingredients

This is usually practiced by milkmen who remove fat from pure milk.

Such adulteration may be carried out primarily by traders or middlemen and occasionally even by some producers.

Apart from deliberate adulteration, the quality of foods may also deteriorate due to improper storage conditions which makes the foods unsuitable for human consumption. For example, fats become rancid on long storage in tropical climate and food grains are subjected to infestation with insects and rodents. However, adulterated foods continue to be sold on a large scale. Housewives and others concerned with the purchase of foods must be aware of the qualities expected in different foods and the ways by which the same can be ascertained.

Cereals and pulses being seasonal crops are usually stored for 6–12 months. During this period degenerative changes may take place affecting their nutritional value because of their liability to be subjected to insect infestation. The changes occurring in them during this process can be summarized as follows:

1. **Loss in weight** with a decrease in the ratio of weight to volume. This happens with insect infestation.
2. As uric acid is the main end product of protein metabolism in insects, contamination with uric acid increases proportionately with the storage period and **insect infestation**.
3. Decrease in organoleptic acceptability.
4. Increase in **hydrolytic rancidity** due to the deterioration of the fat in the grain.
5. Deterioration in the quality of gluten in wheat and its products.

In most cases, the inferior quality of grains is apparent by visual inspection and testing.

Food grains usually sink when steeped in water. If they float it indicates a decrease in the density of the grain, mostly by insect spoilage.

The permitted limit for uric acid is 20 mg% in grains. Market samples that contain more than this is an indication of insect infestation the severity of which is reflected in the uric acid content.

A simple test can be carried out to ascertain the quality of whole grains. A known number of grains (say 100) should be steeped in water for a few hours and allowed to sprout. If the grains are subject to insect-spoilage they will not sprout. In studies carried out in the author's laboratory, the number of sprouts obtained was found to be related to uric acid content. It must be pointed out, however, that while the appearance of good sprouts indicates good quality, its absence does not necessarily indicate insect-infestation as the same may also be due to the immaturity of the seeds. If the grain is of good quality more than 90–95% of the grains are found to sprout well.

The addition of extraneous matter to grains is also widely practiced, especially in times of scarcity. It can be separated from a known weight of grain and weighed.

Pesticide contamination of grains is another factor that affect the quality of food grains. Indiscriminate and unscientific use of pesticides during different stages of grain production, storage and distribution can sometimes lead to the pesticide residues in the grains which are toxic to man. It may perhaps be wise for the housewife who can afford it, to select samples of grain carefully for quality after the harvest season and then buy the grain in bulk. As storage facilities for grains in commercial establishments are strained this may also relieve the pressure in the market on such facilities.

Wheat flour, suji and maida are expected to have a gluten content of at least 7%. As wheat contains 10–12% gluten the permitted limit gives scope for adulteration. Even so, some samples of atta and maida were not found to come up to the standard. Rava is also sometimes contaminated with iron filings which can be detected by combing the same with a small magnet.

Fats and oils

Adulteration of oils and fats is easy as they mix with one another and such mixing cannot be easily identified. Mixing of costly oil with cheaper oil is considered as adulteration.

As mentioned earlier, fats and oils differ from one another in physical and chemical properties and can be distinguished on the basis of the same. Til oil (sesame oil) and coconut oil are often mixed with groundnut or cotton seed oil as the latter are cheaper. Ghee can be adulterated with hydrogenated fat. Adulteration of ghee with hydrogenated fat can be detected by analyzing ghee samples for til (sesame) oil as the law makes it obligatory to add the same to hydrogenated fat in specified proportions. A test known as Baudouin Test detects phenols present in til oil and if this test is positive it can be concluded that ghee is adulterated with hydrogenated fat. During times of the shortage in oils, more harmful practices such as the mixing of vegetable oil with mineral oil and transformer oil have also been reported. Such adulteration is highly injurious to the consumer and can result in death or disability.

Melting point, refractive index and saponification number are used for identifying fat.

The deterioration in fat quality can be measured by measuring free fatty acids(FFA),peroxide value and 2-thiobarbituric acid value (TBA value)of samples. FFA value indicate hydrolytic rancidity where as the latter two tests indicate oxidative rancidity.

Mustard seeds are often mixed with argemone seeds either accidentally or deliberately. Oil prepared in this manner, therefore, contains argemone oil.

Argemone oil contains an alkaloid sanguinarine which is highly toxic and results in dropsy and paralysis which have been found in epidemic proportions in areas where mustard oil is used. It may be advisable to get vegetable oils directly from oil mills.

Milk

Milk is perhaps subjected to more adulteration than any other commodity. The readiness with which water can he added and fat removed and the fact that the demand is greater than supply encourage adulteration.

The composition of milk varies with the breed the season, the time of day, the individuality of the cow, age and feed of the cow, estral period, the part of udder from which milking is done and the period of lactation. Still some reasonable minimum standards can be expected and have been set.

The adulteration of milk consists of either addition of extra water or the removal of fat or both. Sometimes extraneous substances such as ground nut milk are added. The selling of diluted buffalo milk as cow milk after colouring it is a common practice (cow milk has a slight yellowish tinge not found in buffalo milk). To detect adulteration, milk is usually tested for its specific gravity. Milk is a fat-water emulsion and consequently the specific gravity will depend upon the fat content and non-fat solids present in it. The specific gravity of fat is below unity and that of non-fat solids above one which finally brings the specific gravity of milk to 1.029–1.035. As the fat content of milk increases the Specific gravity decreases and conversely, as the non-fat solids increase, the specific gravity increases. Thus added water may not be detected by specific gravity, if water is added and the fat is also removed. Thus specific gravity may not be a reliable criterion. To detect added water another method is to determine the freezing point. As the amount of extraneous water increases, the freezing point decreases. But this requires a special instrument. Analysis of milk for fat, non-fat solids, protein and lactose is more practicable.

The constituents of milk bear a constant relationship with each other and this has led to the formulation of standards such as the percentage of dry solids, protein-fat ratio and lactose-protein ratio which help in detecting abnormalities in the milk sample resulting respectively from addition of water, removal of fat or addition of extraneous matter such as groundnut milk.

A lactometer which measures specific gravity is simple to use by the housewife. Milk adulterated with water when set as curd can also be used as a criterion. Milk adulterated with other substances becomes yellowish and frothy and does not form good curd although it forms sour taste.

A simple method for ascertaining the quality of milk is to heat a known amount of milk with lemon juice, separate the cheese that curdles and remove surface moisture with a blotting paper or cloth. The yield of cheese should be about 1 table spoon or 15-16 g for half a cup of milk (4 ounces) or 14-15 g per 100 g. If the milk is adulterated with groundnut milk, the solid matter that separates out will be smooth, creamy and yellowish and will not have the typical structure of cottage cheese. In a few market samples analyzed the yield of cheese was found to correlate well with values for total solids, fat, protein and lactose obtained by analysis.

Milk should not be sold before the calf is 3 days old. The early or colostrum milk is unacceptable to the human palate. It develops a burnt odour during heating. Sometimes dairy milk is found to be adulterated with colostrum milk.

With practice, the housewife can detect adulteration by taste. The sample tested should not be hot. However, people differ markedly in their ability to detect adulteration by taste. In studies carried out in the author's laboratory most of the people were unable to detect addition of water up to a level of 30% whereas a few were able to detect adulteration at a level of 5–10% or less. We can take a sample of whole milk and dilute it with varying amounts of water and see what each sample tastes like. Similarly we can mix different proportions of skim milk and whole milk to acquire a judgment of fat content by taste.

The yield of butter from a known quantity of milk can also give us an idea of the extent to which fat has been removed.

The following standards have been prescribed by law for milk and milk products

Milk product	Standards specified
Skimmed milk	At least 8.5% non-fat milk solids
Toned milk	8.5% non-fat milk solids and 3% fat
Butter	Milk-fat not less than 80% Condensed skimmed
milk	At least 20% milk solids
Chhanna	At least 15% milk fat
Cream	Not less than 23% milk-fat
Ice-cream solids	Not less than 36% by weight of milk
Khova (mava)	Not more than 10% moisture and not less than 20% fat

Incidentally, many khova samples purchased in the Baroda market were not found to meet these specifications. They are often adulterated with maida which can be detected by testing for the presence of starch.

Salt, sugar and jaggery should be free of insoluble matter. The same can be measured by dissolving the substance in water and filtering the solution. The residue can be dried and weighed. By law, such insoluble matter should be less than 1% in the case of salt, 2% in the case of jaggery and nil in the case of sugar. But some of the samples analyzed were found to contain 4–10% insoluble matter.

Sometime salt and sugar absorb moisture and become heavy. This means that we get less value for money. According to law, the moisture content of salt and sugar should not exceed 6.0 and 1.5% respectively. The same can be determined by weighing the sample before and after drying.

Spices

Turmeric and chillies are coloured with lead pigments in order to give them a brighter colour and the appearance of a produce of good quality.

Small quantities of lead are deposited in the skeleton but a progressive accumulation of the same over the years may result in their release into the blood stream and consequently serious liver damage etc.

Metanil yellow which is a carcinogenic agent is also used for colouring turmeric powder. It is sold as kesar colour and used for the colouring of sweets and beverages very widely and openly although it is prohibited by the law. Its presence can be easily detected as a solution of the same turns magenta in colour with the addition of hydrochloric acid.

Hing (asafoetida) is adulterated with foreign resins. Pure hing dissolves in water to form a milky white liquid and burns with a bright flame on being ignited.

The essential oils are extracted from cloves and cardamoms leaving behind a product without its full fragrance. Cinnamon powder which is cheaper is passed off as nutmeg powder.

Understandably most housewives make their own spice powders. But things would be a lot easier if the same sold in the market can be of guaranteed purity and quality.

Mustard seed is often adulterated with sand which may be as much as 10% or more in some samples. A similar contamination is found in coriander, cumin, etc. with small lumps of clay.

Coffee, tea and cocoa

The quality of tea is affected by malpractices such as addition of saw dust, exhausted leaves, foreign leaves, etc. Microscopic examination of a tea sample discloses a great deal about its purity. Other estimations which should be made when a thorough check up is desired are moisture, total soluble and insoluble ash and nitrogen. In the case of coffee, the raw seeds do not lend themselves to adulteration except by way of mixing inferior seeds with superior ones. But when roasted and ground they are liable to adulteration of various kinds, the most common being powders of chicory and roasted seeds of dates and tamarind. The important constituents of coffee are caffeine, sugars, cellulose, protein and small quantities of fat and essential oils. The ash content of the powder is used as an index of its purity. The ash content of coffee is less than 4-6% of which about half is water soluble, while adulterants like chicory contain a higher amount of insoluble ash.

In the case of cocoa, there is a temptation for the manufacturers to use the finely ground shell as adulterant. Sago flour or starch coloured with red oxide or iron is also used. Chemical analysis includes estimation of moisture, soluble and insoluble ash, alkalinity of ash, fat, fibre, starch, sugar and nitrogen. Microscopic examination is useful in detecting the presence of shell. The contents of theobromine and caffeine are employed as more reliable criteria. Since pentosans are present in cocoa husk and nib in varying amounts (9.5% and 3.3%) their estimation has been proposed as a method for detecting adulteration with shell.

Eggs

The shells of fresh eggs have a glazed appearance. Also the air space between the contents and top of the shell is not more than 1/4' wide. The egg should feel heavy for its size. When opened, the white should be clear and the yolk, yellow and firm without the signs of embryo or a blood spot. Fresh eggs sink in water while spoilt eggs float. The efficiency of this test is improved by using a salt solution containing 2 ozs of salt per pint of water. The eggs can be visually examined by holding them against light or the flame of a candle. Fresh eggs are clear while bad ones show spots. Mechanized means are used in poultry farms for grading the eggs. Eggs must be discarded if there is increase in air space, unpleasant colour, discolouration of yolk, watery white, mold infestation on the shell and blood spots are evident.

The chemical changes found in spoilt eggs are a lowered content of albumin and increase in alkalinity.

Meat

The quality of meat is determined by its tenderness, juiciness, and palatability. It is almost a universal practice to hang the carcass overnight after slaughter of the animals. Thus meat sold to the public is generally hung for 15-24 hours at room temperature. The carcasses become rigid a few hours after the slaughter of the animal and this change is accompanied by changes in pH. The pH of muscle decreases from 6.5 to 5.7 during post rigor change and again increases to 6.1 when stored for 20 hours. The initial drop in pH is explained as due to the formation of lactic acid from glycogen. When meat is hung for some time, certain acids (e.g. sarcolactic acid) develop due to enzyme action and they help to soften the meat tissue. When the tissue glycogen is low, enough lactic acid will not be formed resulting in higher pH giving brownish or purplish black colour and gummy structure to meat.

Inspection of the animal is necessary to ensure that the meat is from a healthy animal in a sound condition at the time of slaughter.

According to the report of the committee appointed by FAO/ WHO in 1955 the following steps should be taken to ensure a safe meat supply:

- examination of animal before slaughter.
- examination of carcass and parts of carcass immediately after slaughter.

- removal of all diseased and unfit materials.
- adoption of environmental conditions to prevent the contamination of edible products.
- hygiene of meat handler.
- transport and distribution of meat under proper conditions.

Vegetables

The quality of vegetables varies considerably and although some variations such as those in tenderness, colour, and moisture content are of no serious concern from the standpoint of hygiene, their cooking quality and acceptability are affected. Also, fresh vegetables contain more ascorbic acid than stored and shriveled up ones. The carotene content of vegetables is sometimes reflected by colour. Vegetables must be checked for mold and worm infestation and also spoilage. Salad vegetables must be fresh, crisp and firm. Tomatoes must be examined for mould spoilage around the stalk. Vegetables and fruits often contain the eggs of intestinal parasites if they have been exposed to contaminated soil and must be thoroughly scrubbed and cleaned if consumed without cooking.

Other foods

It is particularly important to ensure the purity of prepared foods sold in restaurants and sweet-meat shops and ready-to-eat foods such as candy, dates, raisins, etc. Food poisoning often results because of the bacterial contamination of foods, particularly, sweets prepared from milk. Copper poisoning may result from the use of insufficiently tinned copper brass vessels. Milk and prepared foods should be kept in containers made of galvanized iron.

Pesticides

As already mentioned, food grains and vegetables may contain more than safe levels of pesticides. This may result in milk also containing high levels of pesticides. No stringent measures have been introduced in this country to control the use of pesticides and Indians are reported to have the highest levels of pesticides in blood. Great emphasis is given to monitor the pesticide residues in foods in the FSSAI act 2006 to be discussed later. Lack of sophisticated equipments and trained personnel required for pesticide residue analysis in local laboratories is the limiting factor in this regard.

Radiation

Foods such as fish may also become radioactive and, therefore, harmful to man. This is likely to happen in regions where nuclear devices are tested or used.

On the basis of the studies carried out in Baroda in 1967 and 1974 the practice of adulteration seems to have increased enormously because of the current shortages. The figures obtained for the incidence of adulteration of food grains, oils, etc. were of the order of 15–20% in 1967 and 80–90% in 1974.

Theoretically, the law gives the right to the consumer to get a suspected sample analyzed by the Public Analyst, but the procedure is cumbersome and the results delayed. For such a vast country there are only 64 laboratories which are also not adequately staffed and equipped. The number of samples analyzed is less than 0.4 per 1000 of population. The consumers can form their own association and set up a machinery for checking the quality of foods and demanding action if it is not up to specified standards. Students and teachers of nutrition can perhaps play an important role by educating the public and setting up a cell for the detection of adulteration as a consumer service.

A more comprehensive list of common practice of adulteration of foods and practical hints of their detection is given in Appendix IA.

Food Safety and Standards Authority of India (FSSAI)

During the passage of time since the PFA act was passed in 1956 newer knowledge has accumulated in the area of science and technology and many of these newer knowledge has direct relevance to food safety. The laws relating to various categories of foods have been dealt with in different orders such as Fruit Product Order(FPO), Meat Product Order(MPO) etc. and the enforcement of the laws relating to these commodities used to be handled by different departments of the Government of India. A Bill to consolidate the laws relating to food and establish the Food Safety and Standards Authority of India for laying down science based standards for articles of food and to regulate their manufacture, storage,distribution,sale and import, to ensure safe and wholesome food for human consumption was passed in the Indian Parliament and has come into force as Food Safety and Standards Act,2006.

As per the provisions of the act, Food Safety and Standards Authority of India(FSSAI) has been formed with Head Quarters at New Delhi and under the FSSAI Food Standard and Safety commissioners have been appointed for every state for enforcement of the act. Duties and functions of the Food Authority is to:

a) To regulate and monitor the manufacture, processing, distribution, sale and import of foods so as to ensure safe and wholesome food.

b) To set standards and guidelines in relation to articles of food and specify an appropriate system for enforcing various standards notified under this act.

c) To specify limits for use of food additives (substances added to foods during processing), crop contaminants, pesticide residues, residues of veterinary drugs,heavy metals, processing aids, mycotoxins,antibiotics and pharmacologically active substances and irradiation of foods

d) To specify mechanism and guidelines for accreditation of certification bodies engaged in certification food safety management system for food business.

e) To specify procedure and the enforcement of quality control in relation to any article of food imported to India.

f) To specify procedures and guidelines for accreditation of laboratories and notification of accreditation laboratories.

g) To specify method of sampling, analysis and exchange of information among enforcement authorities

h) To conduct survey of enforcement and administration of the act in the country.

i) To set food labeling standards including claims of health, nutrition, special dietary uses and food category system

j) To provide scientific advice and technical support to Central Government and State Government in matters of framing the policy and rules in areas which have a direct or indirect bearing on food safety and nutrition.

k) To implement crisis management procedures

l) To take all steps for dissemination of reliable and objective information about food safety to public, all levels of panchayats and industries.

m) To provide training in food safety and standards to all concerned persons.

To promote coordination of work on food standards undertaken by international, governmental and non-governmental organizations.

The responsibility of enforcing the provisions of the Act in the States is vested with the Commissioner of Food safety appointed by the procedure specified in the Act. The Commissioner of Food Safety in the states will appoint Food Safety Officers for local areas. The Act provides power to the Food Safety Officer to take samples of any food or any substance intended for sale from shops and vendors and send the same for analysis to a food analyst for the local area. Based on the report of analysis decision will be made whether the food article in question conforms to the standards set in the act for that article. There are provisions in the Act for legal proceedings against the offenders of provisions of the act and if proved guilty the offender can be awarded punishments depending on the severity of the offence as mentioned in the Act.

According to the FSSAI Act "Adulterant means any material which is or could be employed for making the food unsafe,sub-standard, misbranded or containing extraneous matter. Contaminant means any substance whether or not added to food, but which is present in such food as a result of production manufacture,processing,preparation,treatment,p ackaging,transport or holding of such food or as a result of environmental contamination and does not include insect fragments, rodent hairs and other extraneous matter."

The FSSAI has constituted Scientific Panels consisting of experts in the following fields to get inputs regarding the risk assessment and safety levels of parameters to be laid down in the standards for foods falling under various categories:-

a)   Food additives, flavouring, processing aid and materials in contact with food;

b)   Pesticides and antibiotics residues;

c)   Genetically modified organisms and foods;

d)   Functional foods, nutraceuticals, dietetic products and other similar products;

e)' Biological hazards;

f)   Contaminants in food chain;

g)   Labeling and

h)   Method of sampling and analysis

The FSSAI endeavour to achieve protection of human life and health and the protection of consumer's interest. The general provisions of the Food Safety and Standards act are the following:-

1.   Food additive or processing aid used in food manufacture of a product should be in accordance with the standards specified in the act. That is to say, that only additives permitted for a specific food and the levels at which they can be permitted in the final product.

2.   Articles of food should not contain any contaminant,naturally occurring toxic substances, toxins , hormones or heavy metals in excess of limits specified in the standards.

3. Articles of food should not contain insecticides, pesticide residue, veterinary drugs residues, antibiotic residues, solvent residues, pharmacologically active substances and microbiological counts in excess of the limits specified in the standards.

4. No insecticide should be used directly on articles of foods except fumigants registered and approved.

5. Labels that appear on the package of the food should be in accordance with The standards specified in the act. The label on the package should not contain statement or claim regarding the contents of the package which is false or misleading the public.

Most of the states of the country have taken steps in the implementation of the Food Standards and Safety Act. To successfully implement the act and achieve the desired result envisaged in the Act it is of paramount importance to increase the facilities in terms of trained personnel, sophisticated analytical equipments and infrastructural facilities in the states.

Part III:
Diets

Chapter 20

Meal-Planning

What are the characteristics of a wisely planned meal ? First of all, we have to remember that food has to be palatable before it can become nutritious as the majority of people will not eat something they do not like even if it has excellent nutritive value. We should remember that appetite is the pleasurable anticipation of food and depends not only on hunger but also on the taste, texture, appearance and attractiveness of the foods, pleasantness of the surroundings and a cheerful frame of mind.

It need not be emphasized that the food must be adequate from the nutritional standpoint while being within the purchasing capacity of the home-maker. This means that the housewife or the dietitian must not only know the cost of foods but also their cost in relation to food value. She must identify a good 'buy' from the nutritional standpoint. For instance, when the diet is lacking in milk, butter and eggs, carotene-rich vegetables such as pumpkin are better choices than those such as bottle gourd even when the two are of the same price, because the former is a good source of carotene. A dietician can always calculate the amount of calories one can get from one rupee of money spent on alternate choices like ground nut, legumes like bengal gram etc. All that is needed for such a calculation is a knowledge of calorie value and existing price of the alternate food choices.

In many cities, toned milk is available at a much cheaper price than whole milk. When the budget is limited it is better to buy the former and supply the nutrients in the fat removed in the form of carotene rich vegetables and fruits.

Thirdly, the housewife must know how the nutritive value of food can be best preserved during cooking so that unnecessary losses can be avoided. She must be aware of food combinations and cooking procedures that will enable her to derive maximum benefit from the foods used.

Next, the housewife must also learn to budget carefully the time spent on cooking and use procedures that will ensure economy of time, labour and fuel.

The attractiveness of meals can be greatly increased by introducing an interesting variety of foods. The housewife must recognize the sources of different nutrients in the Indian dietary, the nutrients contributed by different groups of foodstuffs, the equivalence of foods from the nutritional standpoint and the widely different ways in which the same foodstuff can be used. Such recognition will help to relieve the monotony of meals consisting of roti, dal and rice day after day with minor variations at the time of feasts and festivals. The different ways in which different foodstuffs can be prepared have been described earlier. Processing the same foods in different ways adds to the attractiveness of the meals. Also, different foodstuffs contribute different nutrients and the use of a variety increases the chances of the diet being more adequate. Major deficiency diseases are often associated with the consumption of monotonous diets based on foodstuffs particularly lacking in certain nutrients. The results of exclusive consumption of foods such as polished rice and tapioca have been described earlier.

We must realize that using a variety of foods does not necessarily increase the cost if the meal is well planned. One kg of potatoes, for instance, may not cost more than, say, 500 g of potatoes and reasonable quantities of a leafy vegetable such as spinach and a salad vegetable such as tomatoes or carrots. The three vegetables would make a more desirable combination from the point of view of appearance, variety and nutritive value than only potatoes.

If simple meals are desired varied types of one dish meals combining cereals, legumes and vegetables can be prepared as described in Chapter 13.

It has been shown that the requirements of different nutrients can be met by a varied diet including as many of the different categories of foodstuffs as possible. To summarize, the requirement of calories and protein can be met to a large extent by judicious combinations of cereals and pulses and the inclusion of milk, eggs, meat or fish to the extent possible. Fat can be derived from pure fats such as oils, butter and ghee and also products rich in fat such as whole milk, eggs, nuts, coconut, sesame seeds, groundnut, soya bean, etc. In the absence of adequate supplies of whole milk, eggs etc., vitamin A and carotene requirements can be met by the liberal consumption of dark green leafy vegetables (now abbreviated widely as DGLV) and yellow and red vegetables and fruits rich in carotene. An adequate supply of most of the B vitamins can be had from the consumption of whole grain cereals, pulses and dals. The supply, particularly of riboflavin and vitamin C, can be further augmented by the generous consumption of leafy vegetables, sprouted legumes and fermented foods. Thus one can have a diet rich in quality and nutritive value without going for expensive foods such as oranges, milk, eggs, meat, butter and almonds. A recognition of this fact will go a long way to remove the attitude of frustration among the middle classes arising from a gap between the impossible amounts of expensive foods recommended and encourage the planning of satisfactory meals within the means available.

The inclusion of different kinds of foodstuffs will not only improve the chances of getting adequate nutrition but also result in more interesting meals with an attractive variety of texture, colour, taste and appearance. Individuals brought up on varied diets are more likely to develop healthy tastes and less likely to be victims of food fads and prejudices. A framework in which the interchangeability of foods is taken into account has been suggested in terms of the exchange system propounded in the book 'Modern Nutrition in Health and Disease' edited by Wohl and Goodhart. The principle of this system is to recognize the equivalence of foods from the nutritional standpoint. An attempt is made here to introduce a similar system based on Indian foods.

Food exchange system

Cereals

One exchange to consist of 25 g of one or other of the following and giving 2-3 g of protein and about 90 kcals: rice, wheat, bajra, maize, jowar, kodri, ragi, etc. Macaroni, spaghetti, rava, poha, mumra, tender corn, etc., should also be considered in this group. An appropriate combination of sago or tapioca and pulse can replace cereals. For instance, 20g of bengal gram+30g of tapioca flour or sago can replace 50g of cereals.

Leaf greens

One exchange to consist of 50 g of one or other of the following and giving 900–1200/micro gram of carotene, 15–25 mg of vitamin C and 20–25 kcals: amaranth, spinach, fenugreek, colocasia leaves, coriander leaves, curry leaves, radish, and beet greens.

Starchy roots and tubers

One exchange to consist of 50 g of one or other of the following and giving 50 kcals: potatoes, yams, sweet potatoes, colocasia, etc. Bananas (both raw and ripe) can be included in this group. Hundred grams of other roots and tubers such as beets, turnips, carrots, radish, etc. can replace 50 g of the above.

Other vegetables

One exchange to consist of 50 g of one or other of the following and giving 20 mg of vitamin C, about 5–10 mg of calcium and 20–30 Calories: brinjal, bitter gourd, cucumber, cauliflower, beans, drumstick, cow peas, cluster beans, double beans, parwar, tindola, kankoda, french beans, ladies fingers, green legumes, snake gourd, pumpkin, pink beans, knol-khol, capsicum, bottle gourd, tomato (green), etc.

Fruit

(a) Those rich in carbohydrate:

One exchange to consist of 50 g of one or other of the following and giving 40–50 kcals: bananas, chikku, wood apple, jack fruit, mangoes, rayan, etc.

(b) Those low in carbohydrate:

One exchange to consist of 100 g and giving 40–50 kcals: apples, papaya, guava, watermelon, rock melon, oranges, etc.

Sugar

One exchange to consist of 5 g of one or other of the following and giving about 20 kcals: cane sugar, jaggery, palm gur, molasses, honey, etc.

Legumes

One exchange to consist of 25 g of one of the following and giving 5-6 g of protein and 90 kcals: dals, whole legumes.

Fat

One exchange to consist of 5 g of one or other of the following and giving 45 kcals: ghee, hydrogenated oil and vegetable oils.

Milk and milk products

One exchange to consist of 50 ml of whole milk or curd. Fifty ml of skimmed or toned milk or 200–300 ml of buttermilk can be substituted for the above with appropriate inclusion of vegetables or fruits which can supply carotene and calcium.

Flesh foods

One exchange to consist of 50 g of one or other of the following providing 10g of protein and 100 kcals: fish, mutton, chicken, pork, etc. A couple of eggs can replace one meat exchange.

The dietary allowances recommended in chapter 7 are given in terms of exchanges in **Table 52**. One can easily train oneself to include 1/4-1 exchange of various foods in different dishes at the same meal and in different meals. For instance, approximately one cereal exchange will be provided by one slice of bread, one chapati, half cup rice, khichri or pongal, one serving of upma, one idli or dosa, etc. a serving of poha dishes, 2-3 biscuits, etc.

The amount of cooked foods corresponding to exchanges are shown in **Table 53**.

It can be seen from the foregoing that once the basic principle involved in the exchange system is grasped it will be easy to plan menus and to introduce a good variety in meals as the equivalence of different preparations from the nutritional standpoint.

This system saves dietitians and others concerned with the planning of diets whether for self, family or institution the trouble of referring to the chemical composition of individual ingredients in order to assess the nutritional adequacy of diets.

It should also be recognized that introducing a variety from day to day or at each meal does not necessarily require more work or finance, but does require advance planning. In most south Indian homes, for instance, the house-wife puts the pots on for rice and dal even before planning the menu and this limits the choices available to her. It is better to plan the menu before starting the cooking and preferably at least one meal ahead of time. For instance, many people do not use sprouted legumes, whole legumes and fermented foods frequently, although these foods are very popular and do not involve more of labour or cost, because they have to be planned ahead of time. The left-overs from the previous meal should be taken into account while planning the next meal. For instance, if some rice is already left, khichri or pongal may be a more interesting addition instead of more cooked rice.

In a family a growing adolescent boy may need rich foods to whet his ravenous appetite whereas the not so active housewife may need more of vegetables etc. A young child may require soft and bland foods. The family meal should cater to the needs of its different members.

Similarly a party meal should cater to the needs of both people who prefer rich and spiced foods and those who prefer simple and bland foods. Very often, all the items on the menu are highly spiced or sweet or rich in fat leaving people who are not used to such foods to suffer rather than enjoy the party.

It may be a good exercise for the housewife to record what the family eats for a week and find out how the meals could have been made more attractive without increasing the cost. Similarly if she plans the meals in

Table 52. Dietary allowances in terms of exchange.

Age (yrs)	Economic Level	No. of exchanges								
		Cereals (25 g)	Pulse (10 g)	Milk (50 g)	Leafy vegetable (50 g)	Root vegetable (50 g)	Other vegetable (50 g)	Fruits (50 g)	Fats and oil (5 g)	Sugar (5 g)
1	I	4-6	4	4	less than ½	½	½	½	2	5-8
	II	2-3	2	10-12	les than ½	½	½	½	2	5-8
2-4	I	6-7	4-5	3-4	1	½-1	1	1	3-5	5-8
	II	3-4	2-4	8-10	½	1	1	1	3-5	5-8
5-6	I	7-8	4-5	2-4	1	½-1	1	1	5	5-8
	II	4-6	2-4	8-10	1	½-1	1	1	5	5-8
7-10	I	10-12	5-6	2-4	1	1	1	1	5-8	5-8
	II	6-8	4	8-10	1	1	1	1	5-8	5-8
11-12	I	11-15	5-6	2-4	1-2	1-1½	1-1½	1	5-8	5-8
	II	9-11	4	8-10	1	1-1½	1-1½	1	5-8	5-8
13-15	I	12-18	6	2-4	1-2	1-1½	1-1½	1	5-10	5-8
	II	12-13	5-6	8-10	1	1-1½	1-1½	1	5-10	5-8
16-19	I	15-19	6	2-4	1-2	1-1½	1-1½	1	5-10	5-10
	II	13-15	5-6	8-10	1	1-1½	1-1½	1	5-10	5-10
20-40	I	15-22	6	2-4	1-2	1-1½	1-1½	1	5-10	5-10
	II	14-15	5-6	8-10	1	1-1½	1-1½	1	5-10	5-10
per capita	I	14	6	3	1.1	1.3	1.4	1.0	9.2	5.4
	II	10	5	10	0.9	1.3	1.4	1.0	6.8	5.6

1   The figures in parantheses indicate the amount in one exchange

I   Low income

II   Middle and high income

Table 53. Composition of selected foods in terms of exchange.

	Amount from 1 exchange	other food stuffs used
Cereal foods: Cooked rice	½ cup	
Khichri	¾ cup	½ legume exchange
Pongal	¾ cup	½ -1 fat exchange + ½ -1 legume exchange
Sweet pongal	¾ cup	½ - 1 legume exchange + ½ - 1 fat exchanges + 5 sugar exchanges
Poha dishes (cooked)	¼ - ½ cup	½ fat exchange
Chapatis	1	¼ - ½ fat exchange
Poories	2-3	1 – 1½ fat exchange
Parathas	¾ - 1	½ - 1 fat exchange
Idlis	¾ - 1	¾ - 1 legume exchange
Dosas	1 – 1 ½	¾ - 1 legume exchange + ½ - 1 fat exchange
Upma	¼ - ½ cup	½ fat exchange
Rava idli	1	½ milk exchange
Sakkarpara	½ serving	1 fat exchange
Bread with butter	1 slice	½ - 1 fat exchange
Biscuits	2 – 3	1 -2 sugar exchanges + ½ - 1 fat exchange
Legume dishes: Liquid dal	½ cup	¼ fat exchange
Sambhar	½ cup	¼ fat exchange
Usal	¼ cup	½ vegetable exchange
Khaman	1 serving	¼ fat exchange
Vadas	1	1-1½ fat exchange
Sev	½ serving	1 fat exchange
Vegetable: Vegetable (gravy type)	½ - ¾ cup	½ fat exchange
Vegetable dry type	½ cup	½ fat exchange
Drinks for milk: Butter milk	1 cup	
Curd	¼ cup	
Milk (sweetened)	½ cup	½ sugar exchange
Tea	1 cup	2 sugar exchanges
Coffee	½ cup	1 sugar exchange
Other milk drinks	½ cup	½ sugar exchange

advance for a week or two, she may get into the habit of using the different foods in different ways.

Left over foods can also be dressed up differently and served as attractive dishes. For instance, left over rice can be steamed and converted to lemon rice, coconut rice, onion rice, etc. Leftover bread can be fried as bread crumbs or the crumbs made into upma, cutlets, dosa (make a batter with a little flour, buttermilk, onions and seasoning).

Often, when unexpected company presents itself for a meal, the housewife starts cooking more of chapatis or rice. It would be much more sensible to make instead additional dishes which can be prepared quickly such as poha or rava idli or debra, or dosa, salads, raita, khadi, etc.

Incidentally, a few comments may be offered here regarding the avoidance of wastage of food, particularly at parties and the like. The ordinary housewife giving a party generally tends to overestimate the foods required. She can avoid this by finding out how much total food her family eats normally per head and making a similar allowance for guests. This quota she can use for preparing diversified items. For instance, if one consumes 500–700 kcals at a meal, one is not likely to consume much more than this or at any rate 700–1000 Calories at a party. The quantities cooked must be adjusted so that the amount per capita of cereals, pulses, oil, vegetables, milk, etc. does not exceed more than 100–150% of the amounts usually consumed. As such meals include much more than the usual amount of fat and sugar, the consumption of rice, dal, chapatis, etc. is generally less than the usual amounts. If the home does not have refrigerator, we should avoid preparing excessive quantities of highly perishable foods. Attempts should be made to preserve the leftovers by the methods suggested earlier (chapter 18). Avoidance of wastage is particularly necessary in a poor country such as India where so many people do not have enough to eat.

Chapter 21

Nutritional Care of Particular Groups

Although adequate nutrition is important for every one at all ages, some groups are more likely to be affected by malnutrition than others because of various factors. Nutritional requirements are increased in groups such as young children, adolescent boys and expectant and nursing mothers because of the increased demand for nutrients during periods of rapid growth in the former two groups and the growth of the unborn child and growing infant in the latter case (the nursing mother has to nourish a rapidly growing infant). The rate at which tissue is formed during different stages can be seen from **Table 54**.

Apart from a general increase in nutritional requirements, the need for specific nutrients may also increase in relation to nutritional requirements. For instance, a child needs more calcium in relation to energy intake than the adult. This means that even when the diet does not include much of foods rich in calcium such as milk an adult eating a greater amount of foods so as to get 2500–3000 kcals is likely to get the calcium he needs than the child who eats less (say 1000 kcals). Unless his food provides adequate amounts of foods rich in nutrients such as calcium, vitamin A, iron, etc., he is likely to become more deficient than the adult. Further, the young child is not always in a position to choose the foods he wants to eat and is often subject to restrictions imposed by the mother. The mother is often guided by the size of the child and fails to recognize that the child needs much more food in relation to body weight than herself. For instance, a one year old child needs nearly half as much food as his mother.

Also, all the foods prepared for the family are not given to the young child in the mistaken belief that some of them are not suitable.

Table 54. Body weight increments at different ages*.

Age (yrs)	% increments in body weight per year	
	Western subjects	Upper class subjects in Boroda
0-1	200	220
1-2	29	20
2-3	17	16
3-4	10	10
4-5	9	10
5–8	15	11
8–10	10	8
10–12	9	10
12–15	13	14
15–17	7	4
17–19	3	2

* Calculate from body weight norms given for western subject by Mitchell, H.H. 1964. Comparative Nutrition of man and Domestic Animals, Volume 11, Academic Press, New York and those obtained for Indian Subjects in the Biochemistry Department of Baroda University, Baroda.

Often, when appetite is affected for some reason, the older and the more privileged individual substitutes foods he prefers (e.g. fruits, beverages) whereas the young children just forego their usual food.

Food sharing practices also may not operate according to nutritional need. The adolescent boy needs more calcium than his father, but the latter is more likely to get that extra cup of milk when milk is in short supply.

Even when the supply of rich foods such as milk, eggs, fruits, etc. is not a problem deficiencies may develop because of capricious appetites or wrong beliefs. For instance, adolescent boys and girls in the affluent west and in the upper classes in this country choose foods and drinks such as coca cola and sweets in preference to more healthy foods such as milk and fruit. The expectant or nursing mother often eats unwisely and she may also eat expensive foods (e.g. almonds, ghee, saffron) which have no particular value and avoid foods which are valuable sources of critical nutrients (e.g. curd, papaya, leafy vegetables and fruits) because of mistaken notions regarding their merits and demerits. Special attempts have to be made to create an awareness of the special nutritional needs of particular groups and the way they can be met.

Infants

Every mother is aware that foods prepared for the adult are not always suitable for the young child. But most mothers do not realize that foods suitable for them can be easily prepared without going in for expensive baby foods which are beyond their reach. Although milk is the most natural food for babies, advances in nutrition have enabled the planning of satisfactory meals for young children even without this commodity.

If the child does not get adequate nutrition during this period, the growth of the child is affected. Often children in the poor class who grow satisfactorily during the period they are breastfed almost stop growing during the weaning period because they do not get suitable weaning foods such as milk. The difference in growth rate of well-nourished and poorly nourished children can be seen from **Fig. 8** When the diet is deficient in calcium or vitamin D or both, they suffer from rickets.

Sometimes the mothers feed them enough calories in the form of starchy foods such as sago, tapioca or rice but they do not get enough of protein and other nutrients. Such children develop 'kwashiorkor' because of protein deficiency, and severe eye symptoms culminating in blindness, because of vitamin A deficiency. Children who do not eat enough because of the unsuitable nature of the foods available suffer from severe undernutrition or marasmus. Thus it is clear that good nutrition during childhood is important for the proper development of the child. We will now consider the care of the young child at different stages.

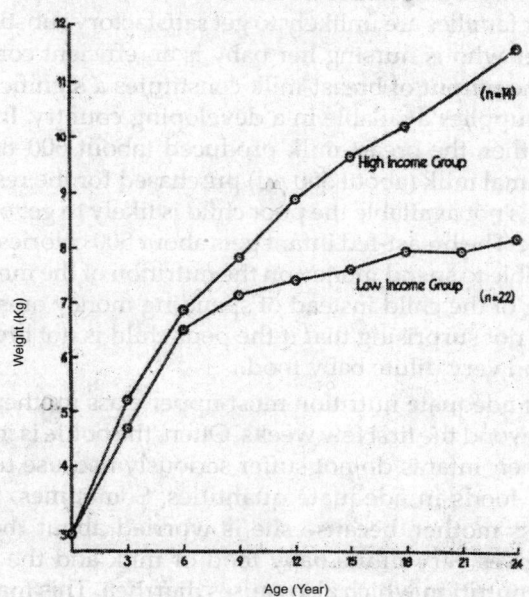

Figure 8. Longitudinal data on the growth of poor and middle class children.

Birth to three months

The food par excellence for the newborn baby is mother's milk. Fortunately, even the poorly nourished mother is able to nurse her child satisfactorily at least during the first few months of life.

The composition of breast-milk with regard to carbohydrate, fat, protein and minerals is not seriously affected by the diet of the mother under ordinary conditions. Deficiency diseases such as infantile scurvy or rickets are not found in breast-fed babies.

The milk of poorly nourished mothers may contain less of water-soluble vitamins but the infant usually gets enough for its requirements and vitamin deficiencies are also rare in breast-fed infants except in areas where polished rice is the staple. Bottle-fed babies getting the best baby foods and getting more of protein, calcium, etc. are not found to grow faster than breast-fed babies.

Breast-feeding has several advantages over bottle-feeding as breast-milk is free from contamination and adulteration and supplies the nutrients in the amounts needed by the infant. It also provides an opportunity for close contact and emotional satisfaction of mother and child. Breast-milk also contains immuno-proteins which protect the child to some extent against infections. An important consideration is that in the absence of breast milk, infants in poor families are unlikely to get satisfactory substitute foods. The human mother who is nursing her baby is an efficient converter of food to milk and the output of breast-milk constitutes a significant proportion of total milk supplies available in a developing country. In a family with a nursing mother, the breast-milk produced (about 600–800 ml) may be more than animal milk (about 500 ml) purchased for the rest of the family. If breast-milk is not available the poor child is likely to get only 100–150 ml of animal milk. The breast-fed infant gets about 500 calories. Economically it is more feasible to spend money on the nutrition of the mother and adopt breast feeding of the child instead of spending money on animal milk for the child. It is not surprising that if the poor child is not breast-fed he gets dilute milk and very dilute baby food.

In spite of adequate nutrition most upper class mothers do not nurse their babies beyond the first few weeks. Often, the bottle is introduced right from birth. Their infants do not suffer seriously because usually they get milk or baby foods in adequate quantities. Sometimes, however, even an upper class mother, because she is worried about the child getting indigestion, gives very dilute baby food or milk and the child develops serious undernutrition which also causes diarrhea. This makes the mother dilute the formula even more and the child gets even more severely undernourished.

The more unfortunate phenomenon is that some poor women, particularly in urban areas, take to bottle-feeding in imitation of the upper class women. As they are not able to give milk or baby food in adequate quantities and are also more ignorant about the significance of diarrhea, their children suffer. Mothers, especially those from the low income group, should be educated on the advantages of breast-feeding. They must also be enabled to realize that diarrhea especially in young children, may not always signify indigestion. It is unfortunate that many children with chronic undernutrition diarrhea are given barley water and glucose by the mothers for prolonged periods either out of ignorance or wrong advice. Fortunately this trend seems to be declining. Whether the child is breast-fed or bottle-fed, the best way to make sure that he is adequately nourished is to see whether he is growing satisfactorily. The well-nourished infant doubles his birth weight by 3.5 to 4 months of age. He can be weighed or measured for length, and the circumference of chest (around the nipples, abdomen (around the navel) and hips. The norms for heights, and weights at different ages and other measurements are given in **Table 55**. The circumference of the abdomen is usually about 2 cm less than of the chest. It does not matter if he is smaller than the average child if be is growing satisfactorily. For instance, a child may be 7 kg at 6 months and 8 kg at 8 months. Another child may be 8 kg at 6 months and the same weight 8 months. Although both are of the same weight at 8 months, it is the latter child we have to worry about.

Table 55. Anthropometric measurements for children at different ages.

Age	Sitting height[1] (cm)	Standing height[1] (cm)	Sitting height[1] — Standing Height	Body weight (kg)[2]	Circumference of — chest (cm)	Circumference of — head (cm)
Birth	32.4	48.3	0.67	2.9	31.1	34.0
3 months	41.5	60.2	0.68	5.7	38.8	40.1
6 months	42.8	65.0	0.66	7.0	42.1	42.4
9 months	44.8	68.7	0.65	7.9	43.9	44.4
12 months	46.7	73.4	0.63	9.0	45.8	45.5
2 years	51.5	84.2	0.61	11.5	49.3	48.2
3 years	52.0	89.7	0.57	12.5	49.4	48.8
4 years	55.3	96.2	0.57	14.9	51.6	49.8
5 years	57.3	105.0	0.54	17.7	53.6	50.0

[1] Crown to rump and crown to heal lengths in the case of young children.
[2] Data reported for boys except for birth weight, taken from Ghai, O.P. and R.K. Sandhu. 1968. *Ind. J. Paediatrics*, 35.91. The vales for height and weight correspond to those obtained for upper class children in Baroda. The values for girls are slightly lower.

As cow-milk is thicker than breast-milk, it is diluted and given. However, the dilution should not be so great as to make the child severely undernourished. In the case of the very young infant, one can begin with 50% diluted milk and decrease the dilution to 25% after a week or so. After a month or two the child can be given whole milk. The utilization of the proteins of breast-milk is nearly 100% whereas that of cow milk proteins is only 80% so that it is necessary for the milk formula to provide more protein than breast-milk. The composition of breast-milk, is compared with that of substitute formulas in **Table 56.**

In any case, young children, after the first few weeks, are able to tolerate whole milk or slightly diluted milk quite well. The young child needs about 100–120 Calories per kg of body weight.

This means that if he is bottle-fed he should get the amounts of cow milk or its equivalent in the form of baby food according to information given in Tables 55 and 56.

The composition of goat milk is closer to that of human milk and the same is considered by some to be more suitable for infant feeding.

Buffalo milk is richer than cow milk because of its greater fat content. It can be partially skimmed by removing the cream, diluted with water and sugar added. The removal of cream will decrease the amount of vitamin

Table 56. Composition of different milk formulas.

	Amount per 100 g			
	Calories (kcal)	Protein (g)	Carbohydrate (g)	Calcium (mg)
Breast milk	65	1-1.2	7-8	28
Cow milk	67	3.2	4.4	120
Buffalo milk (7% fat)	95	3.5	4.5	210
Dairy milk (5% fat)	77	3.5	4.5	190
Toned milk (3% fat)	59	3.5	4.5	190
Milk (50g) + water (50g) + sugar (5g)				
Cow milk	53	1.8	6.3	60
Buffalo milk (7% fat)	68	1.8	6.3	105
Dairy milk	59	1.8	6.3	95
Toned milk	50	1.8	6.3	95
Milk (75 g) + water (25 g) + sugar (5g)				
Cow milk	71	2.5	7.4	90
Buffalo milk	91	2.6	7.4	158
Dairy milk	76	2.6	7.4	143
Toned milk	64	2.6	7.4	143

A available, but this can be met by vitamin A or cod-liver oil supplements. Some children are not able to tolerate buffalo milk because it forms thick curds in the stomach which are not as easily digested as those formed from breast-milk or cow-milk. It has been suggested that animal milk is better tolerated by such children if the same is given in the form of curd (dahi) which can be churned with a little water to make thick buttermilk (The water used should be boiled).

Baby foods such as 'Glaxo' are generally prepared from cow milk. 'Amul' is prepared from buffalo milk. They are claimed to be processed in such a way that they approach breast-milk in digestibility. They are useful when the child is unable to tolerate animal milk as such composition of different milk formulas or when unadulterated fresh milk is not available in the market. Also milk does not stay fresh for many hours. But baby foods are not really necessary if good milk is available and is tolerated by the child. It is unfortunate that many poor mothers have taken to baby foods because of prestige considerations. Because they cannot afford them, they give a diluted baby food with the result that the child suffers from undernutrition.

Some infants are not able to tolerate animal milk. In other words they are 'allergic' to the same. Such children can be given groundnut milk or soya bean milk. The latter is much more satisfactory from the nutritional standpoint. It has been found that infants brought up on soya bean milk enriched with suitable supplements of minerals and vitamins can thrive quite well. Such milk is usually fortified with minerals and vitamins.

Vitamin C

Breast-milk contains liberal amounts of vitamin C and the breast-fed child gets about 20–25 mg of vitamin C per day. Cow or buffalo-milk contains only small quantities of vitamin C most of which is lost when the milk is boiled. Bottle-fed infants may therefore suffer from vitamin C deficiency. Infantile scurvy used to be a dreaded disease in the west. Now it has practically disappeared as most mothers give orange juice to the babies, particularly if they are bottle-fed.

Jelliffe in his report to the World Health Organization has remarked that in this country and other tropical countries infantile scurvy is rare even in the case of bottle-fed babies. He considers that the dangers of giving contaminated fruit juice to the child are greater than those resulting from a lack of vitamin C in the diet. All the same, it may be wise to give some source of vitamin C to the child not receiving breast-milk. Care must be taken that the fruit juice or vegetable extract given is free from contamination as fruits are usually infested with flies. Orange juice is a popular choice but juices from other fruits such as tomatoes, chani bor, etc. can be prepared as described earlier. A sweetened extract prepared from drumstick leaves should be quite safe as the same is prepared by boiling. Extracts of boiled vegetables can also be given.

Often the growth of child becomes slower when the breast-milk supply is deficient. The mother must learn to recognize this. Even illiterate mothers try to keep track of body measurements by using traditional waist bands and arm bands and the like. They can be easily trained to note the length of the same required every month (For instance the bands can be stretched out on a wall and their lengths marked).

As long as the child shows a satisfactory gain in weight and seems cheerful there is no need to worry about his nutrition. The healthy and well-nourished baby sleeps and plays well and is restful. If he is irritable, fretful and cries often, it is necessary to make sure that he is getting enough food. Further, the regulation of appetite is quite efficient on the young child and he is quite unlikely to accept more food than he needs (he will not drink that last drop in spite of mamma's best efforts). There is, therefore, no need for the mother to restrict the supply.

The adequately breast-fed infant does not need supplements during the first few months of life but is likely to need water, particularly under the climatic conditions prevailing in this country. Also, the regulation of water balance and water loss in urine is not very efficient in the young infant and he loses relatively more water in proportion to body weight than adults. In the tropics and subtropics the infant is reported to require more than 175 ml of water per kilogram of body weight. The breast-fed infant gets 600–800 ml of milk in established lactation. As breast milk contains 88% of water this would give 525–700 ml of water for an infant weighing 4-5 kg and needing 700–900 ml or more. The need for water may be greater during the first month when milk yield is much less. The need is also increased in conditions such as diarrhea and vomiting.

It is important to educate mothers on the desirability of giving water when needed or at least once a day. Many mothers believe that this practice is harmful. The water given must be boiled and cooled under cover. It is common practice to give water with glucose or sugar, but this is not necessary. Incidentally, glucose is often given in the belief that it is more readily absorbed than sucrose which has to be digested. The enzyme sucrase is found in the intestine of the child (fetus) several weeks before birth and the digestion of sucrose is quite efficient in the new born child. In any case the water must not be so sweet that the child develops a sweet tooth. If the child is thirsty, sugar may only aggravate his thirst. Also, the excessive consumption of sugar may interfere with his intake of milk. In hot weather, the baby often cries of thirst and will accept the breast if offered but will only cry more after a while. If the baby cries soon after a full feed and well before the next feed is due, it could be due to several factors causing discomfort including thirst. If the baby is thirsty, he will accept the water with gusto giving squeals of delight. The water can be offered with a spoon or a small cup. If the rim of the cup is pressed on his lower lip he will soon learn to sip from the cup like adults.

3–6 months

It has become increasingly common in western countries to introduce starchy and solid foods well before the age of three months. It used to be common practice to defer the same till the child is six months old as it was believed that the synthesis of amylase which is necessary for starch digestion is not efficient before this age. Under conditions prevailing in this country, with the danger of substituting too much cereal for milk too easily, it may not be wise for us to follow current practice in the west.

Non-starchy soups and creamy and smooth solid foods such as mashed vegetables and fruits may be gradually introduced after the age of 3-4 months. The fresh juice of the tender coconut or coconut water (as well as coconut milk) can be given even to very young children. The former contains free sugars, free amino acids, minerals and vitamins in freely assimilable form. It also contains substances (growth factors) which are found to stimulate the growth of plants,

The introduction of fruits and vegetables will correct the deficiency of iron in breast-milk and both iron and vitamin C in bottle-milk.

Soups prepared from vegetables and mashed bananas, plain or mixed with a little honey can be gradually introduced. Only firm but fully ripe fruit must be used. It can be mashed with a fork or a spoon. Similarly, fruits such as papaya can also be given. Orange segments can be given after removing the seed. The baby will spit out the skin after sucking in the juice.

6–12 months

At the age of about six months or even earlier, most babies are ready to accept easily digestible starchy foods and begin to crave for solid foods.

The child can also be given boiled and mashed potatoes as such or with a little salt and lemon juice and other vegetables such as carrots, pumpkin, cauliflower and spinach which can be similarly treated. The vegetables can also be cooked with milk or buttermilk. Sweet potatoes, carrots and pumpkin can be boiled, mashed and then cooked with a little jaggery. Brinjals can be roasted and peeled and seasoned with lemon juice and salt. Raw carrots and cucumber sticks will improve chewing habits.

Gruels and puddings prepared from cereals with or without legumes can be gradually introduced. The ways in which they can be processed for infant feeding have been described earlier (Chapter 10).

Commercially available branded foods can be given if the mother can afford them and the child likes them, but they are not a 'must'. But the money spent can be stretched much further if used for locally available foods. For instance, puffed rice obtained from the bazaar can be used after re-roasting at home to make it crisp and to prevent infection. It can be ground to a coarse texture and cooked in milk to form a thick paste.

The other parched grains, sprouted and roasted grains and roasted dals can be used as described earlier (Chapter 10).

Other preparations such as the following may be given:

(1) Softly cooked rice and dal or khichri with home-made curd or liquid dal or rasam, (2) wheat chapatis can be toasted on a tava on slow heat on both sides till they are crisp like biscuits. They can then be crushed into crumbs and soaked in hot milk and sugar, (3) fermented foods such as idli, khaman and dhokla, (4) puddings or gruels made from sago, suji (rava), arrow root, flaked rice, bread crumbs, rice (whole grain or coarsely ground) etc. Sago must be allowed to simmer on slow heat till it is quite transparent, (5) steamed breads, (6) rusks, yeast breads, buns and biscuits. Some recipe suggestions are given in Appendix II.

Boiled eggs and tenderly cooked meat and fish can be given if the child likes and tolerates them and the ordinary home diet includes them. But they need not be given as a result of parental anxiety to prevent protein malnutrition which occurs only in children given a predominantly carbohydrate diet based on rice, tapioca, etc. without adequate intake of milk and legumes. The newspapers raise such a bogey about the paucity of animal food in our diet and the resulting protein malnutrition that vegetarian parents of perfectly well-nourished children feel guilty about not giving their children animal foods forgetting that they themselves have grown up satisfactorily without such foods.

The above suggestions can be extended to include a rich variety of foods which should be soft, acceptable and free from irritant spices such as chillies and pepper. As mentioned earlier, a portion of the dal cooked for the family can be easily removed before spices and chillies are added and simply dressed with lime juice, salt, cumin seed, etc. Similarly, a portion of the cut vegetables may be removed and cooked separately into soups or can be given as mashed vegetables.

The solid foods can be first introduced at lunch and extended gradually to other meals. Milk intake is likely to go down with the introduction of solid foods but as long as the baby takes at least 1/2 to 3/4 litres of milk and is active and gains weight satisfactorily there is nothing to worry about. Many parents in the upper classes have exaggerated fears of protein malnutrition in children if they do not take the prescribed amount of one quart of milk. Children who are brought up on a variety of foods are healthier and have much healthier tastes than those brought up on just milk and biscuits, fruit juice and vitamins. A mixed diet will also prevent the development of iron and vitamin C deficiencies.

As mentioned earlier a cereal-legume-groundnut combination or soya bean can be given if milk is not available.

1–5 years

If solid foods have been gradually introduced before the age of 1 year, feeding the child should be no problem in the subsequent years. Yet diet surveys show that even children in the high income groups particularly those in large families, are undernourished or malnourished or both because of parental indifference or ignorance and the abrupt change to highly spiced foods and tea. The suggestions made earlier are valid for this group also but the child can be exposed to a greater variety of foods as he can tolerate coarse foods better. Also, as part of the growing process, some of the children, particularly those in small families where there is no competition for food, are poor or difficult eaters at times. Their food intake will improve if the food is interesting and attractive. Chapatis and poories cut in interesting shapes, potatoes shaped like 'bunnies', pretty glasses or cups to drink the milk in, and attractive cereal bowl or plate, can all help. One child would not accept curd until the mother thought of setting it in a pretty bowl and presenting it as 'ice-cream curd'. Similarly, a child refusing milk will accept it if coloured yellow with turmeric or other colouring agent and spiced with cardamom etc. (the turmeric should be added when the milk is hot as otherwise it gives a raw flavour). Salads given to children (and others) should have an attractive appearance and appetizing taste.

Adolescents

Teen age boys and girls undergo rapid growth and if their nutrition is not taken care of during this period they become stunted in growth. The differences between poorly nourished and better nourished subjects are most evident during adolescence (**Tables 57 and 58**). In the scarcity areas of Gujarat feeding a good lunch was found to increase the weight of adolescent boys by 4–6 kg whereas younger children were found to show an increase of only 1-2 kg. Much of the difference in physical stature between Indians and Westerners is due to the slowing down of growth during this period.

Normally, the poor diet is inadequate in both calories and calcium but the adolescent boy may not show any obvious evidence of calcium deficiency because of stunted growth resulting in decreased calcium requirement. A deficient supply of calcium may also lead to reduction in food intake and stunted growth. Occasionally a fast growing adolescent may

Table 57. Heights and weights of males in low and high income groups in Gujarat.

Age (yrs)	Height (cm)			Weight (kg)		
	50th percentile Boston norms	H.I.G[2]	L.I.G[2]	50th percentile Boston norms*	H.I.G[2]	L.I.G[2]
Birth	50.6	51	50	3.4	2.9	2.7
1	75.2	74	69	10.1	9.5	7.7
2	87.5	84	74	12.6	11.4	8.6
3	96.2	94	84	14.6	13.2	10.4
4	103.4	102	92	16.5	14.5	11.8
5	111.2	107	97	19.4	16.0	13.2
6	117.7	111	102	21.9	18.2	15.0
7	124.1	116	107	24.5	20.0	16.4
8	130.0	121	112	27.3	21.4	17.3
9	135.5	125	115	29.9	23.2	19.1
10	140.3	132	119	32.6	25.0	21.4
11	144.2	135	125	35.2	27.5	22.8
12	149.6	140	130	38.2	29.8	24.6
13	155.0	144	135	42.2	34.4	26.9
14	162.7	150	140	48.8	38.2	31.0
15–19	167.8	163	152	54.5–63.1	45–50	40
20–40	172–174	165–170	162	66.5–71.9	55–60	51

* Values for adults taken from Hawkins, W.W. 1964. In Nutrition Volume 1. Ed. Beaton, G.H and E.W. MeHenry, Academic Press. New York.
[2] Values obtained for High and Low Income Groups in Urban Baroda.

have an adequate calorie supply combined with a deficiency of calcium and this results in poor skeletal growth and an uneven gait. Symptoms such as bow legs and flat feet become exaggerated during this period.

Adolescents are physically more active than adults and have a greater metabolic rate. They feel hungry all the time, and, if they can, tend to snack in between meals. This is partly because they don't eat enough at meal time. Often they are so pre-occupied with their friends, games and comics that they don't eat proper meals. As these snacks are often full of fat and sugar contributing empty calories, it is not surprising that even upper class boys often show deficiency symptoms such as glossitis and fissured tongue. Because of faulty food habits many adolescents and children develop dental caries.

The adolescent should be trained to relax and eat properly at meal time. He should have wholesome snacks which he should take at regular times in moderation. The snack should preferably be made from whole grains, dals

Table 58. Heights and weights of females in low and high income groups.

Age (yrs)	Height (cm)			Weight (kg)		
	50th percentile Boston norms*	H.I.G**	L.I.G**	50th percentile Boston norms*	H.I.G**	L.I.G**
birth	50.2	51	50	3.3	2.8	2.6
1	74.2	74	64	9.8	9.2	7.3
2	86.6	84	74	12.2	10.9	8.6
3	95.7	94	81	14.4	12.7	10.9
4	103.2	102	91	16.4	14.1	11.4
5	109.1	109	97	18.4	16.4	12.7
6	115.9	114	102	21.1	18.2	14.1
7	122.3	121	107	23.7	20.4	15.4
8	128.0	107	112	26.3	22.7	17.3
9	132.9	130	114	28.9	25.0	19.1
10	138.6	135	119	31.9	27.0	20.0
11	144.7	140	125	35.7	29.5	20.9
12	151.9	145	129	39.7	31.4	24.5
13	157.1	150	135	45.0	35.0	29.0
14	159.6	152	142	49.2	39.5	32.3
15-19	161.1–162.5	155–158	148	51.4–54.4	45–50	38.6
20-40	160-161	155–158	150	55.9–58.6	45–50	38.0

* Values for adults, taken from Hawkins, W.W. 1964. In nutrition. Volume 1. Ed. G.H. Beaton and E.W. Me Henry. Academic Press New York.
** See Table 57.

etc., e.g., from whole wheat, puffed rice, groundnut, sesame seeds, parched chana, etc. although there is no harm in occasional indulgence of his craving for sweets. Most schools sell snacks such as candy and chocolate rather than those such as parched legumes, fermented foods, sandwiches, etc.

The adolescents in poor families have hardly anything to eat between meals except occasionally 25–50 g of groundnut or parched grains from the street vendor. The health and growth of this group can be substantially improved by giving them a balanced lunch at school.

It is recognized that severe malnutrition in infancy and early childhood can interfere with the normal maturation of the brain as well as psychological development. It is also thought that malnutrition in later life may not have a similar effect. While no one would question the imperative need for safeguarding the health of young children, it is dangerous to conclude that older children do not need proper nutrition as malnutrition during any stage of life can impair function, work performance, etc., and that, during the period of growth, it can impair physical growth and skeletal development and interfere with school performance. School boys constitute a vulnerable group unable to look after their nutritional needs because of economic dependence. Further, work habits and traits such as inertia and apathy resulting from undernutrition tend to persist in later life. Also several studies in Israel and elsewhere have demonstrated that school boys who participate in the organization of school lunch programmes etc. and are given nutrition education as part of the process form an effective channel for the education of the community.

Expectant and nursing mothers

The expectant or nursing mother has not only to nourish herself but also the growing fetus or the nursing infant. During pregnancy a woman gains about 7–10 kg in weight. The baby is born with liberal stores of iron, protein, vitamin C and other vitamins and these have to be supplied either from the mother's diet or her tissues. If the diet is lacking in the nutrients needed by the fetus, they are removed from maternal stores.

The weight of a healthy infant at birth is about 3-3.5 kg. About 10% of the infants born to poor mothers in this country have birth weights below 2 kg in spite of being full-term babies. Also, the incidence of still births is higher among the poor than in the upper class. Such low birth weights are found to be associated with a poor weight gain during pregnancy associated with a poor food intake.

Poor food intake during pregnancy is not just a result of poverty. Often, the poor woman is anaemic to begin with and becomes more so during pregnancy. Symptoms such as loss of appetite, nausea and vomiting which are prevalent to some extent in pregnancy become exaggerated perhaps because of this. Also, cultural patterns seem to subtly influence such traits as these symptoms are much less evident in the upper class woman having a job than the one staying at home. The nausea of pregnancy can be relieved to some extent by toning up the general health of the mother, if necessary, by iron and vitamin supplementation. Also, pregnant women should be advised regarding the need for fresh air and exercise and for simple and appetizing foods such as citrus and other fruits buttermilk, sweet-sour salads etc. Heavily spiced and greasy foods should be avoided. The flavanoids in the peel of citrus fruits may have a beneficial effect in such conditions as candied orange peel and relishes and sauces prepared from orange and lemon peel are found to be highly acceptable. Incidentally, orange peel flavanoids are found to delay the onset of scurvy in guinea-pigs deprived of vitamin C.

The pregnant woman is not able to eat much at a time and must space her meals suitably and provide for drinks such as buttermilk, milk, or lemon juice and simple snacks between meals. Taking lemon juice or orange juice in the mornings and before meals helps relieve the nausea of pregnancy.

The pregnant woman is sometimes pampered with unwholesome snacks such as very rich sweets, fried foods, etc. These only aggravate the symptoms and it would be better to take simple wholesome, easily digestible and appetizing foods.

Sometimes, a restriction of salt is advised specially if there is a tendency to edema. In any case excessive consumption of pickles, chutneys, etc. rich in salt must be avoided.

While, undernutrition in pregnancy may be a problem among the poor the reverse problem is often found in the high income group. The common saying that a pregnant mother must eat for two is not tenable as the requirements of the growing fetus are small as compared to those of the mother. Many women in the upper class load themselves with rich foods such as ghee and almonds during pregnancy and put on a lot of weight. It is not desirable to gain more than about 8–10 kg during pregnancy for the stature of an Indian woman. Moreover, normally, some of the 'stores' acquired during pregnancy are lost after delivery when the mother nurses her child. But many upper class mothers do not breast-feed their babies with the result that they are stuck with part of the extra weight acquired during pregnancy. Further, it has been traditional to enrich the diet of the mother with ghee, milk, etc. after delivery. Again this may be sound practice when the mother is nursing her baby, but will only result in obesity when she is not. These practices are responsible for many young women becoming obese with child birth.

Even when the mother is nursing her baby, the production of milk involves only about 500–600 kcalories and part of this can come from stores acquired during pregnancy. This extra amount can be supplied by whole grain cereals, pulses, milk, curd, etc. and there is no need for her to go in for foods such as ghee and almonds.

The expectant mother needs an additional 150–300 kcalories and 10 g of protein. The nursing mother needs 500–600 kcalories and 10–15 g of protein. Both need more of calcium (300–500 mg) and also perhaps iron (5–10 mg) and vitamin A (600–1000 microgram) deficiencies of which are common during pregnancy and after delivery. These increases can be achieved by either adding about 300–500 g of milk and some 50 g of leafy vegetables and carotene rich fruits to the normal diet or consuming an extra amount of 50–100 g of cereal, 25–50 g of legumes and 50 g of leafy vegetables or other carotene-rich vegetables and fruits and lime-incorporated buttermilk. In the case of poor communities, these can perhaps be provided in the form of suitable snacks or lunches at maternal and child welfare centres. Alternatively, skim milk and vitamin and mineral supplements may be given.

Chapter 22

Diseases Caused by Malnutrition

Inadequate availability of nutrients for metabolic purposes results in nutritional deficiency diseases. The most common cause of deficiency is poor dietary intake. Even when the diet is adequate, a deficiency may arise due to several factors such as those listed below:

Aetiological factor	Examples
Poor absorption	iron in hookworm infection, vitamin A in protein
Protein deficiency	vitamin B12 in pernicious anaemia; all nutrients in diarrhoea.
loss in the alimentary tract	Vitamin A with ingestion of paraffin oil or repeatedly heated fats. Carotene and vitamin A with a relative excess of polyunsaturated fatty acids and a relative deficiency of tocopherols.
excessive loss from the body	nitrogen losses during fever, acute infection following injury; iron and carotene in haemorrhagic and hemolytic conditions.
poor utilization	Vitamin A deficiency in protein malnutrition.
	Iodine deficiency caused by biochemical abnormalities.
increased requirement	as in the case of protein and vitamins during treatment with sulpha drugs, antibiotics, etc., also in conditions such as fever, infections, cold exposure, heat stress, surgery, injury etc.

All these factors must be borne in mind when nutritional deficiencies are encountered.

What follows is a brief discussion of some of the diseases caused primarily by a dietary lack.

When nutrients needed by the body are not available in adequate amounts tissue formation and renewal and metabolic functions are affected resulting in nutritional deficiency diseases.

Undernutrition and malnutrition in children

As stated earlier, even poorly nourished mothers manage to breastfeed their babies satisfactorily during the first few months of life. However, the growth of the child slows down afterwards. While the infant in both the low and high income groups weighs about 7 kg at 6 months of age, at the age of one year, the upper class infant weighs about 10 kg and the poor infant about 7.5 kg. The difference between the two increases between 1 and 3 years of age. Sometimes, the poor infant shows practically no growth during this period. The main reason for this is poor dietary intake. The poor child does not get enough milk and no attempt is made to substitute other foods for milk.

In regions such as Gujarat the child is offered the foods prepared for the family and this consists mainly of tea,thick hard roti and highly spiced dal and vegetables so that the child is unable to eat enough of the foods available. This results in serious undernutrition. Their body weights are often less than two-thirds of expected weights for age. This pattern is prevalent to some extent in the upper class as well. About 60–75% of children in this age group (1–4 years) do not reach their full growth potential. Most of these children do not seem to catch up even afterwards when they have become adapted to the diet and they continue to be shorter and smaller as compared to better nourished children. Their skeletal development is also found to be retarded. They are not as playful and active as they could be and are often 'cry' babies specially between 6-18 months of age because they are hungry.

The situation is complicated by infections and diseases such as dysentery, chicken pox, respiratory infections, etc. The mortality is very high during this period. The children suffer from deficiencies of protein, vitamin A and riboflavin. These deficiencies are more prevalent in rice-eating areas.

Rice is deficient in minerals and vitamins and to make it worse, the surplus cooking water of rice, which contains very little protein, is given in place of rice.

It is important to educate mothers on the need for providing suitable foods based on cereals, legumes and vegetables as suggested earlier.

Kwashiorkor

With the kinds of diets mentioned above, the child first becomes growth-retarded. After severe episodes of diarrhea or other illness, the child becomes further undernourished because the mother substitutes even more unsatisfactory foods for the already poor diet. Glucose water, barley water or conjee prepared from arrow root or sago are given. As all these foods are lacking in protein the child develops severe protein deficiency. This also happens when the ordinary diet consists of rice conjee, tapioca or sago with practically no milk, dal or vegetables.

The child fed such diets may initially present a plump appearance making the mother into thinking that the child is gaining weight. The plump appearance is because of the excess retention of water (See plate). Later, the child develops marked oedema with the swelling of the extremities. This makes muscular movements very difficult and painful and makes the child irritable. The child prefers to sit undisturbed.

In spite of the plump appearance, the kwashiorkor child is often marked by underweight, especially when the weight due to oedema water is taken into account. The child is extremely apathetic. He takes no interest in his surroundings whatsoever and does not show any response when presented with brightly coloured and attractive toys. In fact, some fishermen in the coastal regions of Kerala are found to leave such children on the beach while they go out for fishing feeling assured that the child will stay put till their return.

'Kwashiorkor' in the original African language is reported to mean displaced child. The label owes its origin to the fact that it is common in poor children who are suddenly deprived of breast-milk by the arrival of a sibling. However, only about a quarter of the kwashiorkor cases are found to be 'displaced' children.

In the case of the displaced child the dietary lack probably acts in combination with psychological factors. The sense of rejection by the mother because of the new arrival can be very frustrating. It is interesting that according to Egyptian folklore the treatment recommended is that the mother must put the younger baby to sleep, take the older child suffering from the disease in her lap and gently feed him a preparation made of eggs. Such treatment would naturally take care of both dietary and emotional factors.

In severe kwashiorkor, patches of the skin become inflamed. Both pigmentation (dermatitis) and depigmentation are found. The hair become sparse, soft and discoloured. The liver becomes enlarged because of excessive deposits of fat.

Digestion and absorption are both impaired in kwashiorkor. The secretion of digestive enzymes is poor. The walls of the stomach and intestine become very thin, sometimes paper-thin and diarrhea is frequent.

As the child is also undernourished the kwashiorkor child needs about 200 kcals and 4-5 g of protein per kg of body weight for speedy recovery. This means that the child has to eat more in proportion to body weight. The bulk of the food is greater when nutritional improvement is sought to be made by using cereals and legumes. In the beginning the use of milk powder was popular, but it is now felt that it is better to use milk or milk powder along with cereals and other foods as excessive milk causes diarrhea. It is also found that diets based on natural foods are better than protein hydrolysates and concentrates. When only protein is given, there is a rapid clearance of oedema resulting in dehydration and loss of electrolytes. Further, the metabolism is speeded up and this results in a greater demand for vitamins; and vitamin deficiencies, which were hitherto masked because of the low plane of metabolism, may become aggravated. Five or six small meals given every three hours or so are better than meals given twice or thrice a day. Meals can alternate with simple beverages and snacks. The foods suitable for young children and described earlier,can be used. Fish, eggs and milk can be included in generous quantities. It is better to base the treatment in the hospital on the kind of foods the mother can use at home so that the child will continue to get a good diet after discharge. The mothers can be associated with the purchase and preparation of food, where possible, so that she gets educated about their nutritional care.

Marasmus

An inadequate diet in early life results in another disease syndrome known as marasmus characterized by dehydration and extreme wasting. The skin is loose and wrinkled as in old people and the child is all skin and bone (See plate).

Although both kwashiorkor and marasmus may occur with the same type of diet, there are some differences between the two. Kwashiorkor is invariably associated with a protein deficient diet and lowered levels of serum protein and albumin. Marasmus is also found when children are given insufficient amounts of a good diet. Kwashiorkor seldom occurs before the age of six months when the child is either breast-fed or bottle-fed. Marasmus is found even in very young babies when they do not get enough milk. Intestinal absorption is generally more efficient in marasmus, and blood and serum composition are sometimes more satisfactory. Psychological symptoms such as apathy are less prevalent in the marasmus child which responds readily to environmental stimuli. Mortality is also less in the condition.

The restricted food intake of the marasmus child is sometimes the result of maternally imposed restriction rather than the result of poor appetite and the child is a cry baby, crying all the time for food, but because of symptoms such as diarrhea caused by undernutrition, the mother is afraid to give him enough food. Whereas kwashiorkor occurs generally among the poor, infantile marasmus is occasionally seen in upper class babies because they are given highly diluted milk or baby food. Children who have developed mild marasmus because of insufficient intake of a diet of good quality may not always show retardation in psychological or neuromotor development. More often, however, both marasmus and kwashiorkor occur in children with apparently similar dietary patterns and it is not clear why some children develop kwashiorkor and others, marasmus. In some children marasmus appears to be the result of chronic and prolonged malnutrition beginning from birth or earlier. Many of the children admitted for marasmus have been small at birth and have developed poorly even before the age of six months because of inadequate breast feeding. Symptoms of both kwashiorkor and marasmus (extreme wasting with localized oedema) are found in some cases. The condition is known as marasmic kwashiorkor. Whether the child is suffering from marasmus or from kwashiorkor, he needs a good quality diet in generous amounts and plenty of fluids.

Kwashiorkor, marasmus and marasmic-kwashiorkor are also collectively referred to as protein-calorie malnutrition.

Disorders of the skeleton

Retarded skeletal development is found in most children of the poor, and sometimes, even in upper class children. Deficiencies of protein, calcium, phosphorus or vitamin D can contribute to this condition.

In these children the normal maturation of the bone and the development of ossification centres are delayed. For instance, in the young child, the space between the long bones of the palm and those of the arm is filled with cartilage rather than true bone. As the child matures cartilage is formed into true bone. The motor development of the child depends on a number of factors including skeletal development. Naturally, a child whose cartilaginous areas in the foot have not properly calcified cannot stand up firmly or walk. (This is why young children should not be made to sit, stand or walk before they are ready).

The development of bone requires the formation of a matrix and the mineralization of this matrix. It also involves constant renewal. During growth an outer layer is added and an inner layer removed, so that the bones become longer and larger. This process continues till adult size is achieved. Thereafter, the process consists of replacing old bone by new bone at the same site.

The formation of the matrix requires a supply of protein, vitamin A and vitamin C. Its mineralization requires calcium, phosphorus and vitamin D.

It is not surprising that a deficiency of any of these causes retarded skeletal development.

The state of skeletal maturation at different ages has been studied by X-ray examination of a large number of subjects in each age group. If a three year old child shows the expected skeletal development for his age, his bone age is also considered as 3. Often, however, the child may be 3 years old, but his skeletal development may correspond only to that of a normal 2 year old. In that case, his bone age is said to be 2 and the child is retarded in skeletal development by one year.

Skeletal retardation is difficult to detect by visual examination as the children may look quite normal and can be identified only by X-ray examination. Such retardation may, however, be suspected in children with a 'flabby' appearance.

Among the poor, the main causes of skeletal retardation in young children are a deficiency of protein, calcium and vitamin D. The efficient utilization of both calcium and phosphorus depends on a supply of vitamin D. Often, young children are not allowed to play outdoors in the sun and they also do not get vitamin D in the diet, which is generally lacking in foods which are rich in vitamin D.

Skeletal retardation can be prevented and treated by a nutritionally adequate diet and generous exposure to sunshine.

As already mentioned, in studies carried out by the author's group, administration of a food supplement such as dhokla in which lime and leafy vegetables had been incorporated was found to result in improved skeletal growth. The supplements were given at a play centre where the children were also allowed to play in the sunlight so that their vitamin D supply would have been adequate. Even in the upper class skeletal retardation is sometimes found in young children although their diets are adequate in protein,calcium and vitamin A. A deficiency of vitamin D may be involved in these children. Even milk is only a poor source of vitamin D. Upper class mothers often restrict their children from playing outdoors in the sun resulting in poor synthesis of Vitamin D on the skin.

Rickets

Rickets is caused by a deficiency of calcium, phosphorus or vitamin D. In the West, a deficiency of vitamin D is considered to be a crucial factor but vitamin D can only help in the utilization of minerals and a poor supply of calcium may also be a contributory factor.

Rickets is associated with diets lacking in milk and milk fat. In regions such as the Kangra Valley where rickets was found to be widely prevalent, the soil is poor in calcium so that the drinking water as well as foods produced locally is also poor in the same. Also, when local custom such as the Purdah confines the mothers indoors, the children are also likely to spend less time outdoors. This results in lack of adequate exposure to sunlight which is necessary for the synthesis of vitamin D in the body. Common symptoms found in rickets are pigeon chest, 'rosary beads' or formation of bead growths in the ribs which look like a bead chain, thickening of the bone-cartilage (costa-chondral) junctions, swollen and painful joints, bow legs etc. (see plate). The child with rickets has flabby toneless muscles. Excessive sweating of the head is found. When the onset of rickets is early, there is delay in the eruption of teeth and failure to sit up, stand, crawl and walk at normal ages. The child with rickets is more prone to infections such as bronchial pneumonia.

In rickets, serum calcium levels may become very low, and as a normal level of calcium in serum is necessary for the regulation of the permeability and irritability of the cell, this results in tetany (convulsion caused by ,the frequent twisting of muscle fibres). Severe tetany may result in death,

Aim of treatment should be to increase the intake of both calcium and vitamin D. It must be remembered that treatment with vitamin D alone when the diet is deficient in calcium is not of much use. Adequate vitamin D synthesis can be ensured by exposure to sunlight without clothes. In South India it is common practice to smear the body with oil before such exposure although this practice has not been proved to be beneficial. In any case it is not harmful and may help in relieving symptoms such as dryness of the skin, phrynoderma and infantile eczema due to EFA deficiency.

In the case of infants, the body may be smeared with oil and the infant laid down on the floor for a few minutes against a window in the morning or evening so that the body lies exposed to sunlight whereas the head is in the shade. The calcium content of diets can be increased by incorporation of lime in sour foods as stated earlier (Chapter 4) if the diet does not include enough milk. Supplements of calcium and vitamin D may also be given.

In this country rickets is not a common disease although every year a few cases may be admitted in any large hospital. In surveys carried out by the authors group in rural areas of Gujarat, rickets was rare but not absent. However, it seems more prevalent in rice-eating areas such as Tamil Nadu and Kerala. The poor mineral content of rice as compared to wheat could be a contributory factor.

Studies carried out by McCarrison and others in the Punjab and Kangra Valley showed a high incidence of rickets in these regions. However, studies carried out by Dr. De Sweemer and her associates in rural Punjab rickets were seldom found. It is possible that social changes such as the absence of purdah in contemporary rural society in these regions have contributed to this.

Rickets which was a dreaded disease in the West practically disappeared before the middle of this century. Occasionally cases are now seen in Scotland, particularly among children of Asian immigrants who tend to clothe their children heavily in winter and not allow them to play outdoors for fear of their catching a cold.

Osteomalacia

It is a disease caused by calcium deficiency in adults, mostly in women in the reproductive years. This disease occurs when the diet is generally poor in calcium and repeated pregnancies deplete the body of calcium. A child is born with about 28 g of calcium which involves a deposit in the fetus of 200–300 mg per day during the last trimester and smaller amounts during the earlier stages of pregnancy. Breast-feeding the child involves an output of about 200 mg per day for another six months and about 100 mg per day for a much longer period. These figures do not take into account the incomplete availability of dietary calcium. A deficiency of vitamin D may also be a contributory factor.

Osteomalacia used to be common in areas such as Kashmir and the Punjab and the purdah areas of the Middle East. It is now found occasionally in Asian immigrants in Britain. Common symptoms are back aches, particularly, pain in the lower vertebrae and the bones of the pelvis and the legs. The gait may be uneven. Tenderness near joints on pressure may be found. Tetany is manifest by spasms and facial twitching. Pseudo-fractures are found on radiological examination.

Treatment should be with supplements of calcium and vitamin D. Large doses given initially help a quicker recovery. When only normal amount of calcium are consumed the response is much slower as the amount needed for cure is much more than that needed for prevention.

Calcium lactate with vitamin D can be given. Lime-incorporated foods as suggested in Chapter 4 can be included in the diet.

Deficiencies of protein, vitamins A and C may also result in skeletal abnormalities as described earlier.

Osteoporosis

Even after skeletal growth has apparently ceased in the adult, the bone constantly undergo a process of renewal consisting of the erosion of old bone and the formation of new bone in its place. In the normal adult the two processes are balanced. However, with increasing age after the middle years, the formation of new bone does not keep pace with the removal of old bone and the bones become somewhat thinner and less dense with increasing age. This process is very slow in the normal adult and is hardly of any consequence.

When, however, the balance between dissolution of old bone and formation of new bone is appreciably disturbed and the latter does not keep pace with the former there is a progressive loss of bone resulting in a condition called osteoporosis. On X-ray examination, the pelvic bone which presents a dense appearance normally may look like a sieve. Large areas of the bone may have disappeared altogether resulting in black patches on the X-rays. Osteoporosis is found generally after middle age and is more common in women than in men. Osteoporosis occurs even when the diets are quite adequate. However, in some elderly individuals living alone and not eating satisfactorily, dietary deficiencies could form a contributory factor.

Hormonal factors are suspected to be involved as the disease occurs more frequently in women after menopause. Treatment with growth hormone and estrogens has been found to help. Lack of exercise may also be a factor as the disease is frequently seen in persons confined to bed for a long-period (e.g. spinal injury). The activity of osteoblasts (cells which form the bone matrix) is stimulated by exercise. Osteoporosis is less common in India although the diets provide less calcium. In studies carried out by Walker in South Africa it was found to be more common among European women than in Bantu women although the former had a greater intake of calcium and other nutrients.

Treatment is difficult but consists of a combination of an adequate diet, administration of hormones (growth hormone, estrogens, testosterone) and physiotherapy (a physiotherapist can train the patient to do systematic exercises which help in arresting or reversing the process). Treatment with fluorides has also been advocated as fluorapatite crystals in bone are less readily eroded than hydroxyapatite crystals.

Undernutrition in adults

Undernutrition in early life is often followed by chronic undernutrition which is found in the majority of the world's population. The food intake of the poor is generally 2/3–3/4 of that of well-nourished individuals and may be as low as 50% or less of normal intake in scarcity and famine conditions.

Sometimes, normally well-nourished people may be suddenly subjected to severe undernutrition because of war, famine, serious food shortage, unemployment, illness, etc. Occasionally volunteers have subjected themselves to undernutrition in order to enable studies on the effects of the same. With sudden undernutrition, as for instance when a person habitually consuming 3000 kcals lives on an 1800 kcals diet there is a rapid loss of weight which may be up to about 25–30% of original weight but the weight stabilizes thereafter. This is perhaps, because, with the decrease in

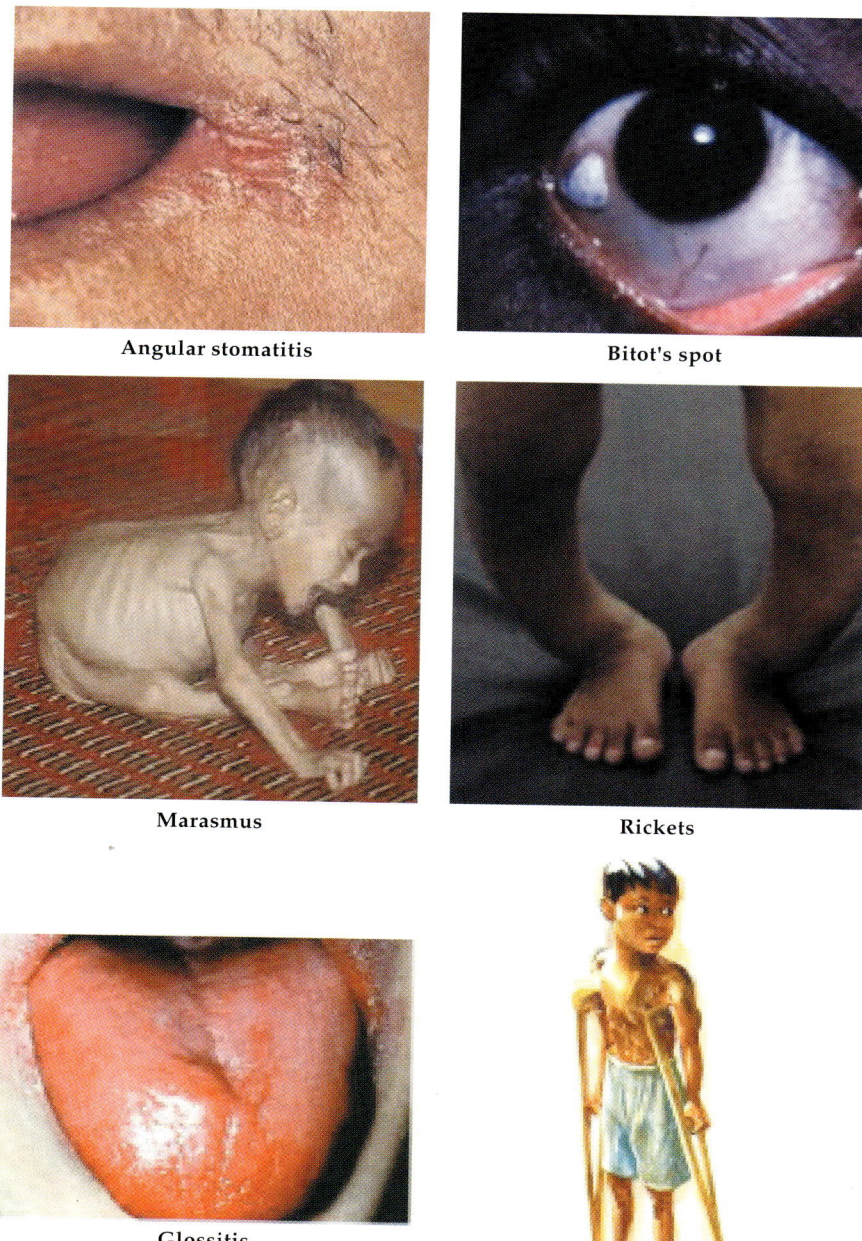

Angular stomatitis

Bitot's spot

Marasmus

Rickets

Glossitis

Lathyrism

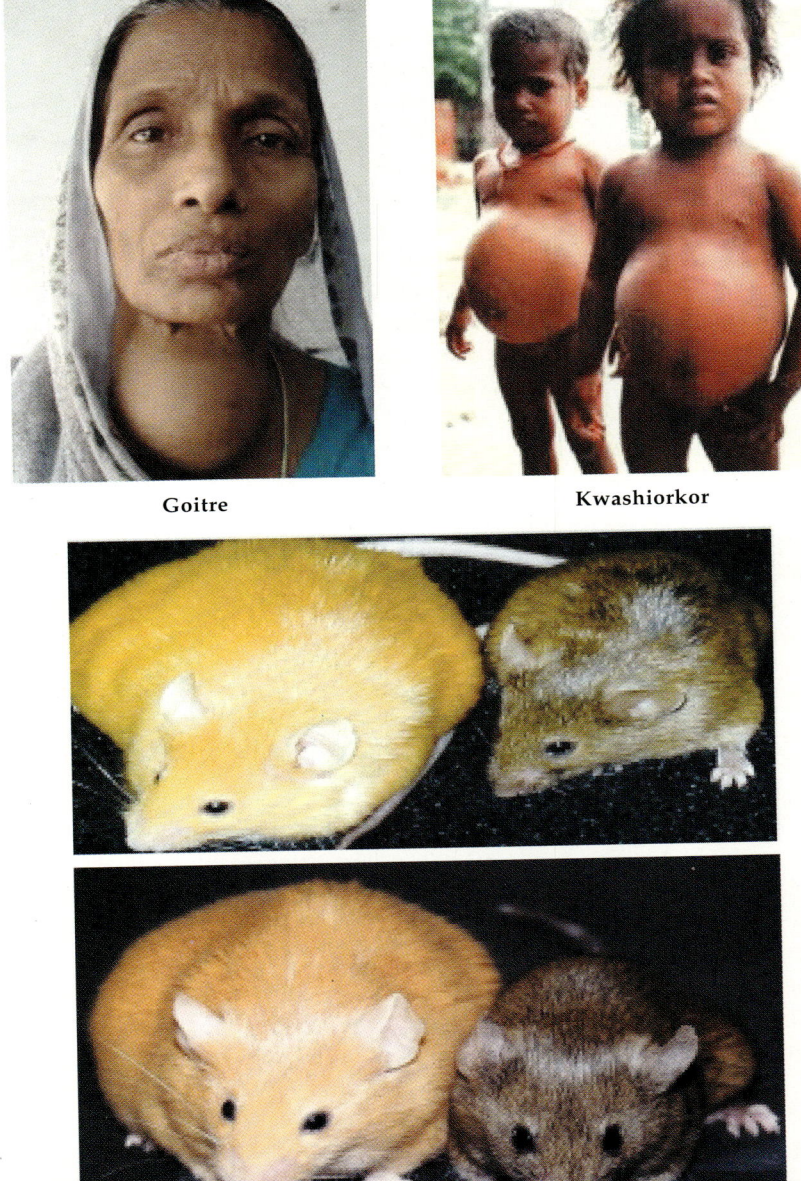

Goitre

Kwashiorkor

Figure 7a. Left Side of both photos—offsprings of mother fed normal diet, Top Right Side—offspring of mother fed normal diet with methyl donors, Bottom Right Side—offspring of mother fed normal diet with genistein.

body weight, energy requirement also decreases. Further, there may be a progressive fall in BMR by more than 25%. With these changes, the energy intakes may just balance requirements so that no further weight loss occurs.

Undernourished individuals also reduce their voluntary activity. They do tasks which must be done in order to earn a living, bull will seldom exert themselves beyond this. Their work generally involves a familiar activity and the energy cost of a practiced activity is less.

Individuals subjected to severe undernutrition are unable to concentrate long enough on a single problem although their intellect is not impaired and they can function normally when adequately fed. They become apathetic and tend to think all the while about food. The attitude of undernourished people towards foods, has been described in a humorous way by P.G. Wodehouse in his book *The performing flea*. Psychologists have found that when hungry subjects are asked to recognize pictures flashed through tachistoscope for a very brief period, they are able to recognize pictures of foods much better than those of other objects.

With acute starvation even family ties break down. Such acute starvation is found in times of famine or when people are stranded in some uninhabited place and are cut off from food supplies. Cases of cannibalism, fortunately rare, were reported during the Bengal famine and during the Irish famine in the 19th century.

The chronically undernourished individual may not show any clinical symptoms apart from a below normal body weight and slowness of movements. Many apparently undernourished individuals may have a normal blood composition.

The effects of acute starvation, however, include extreme wasting, deficiency of adipose tissue, oedema, disturbed kidney function resulting in excessive urination at night, diarrhea etc. The diarrhea is caused by intestinal atrophy. The walls of the stomach become thin and there is an insufficient synthesis of digestive enzymes and increased incidence of infections. Tuberculosis is seen more frequently in undernourished individuals. The diarrhea may result in dehydration resulting in a serious disturbance of water and electrolyte balance and ultimately death.

Most people subjected to acute undernutrition or starvation respond readily to a good diet. The foods given must be those which can be tolerated and easily digested in the initial stages. However, a few persons subjected to acute starvation may become so apathetic that they lose all interest in food even when it becomes available.

Undernutrition may also occur in conditions such as prolonged fever when the basal metabolic rate is increased and nutrient losses from the body are heavy and food intake is restricted. However, the subject usually regains original weight after recovery when fed a suitable diet.

The appetite may be so affected in chronically undernourished individuals that they fail to eat well for sometime even when there is no restriction in the supplies. In studies carried out by the author and her colleagues, undernourished adult men (Bhils in Dohad District of Gujarat) given as much food as they wanted were not found to consume more than 1800 kcals per day during a period of sedentary living. Similarly, pre-school children given a good diet *ad libitum* were found to consume only 400 kcals at breakfast and lunch at the beginning of a feeding programme. The consumption increased to 700 kcals within a few weeks.

Chronic undernutrition also occurs occasionally in the upper classes. Some individuals have poor appetite and are unable to eat large meals. Anaemia and other factors which affect appetite must be ruled out. Psychological tension may be a contributing factor. Pleasant and appetizing meals, a relaxed atmosphere at meal time, beverages and simple snacks in between meals may help.

Protein deficiency in adults

In this country, clinical symptoms of protein deficiency are not usually evident in adults although occasional cases are found in Kerala, when rice and fish are both in short supply and people have to subsist largely on tapioca. Cases of oedema arising from protein deficiency may occasionally be seen just before the harvest when foods are in short supply.

Obesity

Normally, appetite is regulated according to need and a healthy child, allowed to eat as much of a balanced diet as he wants, eats enough to maintain satisfactory growth and function.

We have already seen that 'poor appetites' which can be caused by a variety of reasons, result in inadequate food intakes and undernutrition. Often however, the decreases in energy requirements are not associated with a corresponding reduction in appetite. The individual eats more than he needs and the excess energy is stored as fat in adipose tissue, leading to an accumulation of fat in the body, a condition called obesity.

The amount of fat in the body rather than total body weight should be considered for deciding whether or not a person is obese.

For instance, persons of athletic build may be heavy without being obese. On the other hand an apparently small person may have excessive fat pad in the abdomen, thighs etc. without weighing more than average person. Both body build and body weight should therefore be considered in the assessment of a person for obesity. A person is generally considered over-weight if his weight is more than 10% above the expected weight for age and height and obese if it is more than 20%.

Body Mass Index (BMI) is used as an index for obesity and the same is calculated using the following formula:-

English formula

BMI = Weight in pounds/(Height in inches x Height in inches)x 703

Metric formula

BMI = Weight in Kg/Height in meters x Height in meters

BMI classification

18.5 or less	Underweight
18.5 to 24.99	Normal weight
25.0 to 29.99	overweight
30.0 to 34.99	obesity (class 1)
35.0 to 39.99	obesity (class 2)
40 or greater	Morbid obesity

The obese person is self-conscious and therefore,may have psychological problems. Obesity imposes an extra burden on the skeleton, the heart and the circulatory system. Diabetes mellitus occurring in middle years is more common among obese people. When diabetes runs in the family the best bet against contracting the disease is to maintain below normal body weight. Obese persons move more slowly because of greater body weight and he has to carry this and this result in further reduction in activity and energy expenditure.

Obesity is considered as disease which originates from the changed lifestyle in affluent societies. Both undernutrition and over nutrition are malnutrition. Most of the cases of obesity are due to faulty food habits and in simple logic it is due to the higher intake of calories than expenditure. This can be attributed to life style pattern in modern society and lack of knowledge of basic nutrition. The pattern of eating a major meal once a day either at noon or in the late evening and light meals at other times is sometimes replaced by full meals three times a day and snacks and beverages in between. Further, in most communities sweet dishes were prepared only on special feast days and beverages containing sugar were not common. In Europe sugar was a luxury till the last century and the ordinary diet consisted largely of bread and beans and occasionally meat. The present day European diet includes more than 100g each of butter and sugar. In India an occasional 'kheer' is now replaced by daily cups of tea or coffee, four cups of tea providing more sugar than a cup of kheer.

Food has become more plentiful for people who need it less. The modern European or the upper class Indian hardly indulges in manual labour. In this country the food intake of a white collar worker or a businessman is more than that of a labourer engaged in building construction, for instance, with rather obvious consequences. It is time to heed the injunction, "By the sweat of thy brow, thou shalt eat bread".

Obesity is more common in men and women after the age of 30 years. The Indian adolescent girl weighs only about 45 kg at 18–20 years of age as against a weight of 55 kg for western girls. By 40 years of age she has often caught up with her western counterpart. In contrast,the poor Indian woman maintains a constant body weight of about 45 kg.

The chief causes of obesity after the age of thirty are a reduction in BMR and reduction in activity. But the food habits are already established but if one is accustomed to two slices of toast for breakfast one just has 2 slices and not 1 1/2. It is only young children refuse to eat if they are full. An Excess intake of even 100 calories a day (the equivalent of 1-1 ½ chapattis) can result in an annual gain of about 5 kg. Food intake does decrease with age in most people but often the decrease in energy requirement is greater still so that the intake is excess of requirement. Also, a decrease in requirement is not followed by immediate decrease in intake and it takes some time for new patterns of appetite to be established. In the meantime the person has already acquired some excess weight.

The only treatment for obesity is to decrease the calorie intake and increase the activity. Equally important is to cut down the sugar consumption as sugar level in the blood stimulates insulin secretion which in turn promotes fat synthesis in the body and this aspect is dealt with in detail elsewhere in this book. Special formulae for weight reduction are based on the principle that the same supply a low calorie diet which is otherwise balanced. An equally low calorie diet can be planned at home at much lesser cost.

Sometimes, hormones such as thyroxin are administered in order to increase the basal metabolic rate and hence decrease the energy imbalance, but unless the subject has a thyroid deficiency such treatment are not desirable. Drugs which elevate body temperature and, therefore, basal metabolic rates are sometimes given. Drugs which reduce appetite are also used. All these may be harmful short cuts when the fundamental problem is one of adjusting food intake to body need.

The reduction of calorie intake should be according to the weight loss desired. For instance, the food consumed should contain 250–500 kcalories less than needed if a weight loss of 1-2 kg in a month is desired.

The diet should be planned after calculating the energy requirements of the individual according to height, desirable weight, sex, activity level, etc. The calorie intake should be less than the figure arrived at by the desired value.

The diet planned should provide the calories intended while being adequate in protein and other nutrients. Foodstuffs such as vegetables which provide bulk should be included liberally. Sugar, fat, etc. should be either avoided or taken in minimum quantities. The subject should be educated in adjusting his calorie intake while choosing from a variety of foods. Skimmed milk or partially skimmed milk should be substituted for whole milk.

It is popular belief that obesity can be cured by taking lemon juice with or without honey. The subject should be educated not to believe in such myths.

Exercise also helps in the treatment of obesity. Some surplus calories can be got rid of by exercise, although most activities require much less energy than we think. For instance, one banana (100 kcalories) can finance the energy requirements of a walk for about one hour. This has led a scientist to remark that "the most effective exercise in the control of obesity is to push oneself away from the dinner table in time". However, even an extra 200–400 kcalories used up by exercise should result in a weight loss of about 1-2 kg per month. Further, it is believed that exercise may have a favourable effect on the regulation of appetite. Such regulation is less efficient in individuals leading a sedentary life, It has also been suggested that exercise may increase basal metabolic rate. It is well known that athletes have a higher basal metabolic rate.

One kilogram of adipose tissue represents a store of about 6000–7000 kcalories. The subject should first get an estimate of his energy requirements and decide on the rate at which weight loss is desirable depending on the degree of overweight and cut his food intake accordingly.

The calorie reduction needed for achieving normal weights when excess weight ranges from 5 kg to 20 kg is as follows:-

Excess weight	kcals reduction needed for achieving normal weights in	
	6 months	3 months
20 kg	800	1600
10 kg	400	800
5 kg	200	400

If the subject has been having a stable weight for some time the reduction can be achieved by omitting from the current diet foods whose calorie value is equal to the reduction desired. The amounts of different foodstuffs providing 100 kcals are shown in **Table 59.**

Table 59. Approximate amounts of different foods providing 100 kcals.

	As consumed
Fats and oil	2-2.5 teaspoons
Sugar	5-6 teaspoons
Tea	1 ¼ cup
Coffee	1 cup
Milk with sugar, curd	¾ -1 cup
Dry roasted groundnuts	1 ½-2 cup
Cashew nuts, almonds	1-1 ½ tablespoon
Biscuits	4–6
Rice	½ cup
Chapatis(thin)	1
Parathas	½ -3/4
poories	
liquid dal	¾ - 1
Vegetables: low calories	1-1 ½ cup
high calories	½ -3/4 cup
Sprouted legumes	½ cup
Banana	1
Fried snacks	½ serving (30–40 g)
Halwas	One small piece (20–25 g)
Vadas, bhajya	½ serving (40–50 g)
Khaman	1
Idli	1
Dosa	1
Omelette	1
Boiled egg	1-1 ½
Jam	2 tablespoons

For this approach to succeed, however, it is very important to record carefully the amounts consumed for about a week, make sure that body weight has really remained stable, make planned cuts of the present diet and stick to the modified diet systematically. Often, the temptation is to say just this one dish at one meal will not make a difference. If the subject exceeds his quota at a meal (for instance, at a party) he should cut down his intake the next day. If the subject has been gaining weight, the reduction will have to be more severe.

Alternatively, the person can find out how many calories he needs from information given in chapter 3 and then plan a diet providing 500–1000 kcals less than this depending on the rate at which weight reduction is desired.

For instance, a person having an excess weight of 10 kg can come down to normal weight in six months if he keeps his intake at 400 kcals less than expected requirements. He would have to double the reduction to achieve it in only three months. However, the rate of loss may vary with the nature of the tissue lost and changes, if any, in basal metabolism and activity level.

Let us suppose an overweight woman who has not gained weight recently is consuming the diet shown below:

7 a.m.	Tea	1 cup
	Bread with butter and jam	2 slices
10 a.m.	Tea	1 cup
	Biscuits	4
1 p.m	Chapatis	4
	Rice	1/2 cup
	Dal	1 cup
	Vegetables (potatoes/others)	1 cup
	Curd	1/2 cup
4 p.m	Tea	1 cup
	Snacks (usually fried)	1 service
8 p.m	same as lunch	

The calorie value of the above diet can be reduced appreciably by changes suggested below:-

	Modified	kcals saved
1.	Substitution of dry toast for	45
	Bread with butter and jam	+40
2.	Omission of ghee from chapatis	180
3.	Omission of sugar	120
4.	Omission of biscuits	100
5.	Substitution of toned milk for dry milk	65
6.	Reducing the number of chapattis to 3 at each meal	190
6.	Substitution of low-calorie vegetables for potatoes	60
	Total	800

Many or all of these changes can be made depending on the degree of weight reduction desired. The bulk of the diet can be increased by adding more of fruits and vegetables low in calories.

The general approach should be to cut down or avoid concentrated sources of calories such as foods rich in fat and sugar.

Many people are unable to avoid sugar in tea and coffee and have, in addition, a craving for sweets. One can cultivate a taste for plain dilute tea without sugar, especially if it is flavoured with orange peel and the like, as suggested earlier. Saccharine has been used as a sweetening agent and its acceptability in beverages is enhanced if it is combined with half a teaspoon of sugar. But the excessive use of saccharine is considered undesirable and should be avoided (It is banned in Canada).

Subjects trying to lose weight by dieting may get discouraged first as the tissue loss may be replaced by water initially. Also, weighing too frequently is not likely to be encouraging.

A period of prolonged fasting (often 40 days or more) has been tried with some obese subjects successfully. Complete fasting has the advantage that after the first two or three days, hunger pangs virtually disappear. Also, the weight losses are more rapid and, therefore, reassuring to the subject. Generally, obese people are not found to develop ketosis during fasting. Nevertheless, such prolonged fasting is generally carried out under medical supervision. This is particularly necessary for people with other complications. Restricting the diet is considered better in the long run. Complete fasting once or twice a week has also been tried successfully by some people. Incidentally, in this country, particularly in Gujarat, some Jains observe complete fasting for a period of 30–40 days as part of their religious practice without any ill-effects being apparent although they lose weight as may be expected.

The weight lost during fasting by an obese person is easily gained back unless the diet following the period of fasting is carefully controlled.

Deficiency of vitamin A

As mentioned earlier, common diets in this country are deficient in both carotene and vitamin A.

The chief symptoms of deficiency are night blindness and poor dark light adaptation, dull lusterless eyes and dryness, first of the conjunctiva, and then of the cornea (xerophthalmia). The former is due to the deposit of a light brown substance called keratin on the epithelial surfaces. The invasion of this substance over the cornea which is normally transparent may result in the formation of pigmented spots on the cornea called Bitot's spots (see plate) (these spots may also occur in the absence of vitamin A deficiency in which case treatment with vitamin A does not help). With the progress of deficiency, a film may develop over the whole of cornea resulting in the softening of the cornea. This condition is called keratomalacia. This may lead to the rupture of the cornea resulting in blindness. Keratomalacia if diagnosed must be treated promptly with massive doses of vitamin A by injection.

About 1% of the population in this country is blind and a large proportion of these unfortunate people have become blind in early childhood because of vitamin A deficiency. Even when blindness is the result of infections such as trachoma, vitamin A deficiency may be a contributory factor as the structure of the eye and resistance to infection are both affected by the same.

The disease should have been eradicated several decades ago. It is more common in rice-eating areas where the staple containing neither carotene or carotene-rich vegetables nor animal foods rich in vitamin A are consumed. Among the rice-eating areas it is more prevalent in inland areas such as Madurai than in coastal areas such as Kerala because of the consumption of at least small quantities of fish in the latter. Similar observations were made in Japan several decades ago.

The government and welfare agencies are now alive to the problem and steps are being taken to eradicate deficiency by massive oral doses of the vitamin once or twice a year. Several investigations have shown that normal vitamin A status can be maintained by the consumption of about 30 g of leafy vegetables daily by children and about 50–60 g by adults. Where this is not possible oil enriched with vitamin A so that a teaspoon provides about 300–400/microgram can be made available in villages. There is an urgent need to prevent deficiency in children and such oil should be distributed through panchayats or health centres if alternative measures are not possible.

Scurvy

Scurvy is a disease caused by a deficiency of vitamin C. The most susceptible groups used to be sailors, explorers and soldiers who had to live on diets without fresh vegetables and fruits for long periods and infants fed bottle-milk. The little vitamin C present in cow-milk is mostly destroyed during boiling.

There is an impairment of collagen formation in scurvy. The gums are swollen and there are ulcers which bleed profusely on touch. In chronic cases the teeth may become loose and fall out. Patches of subcutaneous haemorrhages can be seen in the legs, arms, abdomen and buttocks. Anaemia is prevalent in most cases. The obvious remedy is treatment with ascorbic acid and, the response is quick. Drumstick leaf, amla and guava are some of the rich sources of vitamin C. Bleeding gums may be due to factors other than vitamin C deficiency and in that case administration of vitamin C does not help and the condition needs medical attention.

Scurvy is not found either in adults or children in this country and in the latter case mainly because of breast-feeding. In adults scurvy has been found in famine areas. Scurvy has been seldom found in pregnant and lactating women anywhere in the world although one would expect some incidence as the requirements are increased and dietary intakes are low. However, in view of the several important roles played by ascorbic acid and the readiness with which it can be obtained and its possible role in iron absorption, it would seem prudent to ensure a reasonable supply in the diet.

Ariboflavinosis

As mentioned earlier, riboflavin deficiency is another common nutritional deficiency in diets lacking in animal foods, milk and leafy vegetables. Persons suffering from amoebic infections are also found to show these symptoms. A large proportion of adolescent boys and pregnant women are found to show symptoms of deficiency among the poor. An appreciable incidence is found even in the upper class perhaps because of the excessive consumption of 'empty' calories in the form of sugar and fat. As stated earlier, moderate symptoms are found to respond well to an improved diet. A severe deficiency may have to be corrected by initial supplements of riboflavin followed by an improved diet.

Beriberi

The incidence of beriberi caused by a lack of thiamine associated with exclusive consumption of highly polished rice has been discussed earlier. It is also associated with excessive consumption of either refined flour or alcohol. A deficiency in the maternal diet leads to infantile beriberi in the breast-fed infant. Beriberi may be associated with oedema (wet beriberi) or dehydration (dry beriberi). With moderate deficiency in the diets the symptoms found include:

loss of appetite, vomiting, constipation, mental depression and vague fears. With more severe deficiency, soreness and weakness of the muscle, loss of muscle tone, specially in the calf muscle, poor limb co-ordination, loss of sensitivity to touch and temperature, stinging and crawling sensations, difficulty in squatting on the floor and dizziness on getting up, and finally foot drops and paralysis of the lower limb, may occur.

Other symptoms are shortness of breath, irregular heart beat, palpitation, especially after exercise, slow pulse and quickening after exertion, enlargement of the heart and ECG changes.

The symptoms in infantile beriberi include vomiting, restlessness and sleeplessness. Running pulse, difficulty in breathing and cyanosis are found in acute deficiency and sudden death may result. In chronic and sub-acute deficiency, poor food intake, vomiting, oedema, wasting, constipation, excessive urination, neck retraction, puffiness of the face, abdominal pain and aphonia (crying without sound) are found. Convulsions may also occur.

A high prevalence of beriberi was found in Andhra Pradesh till the 1950's, For instance in 1938, the incidence was 32717 in the northern circars (districts) as against 649 in the rest of the then Madras State. Mortality figures were 64 and 4 respectively and population 13.9 and 32.9 million. A similar difference in incidence was found as late as 1949.

In studies carried out in Andhra during 1935–39 peak incidence of infant mortality occurring between birth and 12 months of age was found between 2–5 months. Thiamine deficiency is likely to have been a contributory factor.

Pellagra

Although pellagra has been reported in association with maize consumption in the West and with jowar consumption in Andhra Pradesh, it is relatively rare.

Although pellagra has been found in association with maize consumption in the West it is rare among the Bhils living on maize or jowar in Gujarat and Madhya Pradesh. The urinary excretion of N' Methyl Nicotinamide which is considered as an index of niacin status is also in the normal range although the excretion of the metabolite is reported to be enhanced in some pellagrins because of impaired synthesis of nicotinamide derivatives. Very occasionally "butterfly patches" are seen on the face. However pellagra has been reported in Hyderabad in people consuming maize and jowar. It would seem desirable to supplement maize and jowar with legumes as such supplementation improves the protein quality of the grain which is linked to the etiology of pellagra, as described earlier.

Nutritional anaemia

The incidence of anaemia is quite high in this country even in the upper classes particularly among young children and women during the reproductive period. Anaemia is highly prevalent even among the men in rural areas because of hook worm infestation. The Bhils Subsisting on maize are found to show a higher incidence perhaps because of the low iron content of maize as compared to other grains.

Although the infant at birth is born with adequate stores of iron, these are largely used up in the first six months and thereafter the child becomes anaemic if the diet does not include enough iron. Infants born of anaemic mothers are found to become anaemic much earlier. Breast-milk contains twice as much iron as bottle-milk so that bottle-fed infants need even more of supplements.

It has also been suggested that excess of calcium in the diet interferes with the absorption of iron. Cow-milk and buffalo-milk contain 120 and 210 mg of calcium per litre as against 30 mg in human milk. Anaemia is more common in young children who are brought up on milk and biscuits rather than in those consuming a mixed diet.

The excessive intake of milk in conditions such as ulcers is also sometimes found to be associated with anaemia. Anaemia may be caused by a deficiency of either iron, protein or B-vitamins such as folic acid and vitamin B12. The symptoms are pallor of the mucus membrane, poor appetite and fatigue, shortness of breath, and panting on even slight exertion.

Most cases of anaemia in this country are found to be of the hypochromic variety and respond to treatment with ferrous sulphate. An overall improvement of the diet is necessary. If the anaemia is of complex origin, treatment with iron, B-vitamins, and vitamin C along with liberal intakes of protein is called for. Some iron preparations contain copper and cobalt but there is no evidence that the ordinary diet is lacking in these nutrients. However, when the deficiency is purely due to lack of iron there is no point in giving complex preparations containing vitamins as the cost is increased 5–10 times by such additions. Several studies in this country have shown that treatment with iron salts such as ferrous sulphate is found to be as effective as administration of the same along with vitamins.

Anaemia found in conditions such as asthma, rheumatism and pathological blood loss is not generally due to iron deficiency although the same could be a contributory factor. In these conditions, the red blood cells undergo rapid destruction and the reutilization of the iron released during the process for haemoglobin synthesis is not efficient. Such patients may have more than adequate stores of iron in the tissues.

As hookworm or other parasite infection is often a contributory factor for the deficiency of iron, the stools should be examined and the patient treated if necessary. However, the subject becomes reinfested again if there is no improvement of environmental hygiene. Administration of extra iron is found to compensate for the adverse effects of hookworm infestation.

Pathological blood loss and organic disease and conditions such as rheumatism and asthma are associated with anaemia. This appears to be so because the rate at which blood cells are destroyed is faster than that at which new cells are synthesized.

Lathyrism

Lathyrism is associated with the excessive consumption of the legume kesari dal or *Lathyrus sativus*. The disease starts with weakness of the lower limbs. The movements at the ankle and knee joints become painful. The patient assumes a peculiar posture and stiff gait because the joints are held in a partially flexed position. With the progress of the disease the foot becomes inverted and the patient tends to walk on toes. Soon the patient is unable to walk without crutches (see plate). Ultimately the knees become completely flexed and the patient is unable to stand or walk. In some cases the onset may be sudden.

The severe cases are not found to respond to a good diet. The milder cases take many months. In the areas where the legume is consumed exaggerated knee and ankle reflexes in children and awkward gait while running are quite common.

Goitre

The incidence and aetiology of goitre resulting from hypothyroidism have been described earlier. The distribution of salt or other commodities such as bread or oil enriched with iodine has been advocated and attempted. In the U.S.A. all the common salt sold in the market is iodised. However, more and more people are doing less and less cooking at borne with the increase in the availability of pre-cooked foods. Food manufacturers do not always use iodised salt.

In Tasmania, the enrichment of bread with iodine was not found to eradicate the condition altogether as obese women on reducing diets do not eat any bread.

In this country the distribution of iodised salt has been attempted but only about 25% of the people in susceptible areas seem to be covered. It is necessary to expand the facilities for the production of iodised salt and distribute only iodised salt in areas where goiter is prevalent. Alternatively, other commodities should be iodised, but in this country this may be more difficult. Potassium iodate rather than iodide is preferred as the former is more stable. There is an urgent need to take preventive and remedial measures. Pregnant women, young children and school children need special attention as the development of children may be permanently affected with deficiency in the diet of the mother or in that consumed by the child after birth.

Apart from the Himalayan regions and Assam, small pockets of goitre areas are also found in other regions such as Gujarat.

Fluorosis

As mentioned earlier, excessive amounts of fluorine in the diet or drinking water are toxic and may cause gastroenteritis, nephritis and liver damage. Consumption of moderately high amounts for prolonged periods may result in changes in the teeth and skeleton. With mild fluorosis the teeth become 'mottled'. The enamel loses its lustre and becomes chalky white. This may be followed by brown pigmentation and mottling especially in the incisors of the upper jaw. The condition is found in children usually after eruption of permanent teeth.

Adults who have been living in the region for several years may develop skeletal abnormalities. The first symptom to appear is a tingling sensation all over the body followed by pain and stiffness in the lower regions of the spine. Gradually, the back becomes rigid and the patient loses his ability to bend or turn his head. As the disease progresses during the course of 5–10 years other joints are also affected. As the thorax becomes rigid, abdominal breathing is found. There is progressive loss of appetite and general wasting.

X-ray examination of these cases reveals increased bone density and decrease in the medullary cavity. This may be because, with excessive fluorine, the hydroxyapatite crystals of bone are replaced by fluorapatite crystals which are less readily eroded by osteoclasts. It will be recalled that bone mineral as well as matrix are continually broken down by the osteoclasts and new bone is formed. The balance between these processes is disturbed with excess fluorine resulting in the above abnormalities. The condition is called osteofluorosis. The calcification of normally uncalcified areas of the bone and bony growths are found.

Osteofluorosis has been found in areas such as Nalgonda district in Andhra Pradesh where water contains as much as 11 ppm of fluorine. It has also been reported in the Punjab. Normally, fluorosis is expected only when the fluorine content of water exceeds 5-6 ppm. However, in some endemic areas the fluorine content of water is well below this. The addition of calcium salts or milk powder to the diets of rats fed excess fluorine is found to protect against the development of the condition to some extent. Manual work performed under excessively hot conditions is also suspected to be a pre-disposing condition.

Ascorbic acid has been reported to be beneficial in the treatment of fluorosis and this should be more thoroughly investigated. It seems necessary to defluorinate drinking water in endemic areas. A defluoridation plant has been established in Guntakal. The process is not expensive and yet the expansion of such facilities to other places is yet to be achieved. This approach may also be difficult where drinking water is derived from a number of private wells scattered all over the place. Defluoridation is done by filtering the water through a layer of activated carbon.

Diseases of the skin

Dry and rough skin is very common in young children belonging to the poor families, particularly in the South India. The elasticity of the skin is diminished. This has been attributed to vitamin A deficiency but a dietary deficiency of fat has also been implicated. The poor South Indian diet based on rice is low in fat content as well as essential fatty acids. It is not found in areas such as Malabar where the practice of massaging the skin with vegetable oil is followed. Infantile eczema is found in south India and this may be due to a deficiency of essential fatty acids, as the poor rice diet is low in fat.

Ulcers (boils) in the skin are also found to be more common among poor children in the South. This could be due to a combination of dietary factors and infections. Phrynoderma (or toad skin) is a condition in which the roots of hair follicles become plugged with deposits of keratin. As a result the skin looks horny and hyper pigmented particularly around the elbow and knee joints.

The disease has been found to be associated with vitamin A deficiency in East Africa and Sri Lanka. In this country, the condition is found to respond to treatment with vegetable oil rather than vitamin A suggesting that EFA deficiency may be involved. Treatment with a combination of oil and yeast gave better results suggesting that a deficiency of B-vitamins may also be a contributory factor. People with phrynoderma are more often found to show symptoms of riboflavin deficiency but not those of vitamin A deficiency.

In this connection, some differences have been found between hyper follicular keratosis caused by EFA and vitamin A deficiencies. In the former, the deposits well as the sebaceous glands (glands secreting 'oil') are enlarged.

Chapter 23

Modification of the Normal Diet in Selected Conditions

The normal diet needs to be modified in disorders of nutritional, metabolic or bacterial origin. For instance in diabetes, the amount of carbohydrates should be reduced. The cost of the diet recommended must be consistent with the amount of money spent by the family on food. It must provide enough variety within a framework so that it does not become monotonous. It is better to give the patient a list of foods permitted and those to be avoided so that he can choose a variety for himself. It is important for the patient to understand the principles governing the advice given. The advice given in the case of diabetes or obesity for instance should be in quantitative terms. There is no point in asking a diabetic patient to avoid rice and take wheat without specifying quantities Fifty grams of rice combined with 50 g of meat or fish or chicken contain more protein than 100 g of wheat.

The advice given should be tailored to the individual needs of the patient. An estimate must be made of his calorie requirement from data on height, weight, daily routine, food consumed and recent weight changes if any along with brief medical and dietary history. His likes and dislikes regarding foods must be recorded. It is also advisable to get routine data on blood pressure, haemoglobin content of blood and where possible sugar and serum cholesterol, particularly, for conditions such as diabetes, obesity, etc.

The patient must be followed up and difficulties if any tackled. An evaluation of the diet is also helpful. We shall now consider the principles governing the dietary management of different diseases and how they can be applied to diets commonly consumed in this country.

Diabetes mellitus

The basic defect in diabetes mellitus is a disorder of carbohydrate metabolism caused by a lack of insulin. Insulin is synthesized by specialized cells (beta cells) of the pancreas and a damage to these cells results in impaired synthesis of insulin. The disease may occur in early life in which case it must be attributed generally to hereditary factors. Pancreatic damage in early life because of severe malnutrition has also been implicated. Where the onset of the disease is in middle years, dietary factors, overweight and a sedentary life may all be involved in addition to a familial disposition to the disease.

Since the major disorder in diabetes is one of carbohydrate metabolism, the intake of carbohydrate is restricted. A high protein, low carbohydrate diet is recommended. It has been considered desirable to have carbohydrate and protein in the ratio 2:1 but it is found difficult to achieve this ratio with diets based on vegetable sources and a ratio 3:1 or even 3.5:1 seems a more practicable goal. In Japan a good response has been obtained with diets containing more carbohydrates than are usually recommended in western diets if the carbohydrates are in the form of complex starches which are digested more slowly and result in a slower elevation of blood sugar levels. A practical goal is to cut down carbohydrate to a minimum and to provide this carbohydrate in the form of complex starches. It would be best to avoid sugar.

Among the cereals, whole wheat is preferable to rice, not only because it contains more protein, but also because it contains a hypoglycemic factor, namely, chromium. Also wheat starch is more complex than rice starch.

In the choice of foods to be included in the diabetic diet we are concerned not only with the protein content of the diet but also the percentage of calories derived from protein and the ratio of carbohydrate to protein. Data on protein content and % protein calories in food groups were presented earlier (Table 3). Some additional data on the carbohydrate-protein ratio in selected foods are shown in **Table 60**. It can be seen from the same that foods such as leafy vegetables, no starchy vegetables, animal foods, milk, groundnut and legume are more suitable for inclusion in the diabetic diet. Many cereal dishes can be modified so as to contain more protein and less carbohydrate by using a combination of cereal and legume in place of cereal alone.

Diabetes is often found to be associated with other conditions such as blood pressure, obesity, hypercholesterolemia and cardiovascular disease. The diet must take care of the requirements of these conditions as well. Although a liberal amount of fat is permitted in the diabetic diet it is better if the major part of the fat is derived from vegetable oils high in

Table 60. Carbohydrate-protein ratio of selected foods.

Grams of carbohydrate per g of protein	Selected foods
negligible	Meat, fish, liver, chicken and egg
1-2	Nuts and oilseeds, milk, leafy vegetables, cauliflower, drumstick
2-5	Kopra, low-calorie vegetables, legumes, cereal-legumes mixtures
5-10	Most cereals and millets, beets, radish, onions
above 10	Rice, most roots and tubers, starchy vegetables, fruits

polyunsaturated fatty acids as the condition is often associated with high levels of cholesterol in blood. For the same reason, fish and chicken are to be preferred to meat and eggs. If the patient is overweight some restriction of calories is called for. If he also suffers from high blood pressure, a restriction of sodium is necessary. As exercise stimulates the production of insulin, a diabetic patient should remain as active as possible.

The diet consumed by a selected subject ordinarily and the diet recommended is shown **in Tables 61 and 62.**

Hypercholesterolemia

Although a high level of cholesterol in blood is by itself nothing to worry about, most nutritionists believe that it is desirable to control the level of cholesterol in blood because of its association with heart diseases, specially if the subject is also overweight.

Cholesterol is formed in several tissues but the major site is the liver and the cholesterol in blood is derived from the same. Blood levels are usually elevated because of increased synthesis in the liver, but this may be the case even when the liver concentration is normal. Free cholesterol is a solid insoluble in water. Fatty acids can combine with cholesterol to form cholesterol esters. The excess cholesterol in the body is secreted into the intestine via the bile in the form of cholesterol esters. Cholesterol esters formed from unsaturated fatty acids are more readily transported than free cholesterol and more readily eliminated via the intestine. Part of the cholesterol in blood is in the form of its ester. When the blood contains an excess of cholesterol, particularly, free cholesterol, it forms deposits along with calcium salts in the soft tissues including the blood vessels and forms a crust. This results in the hardening of arteries and a diminution of the elasticity, a condition called arteriosclerosis. Sometimes the smooth inner lining of the arteries degenerates in patches and this is followed by the deposition of fatty materials including cholesterol and calcium salts. The patches spread and weaken the blood vessels (atherosclerosis) and may result in the formation of a clot (coronary thrombosis) which blocks the

Table 61. Diet consumed by a diabetic person.

Age-65 years Height-163 cm Estimate of energy expenditure-1700 kcalories Fasting blood sugar-234 mg per 100 ml Total serum cholesterol-345 mg per 100ml Esterified cholesterol-63 mg per 100 ml	Sex-male Weight -60kg
Diet consumed	
Early morning	1 cup coffee (with saccharine)
Breakfast	Poora or dosa or idli (2) with ghee or oil (10g) and coconut chutney (1 table spoon of grated coconut), 1 cup coffee (with saccharine)
Lunch	Cracked wheat (100 g)
	Sambar (1 cup) (dal, 15 g)
	Vegetable curry(100 g)
	Pickles (1 teaspoon)
	Curd (180 g)
Evening tea	1 cup tea (with saccharine)
	Some snacks such as biscuits, bhajya, dahivada (one serving)
6.30 p.m.	1 cup coffee (with saccharine)
Dinner	Chapatis (3)
	Dal (1 cup 15 g)
	Vegetable curry (60–70g veg.)
	Pickle (1 teaspoon)
	Ghee (1 teaspoon)
	Curd (120 g)

Composition of diet		*Approximate nutritive value*	
Cereals	300 g	kcals	1800
Pulses	50–60 g	Carbohydrate (g)	280
Vegetables	200 g	Protein (g)	60
Milk	600 g	Carbohydrate/protein	4.7:1
Oil or ghee	30 g		

flow of blood to or from the heart. This may result in damage to parts of the heart tissue deprived of a proper blood supply (ischaemic heart disease or myocardial infarction). Although the aetiology of heart disease is complex, it is considered advisable for persons prone to heart disease or with familial incidence of the same to maintain normal levels of serum cholesterol. The

Table 62. Modification of diet described in table 61.

Revised diet		Nutritive value	
Cereals + pulses	300 g	kcals	1700
Leafy vegetables	100 g	Carbohydrate (g)	270
Other low- calorie vegetables	150–200 g	Protein(g)	75
Toned, malai removed or skimmed milk	600 g	Carbohydrate/protein	3.6:1
Low calorie fruit	200 g		
Oil	30 g		

level of cholesterol may be elevated in a variety of conditions including excessive consumption of sugar and fat, specially saturated fat, obesity, psychological tension, a high protein intake, sedentary living, etc.

Aim of therapy

In view of high blood sugar and high serum cholesterol, to reduce the intake of carbohydrate and saturated fats.

Modifications suggested

1. Substitute wheat + legume in the ratio 1:1 or 2:1 in the preparation of cereal dishes. Use cereal-legume combinations such as debra, pongal, khichri.
2. Use malai removed, toned or skimmed milk in place of whole milk.
3. Substitute til oil for ghee.
4. Reduce the consumption of coconut.
5. Omit starchy fruits and vegetables and increase the intake of leafy vegetables.

Studies suggest that an excess of saturated fats increases the liver and serum levels of cholesterol whereas other studies suggest that excess of any fat has a similar result. It would appear that both the amount and type of fat are critical factors and it would, therefore, be prudent to cut down fat and use only fats which are highly unsaturated. Til oil, safflower oil and corn oil are found to be better than groundnut oil. It is considered desirable to avoid or cut down ghee and hydrogenated fat.

Excessive intake of sugar, coffee and alcohol as well as cigarette smoking are also associated with increased levels of serum cholesterol.

Although cholesterol is formed in the body even when the diet contains no cholesterol, foods containing cholesterol such as eggs are found to increase serum cholesterol levels. Similarly, animal foods rich in saturated fat such as mutton and eggs should be avoided as much as possible. Chicken which does not contain much fat, and fish, which has a lot of unsaturated fats are preferable. As milk contains a lot of saturated fat, it should be better to use toned or skimmed, or malai-removed milk.

Foods rich in cellulose and pectin (fruits and vegetables) are found to reduce serum cholesterol levels by preventing its absorption from the intestine. Turmeric contains curcumin which is helpful for decreasing serum cholesterol levels*. In animal studies addition of turmeric even at the level used in cooking is found to do so. About 1/4 teaspoon of turmeric powder can be added to a cup of boiling milk. Its acceptability can be enhanced by flavouring with nutmeg, saffron, cloves or cardamom. Alternatively, fresh turmeric can also be consumed in other ways as suggested earlier.

Similarly, bengal gram, onions and garlic are reported to lower serum cholesterol levels. It must also be remembered that a healthy active person may eat all the cholesterol-forming foods in plenty and still maintain normal levels. Pastoral tribes living in mountains and consuming enormous quantities of milk do not have high levels of serum cholesterol, but such people are active and do not consume much of pure fats, refined sugar, coffee, etc. Sedentary living and obesity also seem to be responsible.

In summary, it would be better for persons with high levels of serum cholesterol to cut down coffee, sugar, alcohol, cigarettes and saturated fats and to increase the consumption of bengal gram, fruits and vegetables and include,in the diet as much turmeric as possible. Exercise and maintaining normal body weight are also important.

Diseases of the digestive system

Inflammation of the intestine

This may result from frequent attacks of bacillary dysentery. Ulceration of the colon (ulcerative colitis) also occurs due to streptococcal and tubercular infections. Intestinal parasites such as *Entamoeba histolytica* and hookworms may also cause inflammation. When the inflammation is severe, the function of the small intestine and consequently absorption are also affected. Both the structure and function of the liver may be impaired.

The first step obviously is to treat for infections if present after careful stool analysis. The dietary problem is one of including only those foods which do not leave much roughage, i.e., foods low in fibre content. Selected foods classified as low, medium and high fibre content are shown in **Table 63**. Those of medium fibre content can be included in moderation whereas those of high fibre content should be avoided.

---

* Aggarwal A., A. Kumar, M.S. Aggarwal and S. Shishodia. 2005. In Phytochemicals in Cancer Chemoprevention,p. 350. CRC Press, LLC.

Table 63. The fibre content of selected foods.

Fibre content (g per 100 g)	Selected foods
nil or negligible	milk and milk products, flesh foods and poultry fats and oils sugar, jaggery and honey, sago, arrowroot flour
0-1	rice, suji, maida, dals, most leafy vegetables, ash gourd, bitter ground, calabash cucumber cucumber, giant chillies, pumpkin, ridge ground tomatoes apple, banana, lichis, mango, orange, melon, papaya, pears and plums
1-2	bajra, jowar, maize, wheat flour, colocasia, coriander, mint leaves, carrots, pink bean, brinjal, broad bean cauliflower, French bean, ladies fingers, green mango, lime, peach phalsa
3–5	ragi, whole legumes, charoli and ground nut, cluster, bean, double bean, parwar, peas and wood apple.
Above	barley, kodri, kopra, figs, guava, pomegranate

When the inflammation is acute, only liquid foods such as milk, buttermilk, sago conjee, etc., which do not leave much residue should be given. Solid foods including fruits and vegetables low in fibre content can be gradually included. The latter can be provided in the form of soups and juices. Frequent meals or beverages may be better than loading the stomach at meal time.

Diarrhea

The above treatment is also appropriate for the treatment of diarrhea. The replacement of milk by curd or buttermilk is found to help. The curd should be prepared at home from boiled milk in order to avoid bacterial contamination. Boiled and cooled water should be used in the preparation of buttermilk. Fenugreek seeds are beneficial in the treatment of diarrhea according to Ayurveda and this is confirmed by experience. Their action could be due to the mucilage in them which forms a 'gel' with water and may thus reduce intestinal irritation. A teaspoon of the seeds can be chewed and swallowed along with curd. They are bitter but the bitterness is not felt if taken along with curd. Alternatively they can be roasted, powdered and added to buttermilk and soups and broth. The skin of the pomegranate fruit dried and powdered can be similarly used. It is considered desirable to avoid very hot or cold foods.

Some people develop diarrhea with emotional stress. Defecation is common in experimental animals placed in strange surroundings.

Chronic diarrhea is sometimes found in women following menopause suggesting the possible role of hormonal factors.

Constipation

Constipation or irregular evacuation of bowels resulting in the accumulation of fecal matter in the intestine may be due to several causes. Not having formed the habit of evacuation at a particular time regularly is one of the chief causes. Foods of low roughage content, poor muscular tone of the rectum, excessive absorption of water from the rectum resulting in the formation of hard stools, inflammation at the anus caused by hard stools which inhibits expulsion of the feces may be responsible and these factors may occur in association with one another.

Formation of regular habits, liberal intake of water, vegetables and fruits combined with sufficient exercise should help. Psychological tension may be a contributory factor. A relaxed state seems to be necessary for normal bowel function.

Ulcers of the stomach and duodenum

The basic reason for development of ulcers in the gastrointestinal tracts is infection due to the bacteria *Helicobacter pylori**. However, there are aggravating dietary factors which have to be controlled in the management of this disease. The walls of the stomach secrete gastric juice which contains hydrochloric acid. Normally, the amount of acid is not large enough to have a corrosive action on the walls of the stomach which, are moreover protected by the mucous membrane. With excess secretion of acid, however, this defense may fail and ulcers may begin to form on the walls of the stomach, resulting in bleeding, pain and poor appetite. If not treated, it may even lead to cancer.

The consumption of tapioca diets is associated with a greater incidence of ulcers than that of rice in animals. This may be due to the low protein content of tapioca as the walls of the stomach are found to become thin in protein deficiency. In Andhra, ulcers are widely prevalent in the lower classes and much less so in the upper classes although both groups take liberal amounts of chillies which are irritant and stimulate gastric secretion. The diet of the upper classes contains more legumes, milk and fat than that of the poor and the resulting difference in the fat and protein content of the diet could be responsible for this difference.

It would seem, therefore, that two factors are involved, namely, the integrity of the walls of the stomach and the secretion of hydrochloric acid. A diet adequate in protein content is necessary for the former.

The secretion of hydrochloric acid is increased by spices, tobacco, coffee, tea and alcohol. Meats also have a stimulating effect on gastric secretion whereas fats have a depressing effect. Foods which stimulate gastric secretion should be restricted or avoided. A bland diet is called for.

---

* Bacterial infection of Helicobacter pylori **missing text** ministering appropriate antibiotics along ith dietary intervention in the **missing text** of ulcer of stomach and ducdenum.

The high intake of chillies and spices is often necessitated because of the need to achieve satiety on monotonous and ill balanced diets consisting mainly of rice or roti. A better balance and more variety in the diet should help cut down the intake of spices to more judicious levels. Because of the paucity of suitable weaning diets, the infant in this country first struggles against and then adapts itself to the high spice content of the diet and gradually acquires a permanent taste for it. Practical demonstrations can be given in Mahila Mandals and like organizations on the preparation of simple but varied and appetizing meals at low cost and the women educated in the judicious use of spices.

Business executives and others in similar positions are often found to suffer from ulcers. This is believed to be due to excess acid secretion because of psychological tension associated with the constant making of decisions and meeting of deadlines.

The acidity gives a burning sensation which is relieved by the ingestion of milk, buttermilk, or other suitable food like coconut milk. Fresh buttermilk which is not sour is found to relieve acidity more rapidly than milk and can be taken more frequently. In severe ulcers, the patient should be put on a liquid diet consisting of milk or cream or egg. Coconut water has been found to reduce gastric acidity.

The treatment of ulcers or hyperacidity in the presence of hypercholesterolemia presents problems as the liberal consumption of whole milk will increase the content of saturated fats in the diet. Skimmed milk on the other hand does not have the same soothing effect. In such cases, skim milk can be mixed with soya milk or with the milk or paste of poppy seeds, charoli or almonds so that the resulting mixture contains a 'normal' fat content but is low in saturated fatty acids.

Many ulcer patients are also obese and their dietary management presents problems as they need some fat in the diet because of ulcers and need to reduce it because of their obesity. Treatment with alkalis may be a solution.

Soluble alkalis are absorbed and combine with calcium to form insoluble salts which are deposited in the kidney and cornea of eyes. The condition is referred to as milk-alkali syndrome which is not generally found when either is used alone. If alkali treatment is combined with liberal consumption of milk, alkalis such as aluminium hydroxide which are not absorbed should be used. They should be taken an hour or so after meals rather than immediately after as the contents of the stomach reach their maximum acidity at about this time. This will prevent the destruction of vitamins owing to the presence of alkali.

Rarely, excessive intake of soluble alkalis is found to result in other undesirable effects such as alkalosis, weakness, lethargy and psychological disturbances.

It is believed that foods rich in pectin such as jams and jellies may have a soothing effect. Coarse and indigestible foods are to be avoided.

Bed rest is found to help in the treatment of acute ulcers. Sedatives and tranquillizers are sometimes used as they make the patient more relaxed. Drugs such as belladonna which inhibit the secretion of pepsin and hydrochloric acid are also used. They decrease the motility of the stomach which is desirable because rapid movements in the stomach may aggravate the ulcers as excessive contractions force the food to exert pressure against the walls of the stomach. However, they may have other undesirable side effects.

Gastritis

Inflammation of the stomach is also found, usually in association with either ulcers or cancer of the stomach. This may also be due to infection and ingestion of toxic factors. Appropriate treatment with antibiotics needs to be given for infection. The dietary management should be as in ulcers.

Disease of the liver

The liver has important functions including the production of bile, storage of glycogen, iron and vitamins and their release as needed. It is an active metabolic site which carries out the synthesis and transformation of many body compounds. For instance, amino acids are deaminated and converted to organic acids which can be used for respiratory purposes. Glycerol is converted to glucose and vice-versa. Nonessential amino acids are formed from other amino acids or products of glucose metabolism. One of its most important functions is the conversion of substances, which will prove toxic if they accumulate in the blood or body in excessive amounts, into products which can be excreted via the urine or gut. The end products of nitrogen metabolism such as ammonia will prove toxic if they are not eliminated through the kidneys after suitable transformation by the liver.

When the liver is damaged, which may happen because of malnutrition, bacterial or viral infections or ingestion of toxic substances, some of these functions may be affected resulting in serious impairment of body functions. Excessive consumption of alcohol is also a contributory factor. Fortunately, liver cells regenerate quickly and the damage done can be reversed in most cases. For this regeneration, a careful dietary management is necessary.

In conditions such as severe protein malnutrition, there is an excessive deposit of fat in the liver referred to as fatty infiltration of the liver. Such fatty infiltration can also be caused by chemical poisons and it can be prevented or reduced by choline and methionine. Fatty infiltration in protein malnutrition may be due to a deficiency of methionine resulting from the low protein content and poor protein quality of the diet.

In some cases, fatty infiltration is followed by a degeneration of the liver cells, a condition described as necrosis. Sometimes these cells are replaced by fibrous scar tissue, resulting in cirrhosis of the liver. In many areas of the world where fatty infiltration of the liver is common, cirrhosis is also common and vice-versa. However, high prevalence of either without the other is found in a few areas. Cirrhosis of the liver without such heavy infiltration and arising from non-nutritional factors is found in young children in Tamil Nadu and other areas.

It is not surprising that liver disease is much more common in the tropical countries of Asia and Africa as factors favouring the same such as protein malnutrition, food adulteration and poor environmental hygiene are all present.

Bile is produced by the liver and stored in the gall bladder. The production of bile is impaired in serious liver damage. The secretion of bile into the gut may be prevented by the formation of cholesterol stones which block the entrance to the gall bladder. In both conditions, the accumulation of bile or bile salts in the blood results in a condition known as jaundice. The latter condition can be treated surgically by removing the stone. Treatment of the former condition depends on the regeneration of the liver.

Hepatic coma may result from the accumulation of end products of nitrogen metabolism when they are not detoxified by the liver. The subject is confused and semi-conscious.

Agents such as sulphonamides, arsenic, phosphorus, and bacterial poisons or contaminants such as heavy metals present in food also seriously impair liver function. Treatment should be in the form of antibiotics or antitoxins, if necessary. In acute damage a high carbohydrate diet with moderate protein (20–30 g) is necessary. Frequent feedings in the form of beverages and fruit juices containing glucose or sugar may be necessary as the appetite is poor and there may be a tendency for nausea and vomiting. In sub-acute conditions and in chronic disease a diet adequate in calories, protein and vitamins is necessary. A restriction of fat intake to about 20–30 g seems desirable. Milk fat is better tolerated as it is present in highly emulsified form. Supplements of both fat-soluble and water-soluble vitamins should be given, if necessary. The protein content of milk can be increased by adding extra skim milk powder or preparations of protein hydrolysates and concentrates. In both acute and sub-acute phases of the disease, the meals must be made as appetizing and attractive as possible to counteract the effects of anorexia and nausea. Beverages can be given between meals.

Although administration of choline or methionine has been found to help in the treatment of cirrhosis, when the diet is adequate in protein content and quality, this is not necessary.

Renal disease

The kidney is composed of microscopic structures called nephrons which are composed of glomeruli and tubules. It plays a vital function by eliminating waste products of protein and purine metabolism. The elimination is done efficiently and against a concentration gradient. For instance, urea is expelled against a concentration gradient as its concentration in urine is higher than that of blood. Similarly, several blood constituents are held against a concentration gradient.

The level of blood constituents has to exceed a certain limit in order for the substances to be excreted into the urine. This level is referred to as renal threshold. For instance, unless the level of glucose in blood exceeds about 170 mg/100 ml it is not excreted in the urine. The normal concentration of glucose in blood is far below this so that no glucose is lost through the urine. Ordinarily the composition of blood varies only within certain limits and substances such as protein and sugar are not found in urine. Thus, kidney function enables the body to maintain a stable composition of plasma. The renal threshold is affected in kidney disease.

Metabolic functions can take place normally only when the blood is neither acidic nor markedly alkaline. Conditions such as excessive accumulation of keto acids can result in acidosis. Other conditions can result in alkalosis. However, both these conditions are very rare as the kidney helps in maintaining acid-alkali balance. When the blood tends to become acidic, it produces ammonia which combines with the acids so that the excess acidity is neutralized. When the blood tends to become alkaline it converts $NaHPO4$ which is alkaline to $NaH2P04$ which is acidic. This results in a reduction in the alkalinity of the blood. The regulation of acid-alkali balance may be affected in kidney disease leading to acidosis or alkalosis.

The diffusible substances in plasma are filtered by the glomeruli in the kidney and most of them reabsorbed from the renal tubule with elimination of only the unwanted waste material such as urea and creatinine in the form of urine from the bladder. The substances so reabsorbed include water, glucose, electrolytes, minerals, amino acids and vitamins. If 10 litres of water pass through the glomeruli about 9.8 litres are reabsorbed through the tubules. The reabsorption is more in a state of dehydration and less soon after generous intake of fluids so that the specific gravity of urine varies considerably. The specific gravity of urine ranges under ordinary circumstances from 1.020 to 1.032. However, it may be as low as 1.001 in urine excreted soon after a large quantity of water is drunk. On the other hand, if fluid intake is restricted, specific gravity may be greater than 1.032. This may also happen under hot conditions because of profuse sweating.

When the glomeruli or tubules are damaged by infection or inflammation (nephritis or damage of nephrons or kidney cells) renal function is impaired. This results in impaired function of the tubules as well.

When this happens specific gravity is around 1.010 and does not change with either fluid intake or restriction. A low specific gravity of urine may also be due to hormonal insufficiency.

The capacity of the tubules to reabsorb water is defective when there is an insufficient secretion of the antidiuretic hormone secreted by the pituitary. It results in a condition called diabetes insipidus in which the volume of urine is large and its specific gravity low. The condition is corrected by administration of the hormone.

The reabsorption of sodium and potassium is controlled by certain hormones of the adrenal cortex. When the synthesis of these hormones is impaired there may be excessive loss of potassium and retention of sodium in the tissues and fluids of the body.

The presence of protein in the urine is also an indication of kidney damage. (Normally, only the protein-free plasma is filtered by the kidney). When the inflammation is severe or other chronic symptoms appear. The loss of protein from the plasma and the fall in plasma protein to levels below 5 g per 100 ml upset the normal pressure balance between the capillaries and the surrounding fluids and results in the loss of water from the blood vessels and its accumulation in the tissues resulting in oedema. Normally, the pressure exerted by the fluids in blood on the capillary walls is balanced by the osmotic pressure of protein in plasma. It will be recalled that oedema is also present in other conditions such as kwashiorkor when the protein content of serum is decreased.

Increased blood pressure within the capillaries associated with cardiovascular diseases also results in oedema which is associated with an excessive retention of sodium in the tissues. A similar retention is found in kwashiorkor. There may be retention of phosphates and sulphates. Increased permeability of the capillary walls and the consequent abnormal flow of nutrients into urine may also result from damage to capillaries in the glomeruli because of toxic agents.

In acute nephritis the excretion of the end products of nitrogen metabolism such as urea and uric acid is impaired because of impaired filtration by the glomeruli resulting in a high concentration of urea and metabolites in blood. When the nephrons are severely damaged, they are replaced by fibrous tissue as in liver cirrhosis.

The output of urine is sometimes diminished. When it falls below a critical level there is danger of death. Sometimes the urine is found to contain blood and pus cells. Often nephritis results in increased pressure in the renal capillaries and this, in turn, leads to an elevated blood pressure in all the blood vessels. When the high blood pressure is due to damage or changes in the arteries it is called arterial hypertension and when it is due to kidney damage it is called renal hypertension.

Acute nephritis occurs more frequently in children and young adults following diseases such as tonsillitis and scarlet fever caused by streptococcal infection.

It is obvious that treatment must aim at healing the inflammation in the tissues, getting rid of the infection if present, preventing oedema and sodium retention, restoring normal protein levels in serum and restoring the acid-alkali balance. Infections if present are treated by sulpha drugs and antibiotics. When the nephritis is mild, a liberal protein intake is necessary to replace the protein lost in the urine to help the healing process.

In acute nephritis, on the other hand, kidney function is seriously impaired and a high protein intake will result in an increased formation of end products of nitrogen metabolism resulting in an extra load on the kidney. Feeding a protein-free diet will not solve the problem as in that case tissue proteins will be utilized for metabolic purposes resulting in the formation of nitrogenous constituents such as creatinine and urea. The protein intake must be regulated so that the amount equals the amount of protein that would be metabolized from the tissues if the diet were free from protein. The amount recommended is about 0.50-0.75 g per kilogram of body weight. When the condition improves, the protein content of the diet should be increased gradually. Even with a liberal protein intake it is considered desirable to restrict the consumption of meat and fish to small quantities.

Because of the decreased output of urine, it is often necessary to restrict fluid intake to prevent oedema. It is recommended that the amount of fluid consumed should be adjusted so that it is 0.5 litre more than the volume of urine excreted. This fluid can be given in the form of milk and fruit juices divided into suitable doses. No restriction of fluid intake is necessary if there is no oedema and the blood pressure is normal. In fact, liberal amounts of fluid are sometimes recommended in order to flush out by mechanical pressure the metabolites accumulating in the body. However this is a complicated affair needing treatment by an expert physician and is beyond the scope of this book.

The intake of salt is also restricted and the restriction may vary from moderate to severe according to the nature of the condition. In moderate restriction no salt is permitted at the table and only a minimum amount of salt is used in cooking; with a greater degree of restriction no salt is added during cooking and foods very rich in salt such as meat and cheese are excluded. In severe restriction, the foods permitted must be of low sodium content. Table 64 shows selected foodstuffs classified according to sodium content. Sometimes nephritis may result in the excessive loss of sodium from the body in which case the intake of salt must be liberalized. If the acidity of the urine is increased, fruits and vegetables which leave an alkaline residue should be included liberally whereas meat, fish and eggs which leave an

Table 64. Common foodstuffs as sources of sodium.

Sodium content (mg per 100g)	Foodstuffs
Less than 10	jowar, rice, kodri and maida, colocasia onion, sweet potato and yam, bitter ground brinjal, cucumber, French bean, ladies finger, parwar, peas and pumpkin, guava, orange, papaya, peaches, pears, phalsa, plums, pomegranate and chikku washed cottage cheese
10-25	bajra, barley, maize, ragi, suji, whole wheat, horse gram cabbage, potato, bitter gourd, cucumber green plantain, tomato cow and buffalo milk.
25-50	most dals and whole legumes carrot, radish, broad bean, pink bean snake gourd and tomato apple, banana, jack fruit, mango and pineapple
50-75	coriander leaves, lettuce, spinach, beet root, radish, cauliflower, tender field beans fish, meat
75-100	fenugreek, tender redgram
above 100	cowpeas, amaranth, lichi, rock melon tinned cheese, salted butter.

acid residue should be excluded. At present, however, it is usual practice to restore the acid-alkali balance by administration of soluble alkalis.

In most of these conditions bed rest is necessary. If nephritis is associated with anaemia or obesity, they should be treated by appropriate means.

As fruit juices are rich in potassium they may tend to upset the sodium-potassium balance in the body. They must be diluted and given. Diuretics are substances which increase the flow of urine. Certain, substances increase the flow of urine. Coffee, tea; cocoa and certain salts exert this effect, either by increasing filtration by glomeruli or by decreasing reabsorption from the kidneys. These are given when the urine output is diminished. Substances such as barley, water and an extract prepared from 'variyali' are reputed to have a diuretic effect. In South India, water in which parboiled rice has been boiled for a prolonged time is given.

It is evident that the dietary management of nephritis is a complicated affair. The job of the dietitian is to help plan a diet according to the dietary principles involved in the treatment as enumerated by the physician and the preferences of the patient.

Other conditions associated with uraemia

As mentioned earlier, nephritis may be associated with the accumulation of end products of nitrogen metabolism resulting in increased blood levels of urea and other compounds. This condition, referred to as uraemia, may also result from other causes such as disease of the cells in the kidney, circulatory failure, decreased blood flow to the kidneys, water and salt depletion, shock, haemorrhages, etc. It may also be due to some obstruction in the urinary tract due to stone formation preventing flow of urine. If the nephritis is due to bacterial infections, antibiotic treatment is given. A liberal amount of fluid must be consumed, if antibiotics are given. Treatment should be as in the case of acute nephritis. Kidney damage may occur with excessive consumption of toxic drugs. When treatment with sulpha drugs or antibiotics is taken for any reason, a liberal consumption of fluid is called for in order to flush them out from the body.

Gout

In conditions such as gout there is excessive accumulation of uric acid in blood. As uric acid is formed from nucleic acid metabolism, foods containing high amount of nucleic acid same are avoided, particularly glandular organs and meat. Milk, eggs and cheese, on the other hand, can be included. However, even when the diet is free from nucleic acid, they are synthesized in the body.

Urinary calculi

Substances such as calcium, oxalate, uric acid, phosphate, and carbonate are normally present in urine. They are held in solution by the colloids present in urine. Sometimes these substances combine to form insoluble salts and are excreted as small crystals. In some conditions these salts may be deposited around a nucleus in the bladder, kidney or ureter and form what is known as urinary calculi or stones. The reasons for this are not clear, but the prevalence is much higher in the undernourished areas of the world. The incidence of stone has come down in Europe with the improvement of the diet as well as public sanitation. Stones are found more often in males than in females and more often in children than in adults. Stone formation is believed to be facilitated by infections which result in lesions in the urinary tract. These may provide nuclei for stone formation.

In experimental animals, urinary calculi are produced by diets deficient in vitamin A, magnesium or pyridoxine. There is no evidence as yet that these are critical factors in man.

Disturbances in calcium metabolism associated with prolonged bed rest are also found to facilitate stone formation. Urinary calculi are found to a greater extent in regions such as Rajasthan where there is an extreme variation in daily temperatures. Mostly the stones are composed of oxalate. Excessive consumption of foods containing oxalic acid has been blamed, but oxalate is formed in the body and generally oxalic acid in foods is not absorbed. However, oxalate poisoning has been found to result from excessive consumption of foods very rich in oxalate such as green rhubarb. It would, therefore, seem prudent for those prone to kidney stones to avoid excessive intake of foods rich in oxalic acid. Some physicians impose a total ban on vegetable and fruit intake. This is neither necessary nor desirable and there are enough vegetables and fruits with a low content of oxalic acid **(Table 65)**. Since a derangement of oxalate metabolism has been found in pyridoxine and magnesium deficiencies, it would be advisable to make sure that the diets are adequate with regard to both. Plenty of fluid intake is advisable. It is also necessary to rule out infections in the urinary tract. If the stones contain uric acid or cholesterol, foods leading to the excessive formation of the same should be avoided.

Gluten-free diet

Some subjects are allergic to wheat gluten. Their diets should be free from wheat and wheat products. Restriction of gluten is necessary in celiac disease.

High protein diets

In some conditions such as convalescence after serious illness or injury, protein requirements are increased. This may be associated with an increase in calorie requirements as well, as for example, in kwashiorkor and pulmonary tuberculosis. When the activity of the patient is restricted as in the case of a patient immobilized in bed, a moderate level of protein has to be supplied while keeping the calories low. In the latter case, foods rich in protein and providing a greater percentage of protein calories (Table 3) should be included as in obesity or diabetes. In the former case, foods such as whole milk, eggs, etc., which are rich in both protein and fat, can be included in generous amount.

Table 65. Oxalic acid content of selected food.

Oxalic acid content (mg per 100 g)	Foodstuffs
Nil or negligible	rice, kodri, maida, sugi, ragi, soy bean ground nut, kopra pumpkin, grapes, oranges, papaya, mangoes cowpea pod
below 25	wheat, jowar, maize, bajra and most dals cabbage, fenugreek, carrot, onion, potato, radish, cluster beans, broad beans, cauliflower, cucumber, knoll-khol, tomato, ridge ground, tender redgram, parwar, apple, oranges, pomegranate, banana, peas, guava, pineapple, chikku, lichis watermelon.
25-100	cowpeas, elephant yam, sowasag, kankoda, field beans, radish greens, coriander leaves, French beans, beet root, brinjal, ladies finger, jackfruit, sitaphal
Above 100	til, cashew nut, almond, amaranth, curry leaves, spinah, drumstick leaves, mint, drumstick, phalsa

Part IV:
Community Nutrition

Chapter 24

Diets and Nutrition Surveys

In nutrition work, we are often concerned with making an assessment of the nutritional status of the individual or a group. Various indices serve to give us some idea of the nutritional status of an individual. These include body build, physical stature, general appearance, feeling of health and well-being, the level of activity, etc. A well-built body, a bounce in the step, sparkling eyes, clear skin and ready smile are generally associated with good health. The body measurements of an individual can be compared with expected norms, and a careful note made of his general appearance as well as that of skin, hair, eyes, mouth, tongue, nails, etc.

In the case of population groups, criteria such as general physical stature and appearance, the prevalence of deficiency symptoms, life expectancy and the incidence of low birth weights, still-births and childhood mortality serve as pointers. Whether it be an individual or a group, a careful assessment of dietary intake is needed in order to identify specific deficiencies, if any, and recommend suitable modifications if necessary.

When we are interested in the general nutritional status of a community as a whole, we try to get an idea of the overall dietary pattern and food consumption of the family. However, we may also be interested in the nutritional status of an individual or of specific groups such as young children, adolescent boys, pregnant women, elderly men, etc. In all these cases, we would need information on the food intake of particular individuals.

Different approaches have been made depending on the aim of the survey. Some of these are discussed below:

The oral survey

The most commonly used method of diet survey in a community is the 'Oral Questionnaire' method. The investigator, using this method, goes from door to door and collects information on the kind and amount of foods consumed. As a large number of families can be covered in a relatively short time, the method is suitable where quick information on the general dietary pattern in the group studied is desired. It is usual for the investigator to use a complete check list of the foods likely to be consumed and other information desired so that the recording of important information is not left to the memory of the subject. The answers orally given by the subject may not, however, be accurate as many housewives do not have reliable estimates (of, say, what a kilogram is) in terms of household measures. A more reliable practice is to get the housewife to show how much she uses and to get volume or weight measurements of the same. Another approach to the problem is for the investigator to fake a set of containers of assorted sizes and get the housewife to identify the measure corresponding to the amount she uses. It is desirable to repeat the survey after some interval to check the reliability of the data obtained at least in a few families. Where only a rapid impression of the dietary pattern prevailing in the locality is desired, a day's survey properly carried out should be enough.

The disadvantages of this method are that it relies on the reliability of the responses made by the housewife. We have found that prestige considerations often affect the responses made particularly in the middle and upper classes. To quote an instance, the average fat intake in nursing mothers was found to be about 110 g per day on the basis of the questionnaire method and 80 g per day on analysis of matched collection of the foods consumed. Similarly, figures given for the consumption of fruits etc. are often exaggerated. Generally, the same tends to be underestimated, especially in the upper classes. The author has found that cereal intakes reported for individual members of the family do not add up to the total amount consumed by the family. Similarly, items consumed which are of low prestige value such as cheaper dals and different varieties of animal foods like small fish, crabs, etc. may not be mentioned. The consumption of illicit liquor is not likely to be given out for the record for obvious reasons. Also the housewife may fail to give information on the consumption of articles like betel leaves and special varieties of ash, clay, etc., eaten by pregnant women. If these items are missed some important information is likely to be lost as their consumption may influence mineral nutrition. If the investigator is aware of the above pitfalls and uses his observation and common sense to check the information given by the housewife, without making such checking obvious, the reliability of the survey can be increased. He should also check whether the amount of different foodstuffs such as fat, sugar, and fruits claimed to be consumed is consistent with the total expenditure on food, the income of the family and the overall dietary pattern reported.

A form for use in diet surveys which would help to record information on the diets is used in the author's laboratory and is given in Appendix III.

An oral diet survey can be made more reliable by taking the following measures.

As the major sources of calories in our diet are cereals, pulses, oils and sugar, error in estimating the intakes of these results in distorted picture. Often an error in recording cereal intake creeps in when the housewife gives the amounts purchased per month or year. Generally the quantities purchased for a month do not last exactly for a month. It is better to ascertain how much grain is consumed per meal. The housewife can be asked to show the amount of flour or rice she uses at each meal and this can be measured out. If the family consumes bread, biscuits, poha, puffed rice, breakfast cereals, rava, maida, etc., these should be recorded and taken into account.

A quick check can be made of information obtained on cereal consumption. The middle and upper class families tend to consume 250–350 g per capita per day and the poor families about 400–500 g depending on the amounts of sugar, fat and milk consumed. Any marked deviation from these figures must be considered suspect unless offset by unusual intakes of other foods.

In the case of milk, the calorie value will depend on whether it is buffalo, cow or goat milk and the extent to which it is adulterated. Some idea of the extent of adulteration with water can be had by tasting a small quantity. Also it must be remembered that buffalo-milk obtained from the dairy contains only 5% fat and provides only 85 kcals per 100 g as against 8.8% fat and 117 kcals according to the food tables of ICMR. Similarly, the figures for sugar and fat can be checked from the overall dietary pattern. For instance, if the family consumes sugar only in tea and on, an average, three cups daily, sugar intake cannot be much more than 25–30 g. Likewise, the information on total fat intake can be checked against the amounts used for chapatis, dal, vegetables, etc. and the frequency with which deep fried foods are prepared. As vegetables are the chief sources of carotene in the diet, attempts should be made to ascertain how often carotene-rich vegetables such as pumpkin, carrots, kankoda and leafy vegetables are consumed. This must be translated into amounts per day. For instance, if a family of five consumes 500 g of leafy vegetables twice a week in the winter months; this means a consumption of about 30 g per capita during four months in the year or 10 g per capita per day. Failure to make this translation has resulted in fantastic figures reported even by 'authoritative' sources. For instance, one survey reports the consumption of 200 g of mangoes per capita per day by the rural poor. Ripe mangoes are available only for two months in the year and the poor families, if they are lucky, may get a kilo about once a week when in season or 7 g per day on an average. Even the total production of fruit in the country is estimated to be of the order of 50 g per day per capita and this includes other major fruits such as bananas. As most of the fruit produced is consumed by the well-to-do, the per capita availability for the rest is much less. There is a Tamil proverb which says, "If ragi (a coarse millet) is reported to be dripping with fat, what happened to the discrimination of the listener?" We have to exercise such discrimination.

The figures given for various foods must be consistent with the overall dietary pattern and expected calorie intake. For instance, if a middle class family consists of father, mother and two children aged 8 and 5 years, the calorie intakes of these people can be expected to be of the order of about 2000 for the adults and 1500 for the children so that average calorie intakes can be expected to be of the order of 1800 kcals unless the members of the family deviate markedly from the average with regard to body weight and activity level. This does not mean that calorie intakes are always according to expectation, as we have both undernutrition and over nutrition, but that the reliability of the figures obtained must be ascertained. In one study, for instance, the calorie intakes of middle class women are reported to range from about 700 to 4300. Clearly the lowest value is too low and the highest value too high for this group. Even women engaged in manual labour consume only about 2500 kcals.

If the calorie intakes suggested by the diet survey seem reasonable the survey is more likely to give us a reliable picture regarding dietary pattern. Rough estimates of calorie requirements of different groups are given in Table 9. The average value for the family can be calculated after taking into account age and sex composition and compared with the value obtained by the diet survey. A serious discrepancy calls for a checking of the calculations and a repeat survey, if necessary

A simple way of checking the figures for the major foods (cereal, pulse, sugar and fat) is to measure out known quantities of foods before the first meal of the day (or after the last meal of the previous day) and request the housewife to help herself only from these for the day's cooking. The amount left can be measured and deducted from the amounts issued and the difference taken as the amount consumed.

Similarly, the family can be asked to keep records of vegetables and fruits consumed over a period of time. We have obtained such records for an entire year in the case of some families and been able to arrive at the relative proportions in which different vegetables are consumed.

Weighment of foods

For a more reliable estimation all the foods used for cooking or consumption must be measured. The housewife can be requested either to measure out the ingredients used for cooking or to put a matched quantity in containers provided for the purpose so that the investigator can measure it out at the end of the day. Alternatively, the investigator will have to be present when the meals are being prepared. As mentioned earlier, an easier method is to take out known quantities of all the foods likely to be consumed by the family and request the housewife to help herself only from these stores for the day's cooking and to keep record of any additional food used. This can be done in the case of the major items used such as rice, dal, wheat flour, sugar, jaggery, oil and ghee. The housewife can be requested to either record the quantities of the other foodstuffs used or put away matched quantities. The amount left at the end of the day can be measured and the amount used determined. It is necessary to take into account any leftover foods not consumed during the day as well as consumption of leftovers from the previous day. To simplify the procedure, grains, sugar, fats and legumes can be issued as described whereas milk and vegetable intake can be recorded orally as in most households definite quantities of the latter are purchased and used during the day. The amounts purchased, the amounts used from the previous stores (e.g. curd, potatoes, onions) and the amount remaining at the end of the day would give us the amounts used.

Determination of dietary intake from cooked foods

The above procedure would only give the amounts used for the whole day by the whole family and not the amounts consumed by individual members of the family. For instance, in a family with four adults and a child using a litre of milk daily, 0.5 litre may be for the child and the remaining for the others so that the per capita intake of the adults in the family would actually be only 125 g and not the average value of 200 g. The family survey suffers from the drawback that it gives an idea of the total amount of different foodstuffs consumed by the family but fails to tell us about the availability of these foodstuffs to different members of the family. For instance, a family survey may show quite adequate protein intakes and yet children under 5 may be suffering from moderate or severe protein malnutrition. Also, food sharing practices prevalent in many families make it unlikely that the expectant or nursing mother gets her theoretical share of protective foods as she often feeds her family first and eats only what is left. Convalescents and the toothless aged may consume less and the head of the family more than what is available per capita. The family survey method would thus fail to give us accurate information on the adequacy or otherwise of diets consumed by groups such as children, expectant and nursing mothers, invalids and the aged.

When an individual is surveyed, he can give the information only in terms of foods as consumed. For many foods such as chapatis, rice, vegetables, etc., several households follow similar recipes so that with experience one can calculate the raw ingredients in a known amount of food without weighing before and after cooking. Some of the factors which vary from household to household are : size in the case of chapatis etc., moisture in the case of rice, dal, vegetables, milk, buttermilk, etc. and fat in the case of vegetables, dals, chapatis, etc. The investigator can make a reasonable guess about the composition of foods from their size, appearance and taste if he has first tried out different recipes of the same food. For instance, one can make chapatis of varying sizes with varying amounts of flour and fat so that it is possible to judge the composition of a chapati from its size. Similarly, softly cooked rice contains 3 parts of water to one part of rice whereas rice cooked to a more firm texture contains 2-2.5 parts. Further, different groups have different cooking practices. Poor families in Baroda make chapatis with 35–40 g of flour and no fat added whereas upper class families use 20–25 g of flour with some fat added to the dough and additional fat used as spread. A roti made by the Bhils in Gujarat contains about 70 g of flour.

The composition of selected foods determined by the recipe method is given in Appendix IV.

For data on the food intake of a person, the subject (or the mother in the case of children) can be asked to record all the foods consumed and the amounts in which they are consumed. A specimen record is shown in **Table 66**. The amounts consumed can be indicated in terms of household measures if weighing is not possible.

The foodstuffs provided by the diet can be calculated by using the recipe method. Nutritive value can be calculated from food tables. Most people do this by calculating the nutritive value of each item consumed. The author finds it much more convenient to calculate the total amount of cereal, pulse, oil, sugar, jaggery, milk, vegetables, etc. in the day's diet, especially for making a quick estimate of calories and protein. For instance, in the specimen record given, the diet would provide 120g of wheat, 25 g of rice, 110 g of pulse, 53 g of sugar+jaggery, 450 g of milk, 55 g of ghee+oil, and 100 g of vegetables. The calculations can be done mentally after some experience provided we become familiar with the composition of foods. Anyone concerned with the conduct of diet surveys should acquire such familiarity.

Here again, the value arrived at can be compared with expected value. For instance, a person's record may show less than expected intakes if he has overeaten the previous day (food intake tends to average itself to a standard value over an interval) or the person might be eating less because of illness or diarrhea. It may also be more than expected when a person is recovering from a previous state of semi-starvation because of illness or other reasons. If no reason for the discrepancy can be found and if the individual has not been losing or gaining weight, the reliability of the record must be carefully checked. In practice, a sedentary individual consumes 35-50% over and above his basal calories (which can be calculated). The corresponding figure

Table 66. Specimen diet record of a subject.

Age : 21 years				Height : 170cm		
Sex : Female				Weight : 60 kg		
Occupation : Postgraduate student						
			Cereals + Pulse (g)	Fat (g)	Milk (g)	Sugar + Jaggery (g)
6.30 A.M	Tea	1 cup	--	--	50	10
7.30 A.M	Tea	1 cup	--	--	50	10
	Bread with Butter and jam	2 slices	40	5	--	10
1.00 P.M	Chapatis With ghee	4	20	10	--	--
	vegetable (gravy type)	½ cup	--	5	--	--
	Rice	½ cup	25	--	--	--
	Liquid dal	½ cup	10	1	--	--
	Curd	½ cup	--	--	100	--
4.00 P.M	Tea	1 cup	--	--	50	10
	Biscuits	4	12	4	--	3
	Sev	1 serving	50	10	--	--
8.30 P.M	Poories	6	60	15	--	--
	Sprouted bengalgram	¾ cup	40	5	--	--
	Milk	1 cup	--	--	200	10
	Total		257	55	450	53

for a moderately active person such as a student would-be 50-75% and, for a very active person about 100%.

Where the food is analyzed for various nutrients, the methods for chemical estimation must be reliable. The values arrived at can be checked by comparing them with those derived by the recipe method using food tables. Such comparisons show that calculated values are quite reliable in the case of protein, fairly reliable for minerals and less reliable for fat and vitamins. If the value arrived at deviates markedly from expected value according to food tables, a repeat analysis may be desirable; provided, of course, the food table values are themselves reasonable. Also, when the diets used are analyzed for vitamins, care must be taken to prevent loss of vitamins in the intervals between collection and transportation and between transportation and actual analysis. This applies particularly to vitamin C. The vitamin C content of foods, as analyzed, was found to be 1–10 mg in a study on lactating women although the analysis was made immediately on arrival in the laboratory. But when the food was collected in air-tight containers and transported under ice the intake in similar economic groups was found to be 10–25 mg per day whereas calculation on the basis of raw ingredients gave a value of about 20–50 mg. When data based on analysis of matched collections are reported, these points must be considered in interpreting the results.

When the collection of a matched portion is left to the subject, there is a tendency to under-collect main dishes. The reliability of the collections can be checked by casual visits at meal time. If necessary, the subject can be fed on some pretext in the laboratory (for instance, if they have to come to the laboratory for other investigations or blood collection), and the amount consumed quietly noted and compared with the amount in the matched collection. The meal served must resemble the home meal.

Food intake of particular groups

Often we are interested in assessing the adequacy of particular groups such as young children, adolescent boys, pregnant women etc. We may also be interested in getting information on the intakes of healthy well-nourished persons in different age groups. People are self-conscious when their food intake is recorded individually and this may disturb the pattern of consumption. When we are interested in group values an easier method can be followed. For instance, adolescent boys of the same age can be seated at the same table and the above procedure followed for the group as a whole. A better method is to make available known amounts of the foods prepared and let the subject help himself. The left-overs and plate waste can be measured and the amounts consumed calculated. This can be done unobtrusively. This method is easy to follow in institutions such as hostels attached to schools and colleges. Boys (or girls) of the same age can be seated together so that food intake at different ages can be estimated.

In the above method it is necessary to ensure that all the meals, snacks and beverages are provided and the subjects do not take anything outside during the collection period. The subjects can be requested to record any foods or drinks consumed outside. When we are interested in obtaining norms on food intake of healthy persons, it would be better to ensure that the diets provided fully caters to the needs of the subjects so that they do not feel the need to eat anything outside.

Institution diets

The above method can be used for studying institution diets. However, a few points must be borne in mind. There is often a difference between the amounts ordered and paid for and the amounts delivered so that it is most important to weigh the foods and not place reliance on the amounts claimed to be delivered. Also amounts consumed by servants or taken home by them as well as plate waste must be recorded. In a survey conducted in Baroda it was found that 1/3 of the butter ordered in an institution was consumed by the kitchen staff. Care must be taken to see that the inevitable 'leakage' which occurs in large institutions does not obscure the information obtained. Vegetables must be weighed after cutting, particularly when cooking is done on a large scale, as more of the edible portion is likely to be removed.

Often there is resistance to a systematic diet survey on the part of those managing the institutions as well as those making supplies of foodstuffs, as they may consider this as an attempt to identify sources of leakage. Some tact is required to get their cooperation.

Whatever may he the method of survey used, the problem of human relations is a crucial one and the most challenging part of the survey is perhaps to get the cooperation of the subjects. The investigator must cultivate a pleasant manner and organize his work without intruding more than necessary on the privacy and routine of the family concerned. He must establish a friendly acquaintance and also make the survey useful and meaningful to the individual or family concerned. In the case of poor families the subjects can be told that their survey is to enable them to plan better meals with resources available. If the investigator also shows an interest in the family, better cooperation is likely. For instance, clinical deficiency symptoms, if any, can be pointed out and suggestions made regarding treatment. Children suffering from worms can be given treatment. Very anaemic persons can be given iron supplements. Practical suggestions can be made regarding the nutritional improvement of the undernourished child, or the alleviation of diarrhea or the diet of a diabetic. Severe cases can be helped to get treated at the hospital. This is easier if the institution of the investigator has some liaison with the hospital.

A reference has already been made to the limitations involved in using food tables for estimating nutrient content. When the survey is carefully done fairly reliable estimates can be obtained for protein, fat, carbohydrate and calories. Less reliability must be placed on values obtained for mineral and vitamin intake. Information must be obtained regarding cooking practices as for instance, on how much of the flour is sieved off before making chapatis, whether cooking water is drained off from rice and vegetables, whether bicarbonate is used in cooking, how rice and vegetables are washed before cooking, etc. In the case of vegetables the freshness of the materials obtained, the time interval between preparing them for cooking and actual cooking, and that between cooking and consumption must be recorded. When all this information is obtained, it is possible for an experienced investigator to make reasonable estimates of probable losses during cooking.

Anthropometric measurements

As growth rate, adult stature and body build are all affected by nutrition, body measurements can give us some idea of nutritional status. For instance, a two year old child weighing 8 kg is obviously undernourished as the expected weight at this age is about 12 kg. Heights and weights are the most commonly used measurements. In the case of children, heights and weights can be compared with expected values for their age. Also, even after allowing for a smaller height, undernourished children have low body weights so that the ratio of height to weight can also be considered. With the progress of undernutrition or malnutrition, Weight is first affected and subsequently height as well. For instance, the weights of the undernourished may be less than 70% of the expected values whereas heights may be 90%. However, while a deficit in only weight indicates short-term undernutrition which is more easily reversed, a deficit in height usually indicates chronic and prolonged undernutrition resulting often in permanently stunted physical stature.

The ratio of weight to height also gives some idea of the overall nutritional status of the individual. As mentioned earlier, changes in weight may be more critical than the actual weight. A child who has stopped gaining weight or has been losing weight is more seriously undernourished than one who is still growing. The growth of the child can be monitored if we compare his weight with expected weight at progressive ages. For instance, if his weight was 90% of expected value last year and is only 80% now, this suggests that he is deteriorating. A graph which shows his weight in relation to expected value can be used for the purpose as shown in **Fig. 9.**

Even when an investigator doing a diet and nutrition survey is seeing the subjects only once information on recent changes in the same should be obtained, particularly in the case of children. Apart from height and weight, body build is also affected. The well-nourished child has a broad chest, a flat stomach and square shoulders. In the case of the malnourished child, the chest may be small and the abdomen protruding. A comparison of the circumference of the chest (taken around the nipples) the abdomen (taken around the umbilicus) may give us an idea of body build. Further, in the case of the growth retarded child, the long bones fail to develop satisfactorily whereas the spine is less affected. This means that sitting height is less affected than standing height (for instance, the difference in height between men and women is more due to that in standing height). The ratio of sitting height to standing height can be compared with expected values (Table 55).

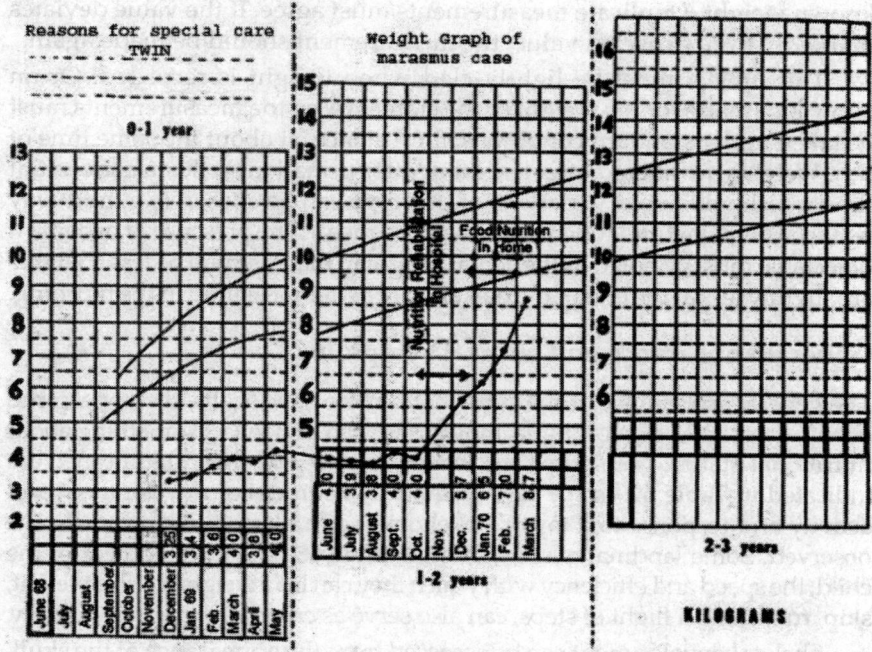

Figure 9. Weight graph (Courtesy: Dr. De Sweemer and associates).

In the very young child, the ratio of chest or arm circumference to head circumference is also used as a measure.

Information on height and weight is easier to obtain than on dietary intake. However, that this is left out in many diet surveys.

These measures not only give us a better idea about the nutritional status of the subject but can also provide an additional check for the reliability of the diet survey. For instance, the per capita calorie intake of a well-nourished family consisting of father, mother and two pre-school children is likely to be of the order of 1500 or more and a value like. 1500 must be considered suspect. On the other hand, a poor family with two growth retarded children is likely to have a per capita intake of at least 1300 calories (if the father is not a manual labourer).

Care must be taken to get reliable measurements of height and weight. For the measurement of height, the subject must stand erect with heels together and his head, shoulders and buttocks touching the wall. The reliability of the measuring instrument (inch tape or height machine) should be checked with standard scales (for instance, 3 inches on different parts of the same inch tape may give different lengths if it is not accurately calibrated). The reliability of a weighing machine must be checked frequently by weighing either a standard weight or an object of known weight. Duplicate measurements must agree. If the value deviates markedly from expected value, the measurement should be made again.

The subject must be lightly clad when weight is recorded. Or an allowance made for the weight of the clothes. Also the measurements must be taken under standard conditions, for instance, at about the same time of day. Weights are altered after a meal or after urination so that a convenient time which will avoid variations of this type can be chosen (e.g. mid-way between breakfast and lunch or just before a meal). The presence of oedema if detectable must be noted as the actual weight in that case will be less. Heights are slightly less at the end of the day and are better measured in the morning.

General appearance and clinical symptoms

The general appearance of the subject and more specifically, the appearance of hair, eyes, nails, skins, tongue, mouth, etc., can also tell us something about nutritional status. The symptoms usually found and their significance are indicated in **Table 67**. In the case of children neuromotor development and activity and response to a toy or novel object or a play situation can also be observed. Some landmarks are shown in **Table 68**. The development of the child, the speed and efficiency with which they can lift a weight, push a weight, skip, run, climb a flight of steps, can also serve as criteria when used skilfully.

Skeletal development can be assessed from the appearance of the skull, chest and legs. The child with past rickets tends to have bow legs, flat feet, pigeon chest and a protruding skull. The ribs are beaded. Symptoms such as fatigue, loss of appetite, dizziness, etc. must also be noted.

Other criteria

Radiological and biochemical examination are also carried out where possible but their detailed discussion is beyond the scope of this book.

Information on other aspects can enable us to assess the status of the community as a whole. Deaths of recent occurrence (say, in the preceding 10 years) and the age at which they occurred can tell us something about the pattern of mortality and the prevalence of childhood mortality. The incidence of still births, miscarriages and low birth-weight babies can give us an idea of maternal nutritional status. The age composition of the population and the percentage of people in the older age groups can tell us something about life-expectancy. The diet survey form used by us seeks to include comprehensive information so that some assessment can be made of the plane of nutrition of the group studied as a whole as compared to another group (for instance, poor families in rural and urban areas; poor and upper class families).

Tact must be exercised in eliciting the information. The questions must be put in such a way that the sensitivity of the subject is not offended. For

Table 67. General clinical symptoms and their significance.

	Symptoms	Possible significance
Tongue	thick and glossy raw and scarlet appearance fissures and ulcers in the tongue	deficiency of B vitamins particularly riboflavin
Lips	Chaffing of lips (cheilosis), ulceration at the corners of lips (angular stomatitis)	"
Eyes	profusion of blood vessels around the cornes very pale appearance dry conjunctiva and corneal white, chalky spots on the conjunctiva (Bitot's spot)	" anaemia deficiency of vitamin A
Hair	clear, moist and glistening dull and lusterless, thick and sparse, hair pulled out easily alternative bands of discoloured and normally coloured hair	normal protein deficiency alternate periods of adequate nutrition and protein deficiency
Skin	smooth and clear rough and dry horny skin (toad skin) symmetrical butterfly patches on the skin inflamed and flaky skin	normal deficiency of vitamin A deficiency of vitamin A or EFA or B vitamins protein, calories or niacin deficiency protein deficiency
extremities	oedema or water retention foot and hand appear swollen and do not bounce back but remain dented when pressed skin wrinkled and shrunk	protein deficiency starvation, kidney disorder dehydration, marasmus
bowel movements	chronic diarrhea constipation	intestinal infections protein calorie malnutrition, niacin deficiency, disorders of digestive system thiamine deficiency.

Table 68. Landmarks in development.

	Average age (months)
Holding the head	3-4
Sitting with support	5-6
Sitting without support	6–8
Standing with support	6-7
Standing without support	8-9
Crawling on belly	6-7
Crawling on knees	8-9
Walking with support	10-11
Walking without support	11–15

instance, in order to get information on infant and childhood mortality it is brutal to ask the mother how many children she lost. Rather the questions should follow the sequence: How many children do you have? Did you have only three? Also the questions should not be asked routinely according to a check-list. For instance, rather than ask a family how much of ghee, hydrogenated fat, oil, butter, etc. they use, it is better to ask what oil do they use mainly, and after getting the answer, ask whether they use any other fats occasionally. Certainly, there is no point in asking a poor family how much of cheese and chocolate drink they consume. Some students when given information on the, dietary pattern, asked in a surprised tone, "Is that all?" Neither the question nor the tone in which it was asked was calculated to obtain further cooperation of the subject. Certainly, a condescending attitude must be avoided. Also, if possible the family can be given helpful, friendly and practical suggestions not only regarding their diet and health but other aspects as well where possible (e.g. medical help, education, job opportunities, etc.).

Chapter 25

Nutrition and Human Development

The importance of nutrition is amply brought out in the title "Food becomes you" by Dr. Ruth Leverton. We should perhaps add, "If you eat the wrong foods, you become the wrong 'you'. As Bertrand Russell observes, the absence of iodine in the diet can turn a genius into an idiot. Although fortunately such conversions have not been attempted, it is possible that many potential geniuses do not reach their full stature because of poor nutrition which affects not only the life of an individual but of those around him. When malnutrition is widespread in a community, the whole community acquires characteristics such as lethargy and inertia and these become more or less a tradition. The drive to improve the home and environment found in the west is not found in poor countries. Even to a casual observer, western society appears to be different from our society. These differences are found in little things such as the pace with which men and women walk and the vigour with which children play. In the west, a substantial part of a man's leisure time is spent in gardening, carpentry, making additions to the home, building a spare cottage in the country, swimming, etc. whereas most of our leisure time is spent in idle gossips or just lazing around. The little patch of land around a western home blooms into a beautiful garden. It seldom does here without the help of a gardener who also does not do a full day's work. A poor man in this country prefers to go without vegetables rather than cultivate a patch of greens. This is not to say that individuals with drive and initiative are absent in our society but their proportion does seem to be far less. These differences may not entirely be due to nutritional factors and well-nourished individuals in the upper class in this country are certainly not models of productivity.

However, most individuals are prevented from making their best efforts if their health is below par.

Physical stature

As stated in chapter 1, the growth of the body as well as adult height depend to a large extent on dietary intake during growth, although heredity also plays a role. In this and other developing countries the effects of undernutrition are dramatically evident when we consider the growth rates of people in the upper classes who have enough to eat and the poor who do not. Both groups come from the same racial stock so that heredity cannot be entirely blamed for the slower growth of the poor. The growth rate of the poor and upper classes in this country, as compared to western norms, are shown in **Figs. 10–13**. The differences in weights between the three groups is not entirely due to that in heights as can be seen from **Figs. 14 and 15**.

Although height and body build are affected by heredity, the difference in physical stature between the poor and upper class in this society is mainly due to differences in nutrition as not much difference is found till the age of six months or so. Further, when children in the poor group are given food supplements they grow as well as those in the upper class. The children of Japanese parents settled down in the U.S.A. were found to be taller and heavier than their cousins at home. The average birth weight in

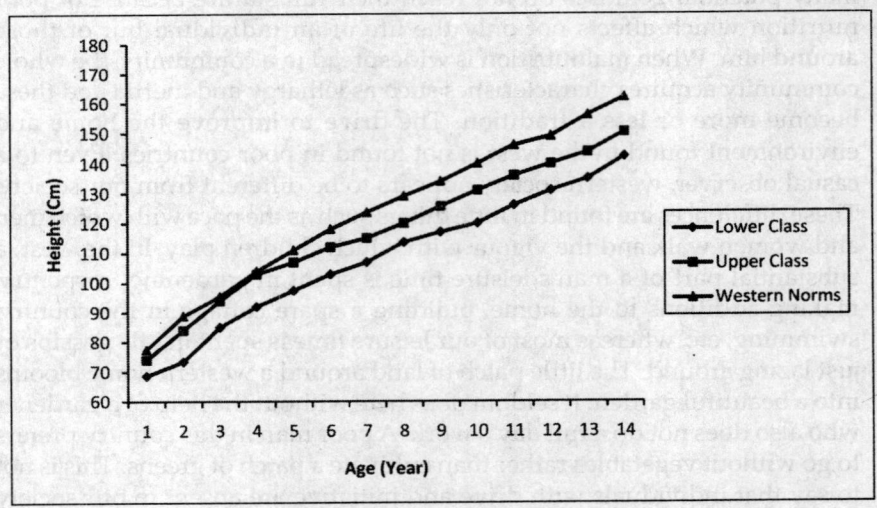

Figure 10. Heights of boys in the lower and upper classes in Gujarat as compared to western norms.

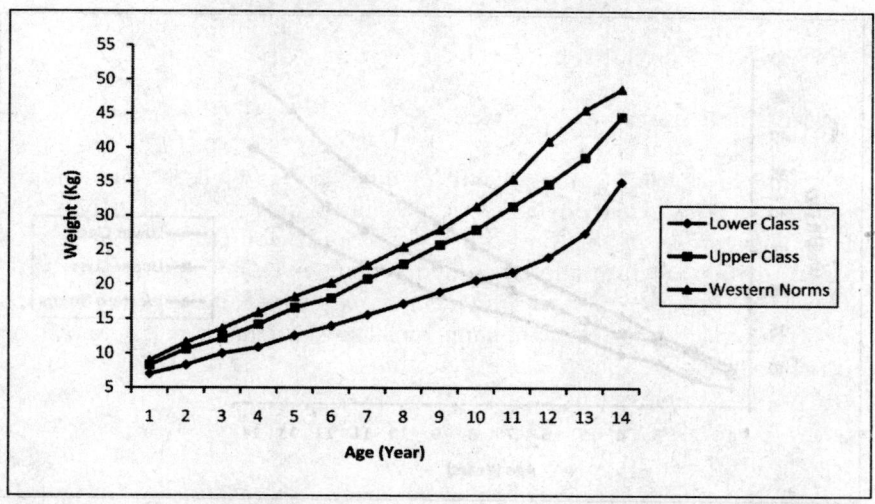

Figure 11. Weights of boys in the lower and upper classes in Gujarat as compared to western norms.

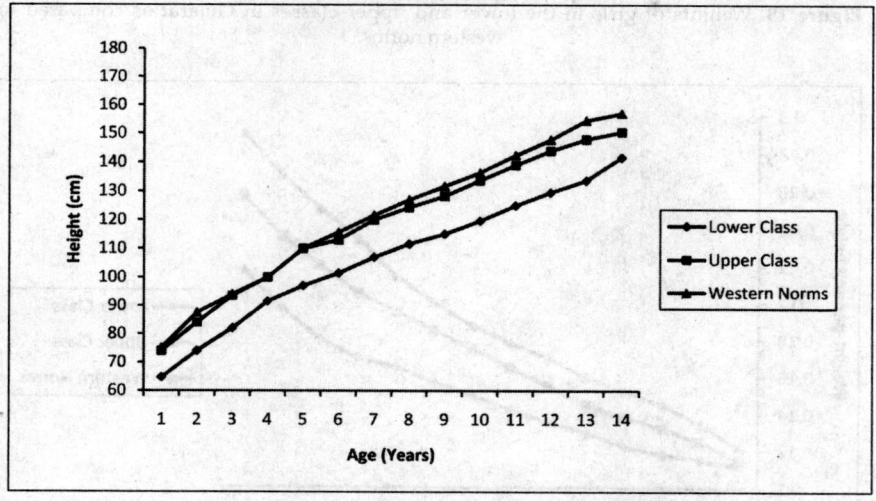

Figure 12. Heights of girls in the lower and upper classes in Gujarat as compared to western norms.

Japan has gone up with improved nutrition during the last few decades. These changes show the role of diet in determining physical stature.

A person with a good body build is better equipped for heavy manual work, athletics, sports, etc. While a well-nourished individual who is small

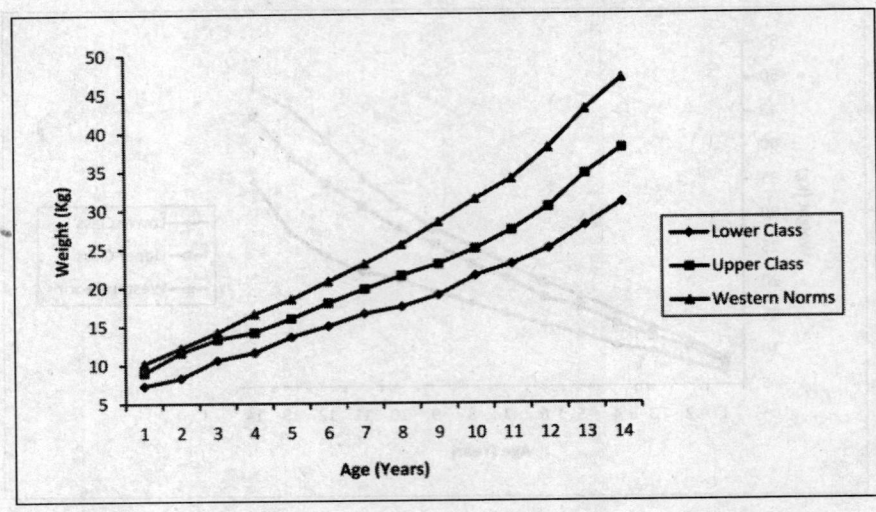

Figure 13. Weights of girls in the lower and upper classes in Gujarat as compared to western norms.

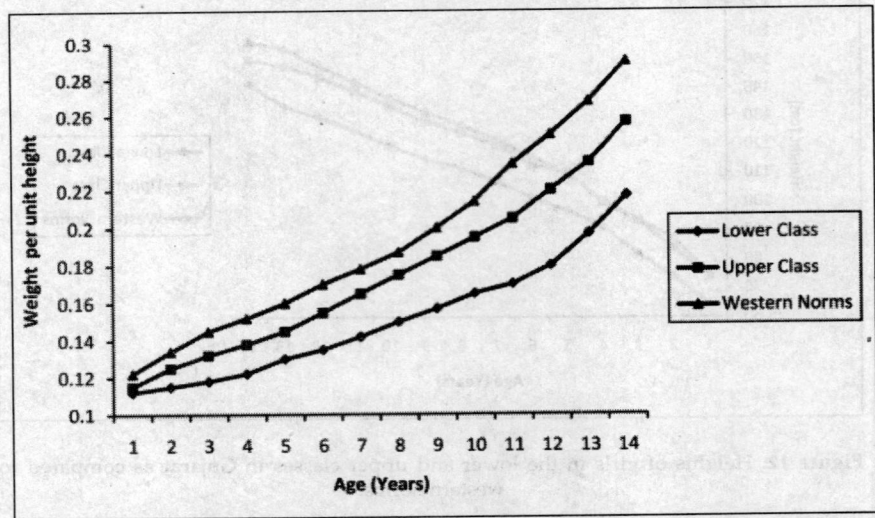

Figure 14. Weight (kg) per unit height (cm) of boys in the lower and upper classes in Gujarat as compared to western norms.

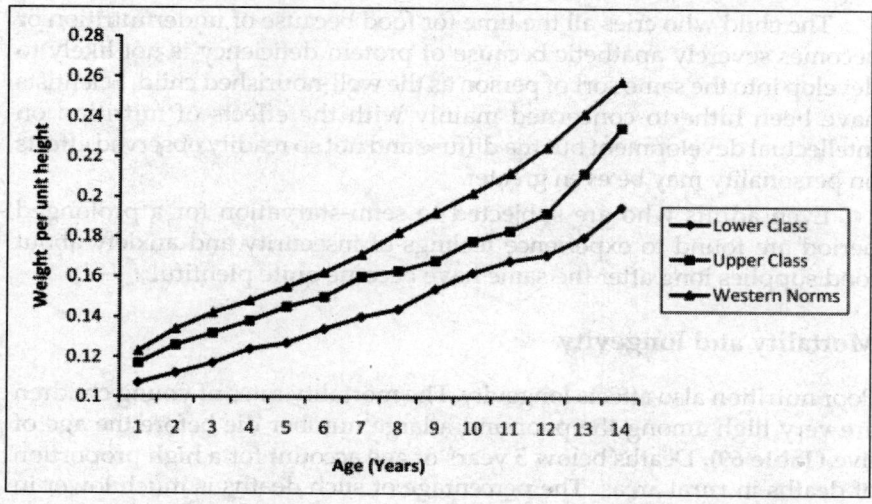

Figure 15. Weight (kg) per unit height (cm) of girls in the lower and upper classes in Gujarat as compared to western norms.

because of hereditary factors functions quite well, the same may not be true of people who have become stunted because of chronic hunger.

Psychological status

The effects of malnutrition on psychological characteristics may be even more serious. Very severe malnutrition in early life has been found to affect intellectual development and this is sometimes reported to be not fully remedied even by a good diet subsequently. Experimental animals undernourished in early life are found to show a number of behavioral changes such as greater emotionality, increase in purposeless activity, decrease in exploratory activity, etc. They also show a tendency to hoard food presumably arising from insecurity about food supplies. In some situations (e.g. severe protein deficiency), learning capacity is also affected. Female rats subjected to malnutrition or undernutrition do not care for their young ones as well as well-nourished animals. Sometimes they show aggressive behaviour instead of maternal behaviour.

An individual who is undernourished has to cut down his activity to a minimum in order to survive. The unfortunate thing is that such an individual becomes permanently attuned to a low level of productivity even when food is available and when more exertion can mean a higher standard of living.

The child who cries all the time for food because of undernutrition or becomes severely apathetic because of protein deficiency is not likely to develop into the same sort of person as the well-nourished child. Scientists have been hitherto concerned mainly with the effects of nutrition on intellectual development but the diffuse and not so readily observed effects on personality may be even greater.

Even adults who are subjected to semi-starvation for a prolonged period are found to experience feelings of insecurity and anxiety about food supplies long after the same have become quite plentiful.

Mortality and longevity

Poor nutrition also affects longevity. The mortality rates of young children are very high among the poor and a large number die before the age of five **(Table 69)**. Deaths below 5 years of age account for a high proportion of deaths in rural areas. The percentage of such deaths is much lower in urban areas, possibly because of improved sanitation and better medical care. The life expectancy of the average man in this country is lesser than that in western countries. In western countries, the percentage of people in the older age groups is much higher.

Nutrition and human development

About 10% of infants born of poorly nourished mothers in urban areas, have low birth weights than well nourished ones. The incidence of premature

Table 69. Morality at different ages in the village of Raipura (Baroda District)*

% of total deaths reported

Age (years) at death	Males (298)	Females (181)
Still born	6.7	5.0
0-5	62.0	66.8
5-10	4.7	7.2
10-15	2.0	1.1
15-20	1.3	0.6
20-40	4.7	9.9
40-60	11.7	5.5
60-80	5.4	3.9
80-100	1.3	----

* The figures are based on deaths reported to have occurred in 307 families
  Surveyed in the village of Raipura during ten years preceding the survey.
  Death rate below 5 years was found to be much lower in urban areas.
  The figures in parentheses indicate the total number of deaths.

births and miscarriages is also somewhat higher. Fortunately for us, the effects of maternal malnutrition do not have consequences as serious as we might expect so that most of the children even in the poor class are healthy for the first 4-6 months when they are adequately breast-fed. However, about 10% of poor infants fail to grow properly during this period because of inadequate lactation.

A high mortality is not only a tragedy but also a waste. In man, an individual depends on others till the age of 15–20 years. An individual dying before maturity has not had a chance to fulfill his potentialities and contribute to the society which has raised him. An individual dying soon after maturity can only make a smaller contribution, generally speaking although a long life by itself does not signify a rich life. After all, as Laski has pointed out,"Antiquity is not experience."

As has been pointed out earlier, malnutrition is associated with clinical symptoms, changes in the composition of blood and tissues. Many of these changes affect the functioning of the individual. For instance, a person with chronic ulceration of the tongue and mouth is unable to eat properly. One with eye symptoms is also handicapped. A person with anaemia is not able to work at his best.

Malnutrition and productivity

The productivity of agricultural and manual labourers is low in communities which are undernourished. This is not surprising as work can be performed by man and animals only at the cost of food energy. If an individual consumes 2000 kcals out of which 1500 are needed for basal matabolism, he can only turn out 500 kcals worth of work. If he consumes 3000 kcals, he can turn out 1500 kcals worth of work. This means that a 50% increase in food supplies can enable him to treble his output. The energy intake of Polish miners is of the order of 5000 kcals as against 3000 kcals in Indian miners. In South America, road building was found to be speeded up when the workers were given a mid-day meal. In Germany, during World War II, production in factories declined when the rations were drastically cut, and rose when they were increased. The productivity of an Indian labourer is reported to be 25–50% of that in affluent countries.

This does not mean, however, that extra calories will be automatically converted to work output. A plate of 'halwa' consumed by a sedentary individual is not followed by an outburst of activity but rather by the acquisition of some more adipose tissue. However, while an individual can remain idle even when food is available in plenty, he cannot be expected to work if he is starving.

Thus, productivity is hampered because of undernutrition; and good nutrition is not possible with low productivity as it results in low living standards. Efforts should be made to evaluate the impact of improved nutrition on the productivity of factory workers and agricultural labourers.

In addition to low productivity the malnourished individual is absent more often from work because of sickness. Because of poor education and environment in early life and also perhaps because of poor nutrition, his capacity to learn new techniques and to benefit from modern innovations is also limited. This means that the contribution of the malnourished person to society is much smaller than it might have been, had he been well-nourished. This means that living standards, in countries where the people are malnourished or poor, are low and this in turn results in poor economic capacity and poor diets. Some idea of the purchasing capacity of the Indian as compared to that of western man can be seen in **Table 70**. It can be seen from the table that in 1974 when the data were collected ,the per capita expenditure on food commodities consumed in India used to be higher. It continues to be higher than many other countries as revealed by the data on Global Food Spending collected by United States Department of Agriculture Economics Research Service in the year 2010.

India's food spending is reported as 35% of income as compared to developed countries which is 7 to 12%. Thus we have a vicious circle of poverty resulting in malnutrition which in turn results in more malnutrition.

Malnutrition among the rich

The poorer classes who are ignorant, illiterate and lack purchasing power have perhaps some excuse for being malnourished. We must not forget that conditions such as obesity, diabetes and heart diseases are more prevalent among the upper classes after middle age and dietary factors and faulty living habits are believed to be partly responsible for these diseases. Diseases such as diabetes showed a lower incidence in England during the war when the intake of fats, sugars, etc. was reduced. The upper classes would also, therefore, appear to need education on sound nutrition.

Even those who have an awareness of the role of dietary factors in the aetiology of these diseases do not always control their diets which underlines the difficulty in changing food habits. Sound food habits must, therefore, be formed at a very early age. In conclusion, malnutrition affects not only the health and well-being of the individual but also the status and progress of the whole communities and nations. The eradication of nutritional deficiency diseases is crucial for the success of our programmes for national development.

Table 70. Comparative cost of food articles in different countries.*

				Approximate cost in rupees per kg				
	India (Baroda)	Australia (Adelaide)	Canada (Montreal)	Israel (Jerusalem)	Malaysia (Kuala lumpur)	Philippines (Manila)	U.K. (Glasgow)	U.S.A. (Los Angeles)
Cereal**	2.0	2.0	2.5	2.5	3.1	2.1	2.4	3.0
Pulse**	2.5	3.8	10.5	5.8	3.0	2.6	10.0	8.3
Cooking Fat**	10.0	8.4	8.8	4.0	10.0	2.1	10.0	9.9
Milk	2.0	1.8	2.8	1.8	—	1.8	2.2	2.5
Potatoes	1.0	3.3	2.6	2.5	2.6	2.5	2.6	3.0
Onions	0.8	3.4	3.0	2.5	2.6	2.4	3.0	1.7
Animal Foods**	8.5	9.0	10.0	18.4	4.3	5.1	14.0	5.7
Annual Income (rupees) per Capita	700	21000	30000	13000	2500	1700	18000	36500

* Compiled from information on price level in the summer of 1974 supplied by Mrs. Hilde Roman (Australia) Prof. F.A. Farmer (Canada), Prof. K. Guggenheim (Israel), Miss L.C. Foo (Malaysia), Dr. Carmon intengan (Philippines), Sir David Cuthbertson (U.K) and Dr. D.B. Jelliffe (U.S.A.).

** The prices listed are those for the cheapest of the locally available foods in each category.

Chapter 26

Improving the Nutrition of the Community

We have seen that poor nutrition is partly or fully responsible for low birth-weights, increased incidence of still-births, high mortality during childhood, stunted physical stature, decreased longevity, increased susceptibility to infection, poor productivity, and perhaps, even poor psychological development. The cost of all this to the individual and society is indeed great. What can we do to arrest and reverse this state of affairs?

Some improvement can be expected when the economic conditions improve. In the meanwhile, it would be tragic to allow more and more children to become so severely malnourished that their potential for development is permanently affected. What can we do about this?

Neonatal period

It is obvious that as poorly nourished mothers produce small babies, good nutrition has to start with the mother. It would be desirable to give poor pregnant women food supplements providing energy, protein, vitamin A, calcium, iron and B-vitamins. But this may not be practicable. A most urgent need is to distribute at least iron supplements to pregnant women as anaemia is a major problem in pregnancy and in young children. They can also be given advice regarding the greater consumption of foods rich in carotene, calcium etc. A simple advice to all the groups would be to increase the consumption of leafy vegetables and pulses. We could have mother and child welfare centres where such advice is given. Such centres may also give advice in family planning. One reason for the mother's reluctance to limit her family is her fear of losing the children. If she knows that her children are well looked after and stand high chances of survival, her attitude towards family planning can be expected to change. This has, in fact been the experience in places where such services have been organized. An example is the rural health centre at Narangwal near Ludhiana in the Punjab where the John Hopkins University has organized such services.

Pre-school children

The care of pre-school children deserves top priority as this group is the one most likely to be malnourished. The group often suffers not only from malnutrition but also from maternal neglect. In rural areas, most of the poor women work in the fields and they leave the child under the care of an older child, who may be only six or seven years of age and not really competent for the job. This also affects the development of the older child who is deprived of schooling as a result of his or her duties as a baby-sitter. Organization of baby creches where the children can be looked after and fed one or two balanced meals or snacks daily, will contribute greatly to an improved nutritional status. We have organized a baby centre for pre-school children in a selected village and helped the village panchayats in 20 villages in Baroda block v to organize similar centres. A simple lunch is provided for children in these villages and is based on cereal or millet 40–50 g, legume 20–25 g, leafy vegetables 30–50 g, and oil 5–10 g. ... A glass of buttermilk can be given wherever possible. A number of one dish meals such as dhokla, debra, khichri, and sambhar-rice can be prepared from the above ingredients as suggested. A supplement or meal based on the above would provide 370 kcals, 12 g of protein, 150 mg of calcium, 2000 microgram of carotene and generous quantities of other critical nutrients. The object of the supplement is to fill in the gaps in their calorie and protein intakes and meet most of their mineral and vitamin requirement. The actual recipe used should be based on local food habits. For instance, parboiled rice cooked with green gram and served with yellow pumpkin is well accepted by children in Kerala and dhokla is well-accepted by those in Gujarat. Sambhar-rice is already used in Tamil Nadu. This is based on rice, red gram dal, and vegetables. We find that the substitution of sprouted red gram for dal, and substitution or addition of leafy vegetables for other vegetables such as brinjal, and the addition of lime powder to the tamarind juice added can appreciably improve taste and nutritive value of this preparation without adding to the cost. These simple changes would increase the amounts provided of calcium, iron, carotene, riboflavin and vitamin C.

Such feeding programmes are found to result in improved weight gain, clearance of deficiency symptoms, and restoration of blood and serum constituents to normal levels, better bone development and sometimes improved psychological performance, specially, when these programmes are organized at play centres where children are exposed to toys and games and looked after by a nursery-trained teacher.

The cost of such supplements compares favourably with that of processed foods, the cost of which is increased by at least 100% during the preparation, packaging and distribution of such foods. It has also been our experience that children accept such foods much more readily than foods like high protein biscuits. In one village where the children were allowed to eat as much as they liked of either high protein biscuits or dhokla, they took only 120 kcals worth of biscuits and about 300–400 kcals worth of dhokla.

However, facilities may not always be available for the preparation and distribution of cooked foods. This is particularly the case in tribal areas where the families are scattered over a wide area. The distribution of ready to eat foods such as biscuits and bread which can be prepared on large scale and which have good keeping quality has been advocated. The use of refined flour in biscuits and breads tend to limit their nutritive value and it would be advisable to use at least half the flour in the form of whole wheat flour in such preparations. These foods should be reinforced with calcium,iron and vitamin A. Better alternatives are foods such as sukdi or prepared mixes, which can be easily cooked and distributed. In some our studies we have distributed prepared mixtures of roasted wheat and Bengal gram described earlier. The mixture was given in packets of 30-50 g each and the mother given a week's supply at two packets daily and asked to give a conjee prepared from the same, in lieu of tea. Supplements of vitamin A, calcium and iron can be added to such mixes. This measure was found to improve the nutritional status of young children in poor urban families in Baroda.

At the end of the study, the mothers were given demonstrations about how to prepare the conjee ingredients. However, some of the mothers said it would be difficult for them to prepare such a mixture on their own but said they would be glad to buy it at nominal cost. If arrangements can be made for the sale of such mixes, the cost being kept down to that of only the ingredients used, this may make an appreciable impact on the health of young children. Initially, they can be given some samples of the product so that the mothers can see for themselves the response of the child and the acceptability of the product. These ready-to-use food mixes can be prepared in rural areas with simple household equipment. The cost of processing and the other ingredients added can be subsidized by the panchayats or others.

Where supplementary feeding programmes are organized, the question arises as to who is to foot the bill. In some villages, in Baroda block, the panchayats have set apart 5–10 acres of land. the produce of which is either used for the feeding programme or sold and the sale proceeds used for the same.

If the play centre or feeding centre is organized in an area where the landed families live, the landless labourers do not send their children there and vice-versa. If it is not possible to persuade both groups to send the children to the same centre, either centres should be organized in both areas or priority should be given to organizing a centre for the landless families.

School boys

The group next deserving our consideration is that of children of the school going age. Most villagers send their children to a primary school and the school can, therefore, be used as an effective centre for improving the nutritional status of school children and their families, through lunch programmes as well as nutrition education.

The meals or snacks can be based on a combination of cereal pulse + leafy vegetables, as in the case of pre-school children. If cooking is not possible, wholesome and simple snacks such as parched grains, puffed rice, parched Bengal gram and roasted groundnut can be made up into packets and sold at nominal cost. The boys can also be given oil enriched with vitamin A. The school lunch can serve as a nucleus for a discussion of the various nutrients needed by the body, the effects of deficiencies of the same, the foodstuffs which can provide these nutrients and the formulation of meals based on the same. The children can be made to record their own heights and weights and observe the clinical symptoms present in the group before the initiation of the programme so that they become more aware of the impact of the same on nutritional status. They can also take turns to help with the preparation and distribution of lunch. They can be encouraged to cultivate in the school garden, the vegetables needed for their lunch. Such an approach was found to be very fruitful in a trial lunch organized by us in a village. This experience can serve as a basis for discussing how their home diets can be improved.

Central Food Technological Research Institute, Mysore has developed "Energy Food" prepared from wheat, gram dal, jaggery, edible ground nut cake, minerals and vitamins which is an easy to cook product to meet the energy and protein needs of school children. Energy food is now being manufactured by Karnataka Agro-Industrial Corporation, a Government of Karnataka undertaking. This is distributed in schools of Karnataka for alleviate protein and calorie malnutrition in school children. Similarly, mid-day meal programmes are underway by establishing anganwadis under the Department of Woman and Child.

In one village, where we attempted nutrition education by holding classes in the school, the mothers were also invited to attend these classes.

The impact was found to be greater in families where both children and mothers attended and with only children than with only mothers. Similar experiences have been recorded in Israel.

Other groups

Other groups such as landless labourers, building construction workers and factory workers are also in need of nutritional improvement. While protein status is not bad, they are undernourished and their productivity will improve with a food supplement provided on the spot. Most of them are also deficient with regard to vitamin A.

Immediate steps are needed at least to eradicate anaemia in women and vitamin A deficiency in children. Suggestions along the above lines have been made by various bodies including certain committees appointed by the Government of India. Organizations such as the UNICEF, FAO and WHO have also contributed to spreading an awareness of the need for nutritional improvement through their Applied Nutrition Programme. Organizations such as CARE have sought to improve the nutritional status of young children and school boys. But these efforts have hardly touched the fringe of the problem and much more extensive and intensive efforts are needed.

Nutrition education

Poor economic condition does stand in the way of improved nutrition, but ignorance regarding nutrients needed by the body and cheap foods which can provide them are also partly responsible. For instance, most mothers are not so poor as not to be able to afford an ounce of leafy vegetables to the child daily if they realize that this may make a difference between blindness and normal vision. Similarly, the mothers of many kwashiorkor children in Kerala were found to have spent quite a lot of money on the treatment of their children, including the purchasing of medicines, tinned barley and glucose, money which was rather disastrously spent when all that the child needed was a greater share of the foods prepared at home in a form suitable for the child.

Information media such as the radio, the news papers and television can help. In many areas such as Tamil Nadu, the farmers' programmes are quite popular and perhaps nutrition education can be attempted along with these. There are channels in television broadcasting educative programmes in health and diseases common remedies for various illnesses. However, programmes on nutrition education are scanty. Regiospecific programmes adaptable in the households in nutrition delivered by experts in the field will go a long way in solving the nutritional problems of the country. News papers can have a regular column on nutrition and perhaps one for answering questions relating to nutrition. School children are found to form an effective medium through which the parents can be educated. Most boys in rural areas have illiterate parents and what they learn in school carries weight with the parents. In this country the views and preferences of sons count for something with the mothers, particularly in rural areas.

Nutrition education should form an integral part of the science curriculum. It can also be integrated with the organization of the school lunch programme.

Till recently, whatever nutrition education is given in schools is in the form of isolated bits of information, or more often, misinformation scattered in science textbooks. Most of the recommendations are impossible and out of date. It is necessary to formulate a systematic syllabus which will emphasize the use of easily available and cheap foods for satisfactory nutrition. Many science textbooks give the impression that good nutrition is not possible without a generous supply of milk, eggs, oranges and meat. As even the upper classes cannot afford these in adequate quantities, the only possible response is to shrug one's shoulders and dismiss all these as so much theoretical. Efforts in these directions are now being made by the, National Council of Education Research (NCERT) the body which decides the syllabi and text books of Schools.

In our attempts at nutrition education in a selected village, we aimed at the education of children with the mothers in the school. We first pointed out the deficiency symptoms they had and explained how they can be prevented and corrected. We showed them how to prepare the foods we recommended and helped them to cultivate vegetables and fruits which can improve their nutritional status. We gave them cyclostyled summaries of the topics taught and objective tests to ascertain how much they had understood after distributing transcripts of the lesson taught (some specimen lessons are given in Appendix V). Needless to mention that these lessons have to be translated in the local language. We repeated the instructions if necessary and gave a repeat test till we were convinced that they had understood the lesson. We carried out diet surveys on their families before and after this course and found that some of these children had influenced food habits for the better in their homes. The effects were greater if both the mothers and children had been participating.

Our practical objectives in the above attempt were as follows:

a) To create an, awareness of the effects of poor nutrition on growth, general health and well-being and of the significance of specific clinical deficiency symptoms.

b) To emphasize that a combination of cereal plus pulse is superior to that of only cereal and that the cost of such a combination need not be more expensive than that of only cereal as the amount of cereal can be reduced correspondingly.

c) To emphasize proper cooking methods such as cooking rice by absorption method, not sieving off the bran from atta or to only use a very coarse sieve, to wash vegetables before cutting and to cook them under cover, etc.

d) To use under milled or parboiled rice and to use jaggery in place of refined sugar.

e) to include regularly leafy vegetables and other carotene rich vegetables and fruits.

f) To use frequently sprouted legumes and fermented foods.

We also found that very poor mothers, belonging to the families of landless labourers, were unable to benefit from such education because of their poverty. Many of these families bought only cereals, salt and spices and negligible quantities of other foods. Nutrition education is much more successful if the family can spend at least a minimum amount per day per capita on food.

Other ways of improving community nutrition have been advocated. Fortifying foods such as flour is one of them. Unless these fortified foods are used by the poor or in feeding programmes organized for them, they are not likely to make a significant impact. Enrichment of flour has met with success in western countries only because the flour is produced and distributed by the food industries organized on a large scale which makes it possible to enforce legislation regarding the enrichment of refined flour. The cost of the flour sold is also well within the purchasing capacity of the people. As stated earlier, conditions are somewhat different in this country. The difficulties in such programmes can be imagined if we consider how far we have succeeded in distributing iodised salt in goitre areas. As compared to cereal whose consumption is 400 g per day per capita, salt consumption is only 10–15 g. The population affected is only 10%. Salt is produced only in selected areas and is supplied to the goitre areas from outside whereas in most parts of the country cereals are locally produced and consumed. Preparation of iodised salt is a much simpler and cheaper process than enrichment of flour. There are no serious problems regarding the keeping quality of salt whereas enriched flours do not have the keeping quality of whole grains. In spite of the relative ease with which salt can be fortified and distributed and in spite of the fact that only 10% of the population living in goitre areas needs iodised salt, we have succeeded in distributing the same, for the entire population affected. If cereals have to be enriched the magnitude of the problem will be at least 250 times that involved in fortification of salt with iodine after taking into account the population affected and the, amount required, not to mention the problems in the collection, storage and distribution of grains.

It has been said that nutrition education is a costly and time consuming process. It can be seen from the foregoing that enrichment schemes are not likely to be less so. If we make a concerted approach at nutrition education through schools, training colleges, village leaders, health personnel, women's organizations and the like, we can make an impact on at least 25% of the people receiving instruction. Nutrition education has to be given only once whereas enriched foods have to be made available on a long-term basis. It would, therefore, appear that nutrition education need not be more expensive in the long run. If at least one teacher in each school receives adequate training in nutrition and is responsible for teaching the subject in the school in a realistic way and also makes efforts to reach the community, an impact should be soon felt.

If panchayat leaders receive similar training it will make the promotion of welfare measures easier. If we wish to reach a large segment of the population, we can attempt this through special workers trained in nutrition. A public health nurse whose opinion on health is respected by the villagers might prove a suitable agent for this purpose. However, her duties are so diverse that unless she has only a small population to cater to, it will not be possible for her to take up nutrition education as well.

Recent attempts in Madurai suggest that even illiterate women in rural areas can be trained to monitor the health and growth of young children and render appropriate advice regarding their nutritional care and treatment of disorders such as diarrhea, dysentery and scabies under the guidance and supervision of a medical team which visits once a week. They are also able to monitor the health and well being of expectant and nursing mothers and to emphasize the need for safe drinking water, boiling the water given for young children and so on. Similar studies have been made in Maharashtra.

It has been argued that we have been trying nutrition education for the last several years and failed. This is primarily because those concerned have been asking the people to do the impossible. We have been proclaiming from our ivory towers the excellent nutritive value of foods such as milk, fish, eggs, oranges, etc., which are beyond the reach of most people. Charts prepared in the sixties by a health department showed prominently cheese and beef as sources of nicotinic acid in a country where either is consumed only by negligible sections of the population. When the author was associated with the Applied Nutrition Programme in 1964, she was shocked to find the gap between diets usually recommended and the purchasing capacity of the people. We have been trying since 1964 to formulate and evaluate diets based on foods available in villages. Our experience has shown that when dietary advice is simple and practicable and requires only minor modifications of the existing diet without increasing the expenditure on foods, it is likely to be accepted by a large proportion of the people.

Food fads

Poor availability of nutritious foods is an important factor in malnutrition. But even available foods are not utilized fully because of wrong beliefs.

Many foods are excluded during late pregnancy and early lactation. The myths surrounding these fads will be evident when we find that the foods avoided by one group are those recommended by another group. In Gujarat, perfectly healthy and valuable foods such as dals, leafy vegetables, rice, curd and fruits are avoided by the nursing mother. In Tamil Nadu, on the other hand, rice, curd, leafy vegetables such as amaranth, and betel leaves are considered a "must". In Gujarat, a halwa (sirrah) prepared from cracked wheat is given soon after delivery where as in Tamil Nadu, wheat is avoided and the mother kept on liquid diet for two days after delivery and given solid foods only on the third day.

Child birth involves loss of body fluids. In addition to the loss of blood most women sweat profusely at the time and suffer from dehydration unless they drink enough water. In both Gujarat and Tamil Nadu, drinking water is considered harmful. The author knows at least one case of a mother developing fever due to dehydration. Many cases of infantile diarrhoea prove fatal because of dehydration. Education is needed on the fact that boiled water is perfectly safe in almost any condition.

Also ghee is associated with mysterious strength giving properties. Although it is all right as an item in the diet, where the money to be spent on food is limited it is not a good buy. The amount of money spent in getting an extra 25–50 g of ghee can be usefully spent in other ways. We can get for much less than the cost of ghee and oil, 50 g of dal and 50–100 g of leafy vegetables. Similarly, honey and almonds are believed to have mysterious qualities and both are expensive. A much better buy can be made for money spent on these items.

Papaya is believed to cause abortions and some women hopefully take kilograms of the stuff without effect. The unfortunate thing is that many women avoid taking this very nutritious fruit during pregnancy. Similarly, jaggery is believed to heat up the system, whatever that may mean. Most foods are burnt in the body giving heat. Our ancestors might have cautioned against the excessive consumption of sugar which in those days was available only in the form of crude sugar or jaggery. They had nothing to say about refined sugar because there was none in their time. This has given rise to the present notion that jaggery is harmful whereas refined sugar is all right. On the basis of their composition, jaggery and palm sugar are preferable to sugar and we have recommended their use in the place of sugar in community feeding programmes.

In South India, wheat is believed to be heat-giving and to be harmful unless it can be taken with large quantities of milk. Wheat is the major component of the diet of the poor in Uttar Pradesh who do not consume much milk and who are not any less healthy than South Indians.

Bananas are believed to result in convulsions in children and even death. The young child does get mild stomach upsets if unripe banana is given, but fully ripe bananas can be mashed and given. Similarly, pulses are excluded from the diet of children whereas many studies have shown they have no difficulty in tolerating well-cooked pulses. Potatoes, pumpkin, etc., are believed to result in flatus (gas) particularly in children and nursing mothers. Potatoes form the staple food of the poor in Ireland and as stated earlier its prolonged consumption is not associated with any harmful effect. The belief regarding pumpkin is prevalent in Tamil Nadu but not in Maharashtra which shows how baseless it is. Yellow pumpkin is a rich source of carotene and many young children, nursing mothers and others will benefit from consuming the same.

Buttermilk is believed to result in sore throats and is avoided by persons having a cold. While very sour buttermilk causes a mild irritation in some people, fresh buttermilk is a refreshing wholesome beverage.

Pepper is believed to stimulate blood formation. It is also believed that a diet lacking in spices is not easily digested. Both these beliefs have no foundation in fact.

To give a classic example of how wrong beliefs can deprive us of valuable foods, tomatoes were once considered poisonous till some one dared to taste it Now it is a vegetable which has versatile uses. Ghee is believed to be more easily digested than til oil, and the latter, more easily digested than groundnut oil. While these fats differ in their fatty acid composition, there is no appreciable difference in their digestibility.

It is popularly believed that ladies' fingers (okra) and fish are good for the brain since they contain liberal amounts of phosphorus needed by the brain. Ordinary diets are certainly not deficient in phosphorus and the phosphorus in these foods can hardly improve brain function. The author is reminded of Mark Twain, who was asked by a young literary aspirant as to how much fish he should take in order to improve his skills as a writer. Mark Twain replied that if fish does improve brain function, a medium-sized whale should be enough for the aspirant, judging from his literary standards.

In South India, buffalo milk is believed to make a person lethargic and dull. The baselessness of this needs is hardly to be pointed out.

It is not surprising that man should have an instinctive suspicion of anything strange (this includes foods, people and other matters) but it is indeed surprising that such beliefs have persisted for such a long time without any basis and in the face of evidence to the contrary.

A nutrition worker should seek to remove erroneous and harmful beliefs regarding foods. The common man deprives himself of healthy foods because of wrong beliefs. We are now witnessing another phenomenon in the educated classes who have become highly concerned about their nutritional status largely because of newspaper features on malnutrition and its high prevalence and consequences. This has made them an easy prey to the designs of the commercial food manufacturing industry. For instance, it is all right to take a malt beverage available in the market if one does not like plain milk and can afford the stuff, but it is not going to help anyone excel in sports or studies. A certain milk food is claimed to contain 24 nutrients as against 9 in milk. Milk is deficient only in iron and vitamin C which can be provided by relatively cheap foods in the ordinary diet. Glucose is advertised as the fuel used by the brain which is true enough. Except when an individual is starving, glucose supply to the brain is no problem as any carbohydrate is converted to glucose in the body. Even the newborn infant can get its glucose from sugar and milk. Glucose biscuits are not more nutritive than chapatis. They may merely be convenient to have around. Corn flakes are advertised in the West as having all the energy of 'sun-soaked' corn which is perfectly true as all the food energy we get is ultimately derived from solar energy trapped enough during photosynthesis, but corn flakes contain no more solar energy than corn or other grains and are in fact less nutritive because of the destruction of lysine. A number of families use high protein beverages and snacks not because they like them but because they consider them good for health although protein deficiency is not a problem in the educated classes who consume enough of milk and pulse and for the cost of these foods, other more palatable and nourishing foods can be obtained. Now the deficiency of lysine in cereals is exploited to popularize lysine-added breads, biscuits and tonics although the upper class diet is more than adequate with regard to lysine. These examples can be multiplied. It would be better for news media to create not only a concern but also knowledge about nutrition so that the public do not spend their hard earned money on foods that they do not need and do not particularly relish.

Chapter 27

Food Production in Relation to Population Growth and Need

No amount of nutrition education can help a population to eat foods that are not available. It is obvious that targets for food production must be based on an assessment of the needs of a balanced diet for the whole of the population after allowing for surplus consumption by its affluent sections.

Agricultural production

In India the population has been growing steadily at the rate of about 2%per annum whereas agricultural production has been fluctuating from year to year as can be seen from **Table 71.** Cereals production has increased from 70 Metric tons per year during the period 1961–66 to 235 Metric ton in the year 2010. There has been a record production of 267 metric ton of cereals in the year 2008. The per capita availability of cereals is not commensurate with cereal production during the period 1961 to 2010. This may be due to two factors namely, population growth and improper accessibility. Starvation has been reported in several parts of the country in spite of buffer stocks of food grains

The National Food Security bill to be passed in the Indian Parliament propose to ensure food security by providing legal right to every Below Poverty Line (BPL) families to gain access to certain minimum quantity of rice,wheat and millets in subsidized prices. The main feature of the Bill is to categorize the households to Priority and Non-priority households. The Priority households would receive rice, wheat and coarse grains at Rs. 3, Rs. 2 and Re. 1 per Kg. The act is now being implemented in the states and aims to cover the entire population by 2014. National Food Security Mission (NFSM) aims at achieving an additional production of 10, 8 and 2 million tons of rice, wheat and pulses by the year 2012.

Table 71.   **Food grain production in different years in India.**

| Year | Population (millions) | production | | | | | |
| | | Per annum (million tons) | | | g per capita per day | | |
		Cereals	Pulses	oilseeds	Cereals	Pulses	oilseeds
1961–66	467	70	11.1	6.6	410	67	40
1966–71	521	83	10.8	7.2	437	57	38
1973–79	613	108	11.1	8.8	484	51	40
1977	625	100	11.2	7.2	447	50	32
1978	638	143	11.8	12.2	614	51	52
1979	651	130	12.0	11.7	543	51	49
1980	688	140	10.6	9.37	557	42	37
1990	833	193	14.3	18.60	634	47	61
2000	1014	235	13.4	18.40	635	36	50
2008	1094	267	14.5	24.30	668	36	60
2010	1170	235	18.2	23.10	550	43	54
2012		165					

Sources: Bulletin of food statistics, 28th issue(1978). Directorate of Economics and statistics, Ministry of Agriculture and irrigation, Government of India. Volumes 22 (1972), 23 (1973), 24 (1974) and 25 (1975).

Agricultural Statistics Division. Dept. of Agriculture & Co-operation, Govt. of India IVth Advanced Estimates (2010-11).

Directorate of Oil Seed Research (ICAR), 2005.

Demand for food grain production in the year 2030 is 345 metric tons and for pulses is 30 million tons based on the the trend in population growth. Production depends on the availability of good quality seeds, soil conditions and availability of water and manure and the productivity of the farmer himself.

Even where irrigation facilities are available, water is not efficiently utilized and only 20% of the water let out for irrigation reaches the crop, the remaining 80% lost through diffusion into the soil during transit. In Israel, where the conditions for such loss are much more favourable because of the sandy soil, 70% is utilized. It is obvious that we can do something about the better conservation of water in irrigation canals and that this will help in better irrigation facilities.

In Israel, even the sandy tracts, typical of a desert region, are very successfully used for cultivation by taking measures to see that only the top layer of soil is used for cultivation and that this top-layer is sectioned off from the layer below by the use of asbestos troughs and the like. Such measures may enable us to increase or introduce cultivation in areas such as Rajasthan and Kathiawar.

The availability of water when needed and in the amounts needed is a major problem. Most of the farmers depend on good and timely rains and have to plan their sowing operations accordingly. Often a good rain in late June and in early July may be taken to herald the onset of monsoon and sowing operations started only to find that the next rain is not forthcoming for days to come. If the farmer can get a steady supply of water during this period so that the crops do not wither away, it would help. But irrigation facilities cover only a fraction of the land and we do not have enough tube wells and the like.

It may also be possible to collect and store rain-water as it is done in Australian homes. Rain water harvesting has received great attention all over India and the methodology for the same is being propagated among the masses.

The possibilities of artificial rain and the exploitation of sea water have been suggested but they may not materialize in the near future.

The other problem is the abundance of water when it is not needed. Every year, we see the spectacle of droughts in some areas and floods in other areas. Sometimes, a period of drought is followed by floods in the same area.

While droughts and floods can be blamed on nature, we certainly have not established conditions for the management of either. It is now accepted that rains depend to some extent on the forests in the area. Similarly, the fury of floods generally caused by the inundation of rivers can also be controlled to a considerable extent by preventing soil erosion near the source and along the course of the rivers and the consequent silting of the mouth of the rivers due to the eroded soil. The denudation of forests near the catchment areas and along the upper reaches of the river, greatly adds to the danger of floods. This problem and the need for afforestation were repeatedly emphasized by Gandhiji.

The denudation of forests is also due in large measure to goats which eat up the young saplings before they can grow into trees. Unless the ravage caused by goats near the upper reaches of the river is prevented, any programme of afforestation is bound to fail.; The catchment areas of some of the Himalayan rivers are in Nepal and these areas will have to be covered. International agreement and legislation within the country must seek to solve this problem. At present the goat-herds, whether in Nepal or India, allow the goats to fend for themselves and this is unlikely to stop unless the poor goat-herd has alternatives.

The interconnecting of all the rivers in India from the Cauveri, in the south to the Ganges in the north was suggested many years ago by a former Diwan of Travancore, the late Sir C.P. Rama-swami Aiyar. It is seldom that floods occur in all parts of the country, and usually they are associated with droughts in other parts of the country. Such interconnection of the rivers will not only act as a safety valve, but also supply water to deficit areas. The proposal is reported to have been found technically feasible by engineers. Other proposals such as the Garland Canal Scheme also involve basically the connection of different rivers. May be, we need to consider the feasibility of these proposals and execute them with international help. The project will no doubt be expensive, but considering the annual losses of human lives, cattle crops, and goods on account of floods, the project may prove profitable in the long run.

Floods and poor rains are not the only problem. Even in a good year the agricultural yields in this country used to be among the lowest in the world. After the advent of the Green Revolution the Scenerio has changed and the productivity has increased substantially due to improved farming practices. The demand for food grains in India is projected at 345 million tons in 2030 and that for pulses at 30 million tons.

Optimum water supply, the poverty of the soil, lack of good quality seeds and poor farming practices are factors affecting agriculture productivity.

Seeds of good quality should be made available to the farmer in time at reasonable prices. The small land-holders have often to borrow money at high interest and buy whatever seeds are available.

The quality of seeds can be tested by sprouting a known sample and counting the number of grains that develop good sprouts. The latter should be at least 90%.

In the case of maize separation of good quality seeds from infected seeds is being done in Gujarat by machines. The machine works on the basis of difference between the density of the good quality seeds and infected seeds as the latter is lighter on account of hollowness.

Good quality seeds must be made available to the farmer at reasonable prices. At present they are about 5–10 times the market prices for whole grains.

Table 72. Projected supply and demand of food grains in India.
(million tons)

Commodity	2004-05		2011-12		2021-22	
	Supply	Demand	Supply	Demand	Supply	Demand
Rice	88	92	96	101	106	113
Wheat	72	70	80	81	92	89
Total cereals	187	190	210	211	242	234
Pulses	15	13	16	16	18	20

Sources: S.Mittal, working Paper No.209 .Demand-Supply Trends and Projections of Food in India, March 2008.

Kumar, P., P.K. Joshi and Pratap Birthal. Agricultural Economics Research Reviews, Vol. 22, July–December 2009. pp. 237–243.

Some efforts have been made to develop hybrid strains of cereals and millets which give very high yields but only a small proportion of total cultivated land are used for the cultivation of such strains as they require a steady supply of water, fertilizers and pesticides, and their yields are less than those of conventional strains if this is not maintained. Also, it is urgent to develop similar strains for legumes.

The qualities sought in hybrid strains are high yield, disease resistance, early maturity, bold and lustrous grains etc. At least five to six years are needed to develop a satisfactory strain. When a promising strain is obtained in the research laboratory, it is tried out in selected fields for two or three years and recommended for general use only after the results have been evaluated and found satisfactory.

Further, care must also be taken to ensure that the nutritive quality of the grain is not affected in the development of the strain. For instance, in some cases, the protein content is high but the quality of protein is poor because of the associated decrease in lysine content. On the other hand, it is also possible to develop strains of better nutritional quality. For instance, a strain of maize, called opaque maize is found to have a satisfactory lysine content and consequently a higher protein quality than the conventional strains.

Next comes enrichment of the soil. Plants are made up of water, varying from 75% in woody plants to 85% in other plants, and organic compounds which are composed mainly of carbon, hydrogen, oxygen, nitrogen, sulphur and phosphorus and also contain potassium, calcium, iron, sodium, chloride and silicon as minor constituents and traces of other elements such as copper and manganese. Thus, in addition to carbon, hydrogen and oxygen, which are derived from carbon dioxide in air and water, they require nitrogen and minerals. Among the latter, nitrogen is the most important single element

Sources of nitrogen

The nitrogen required by plants is available in the form of nitrates and ammonium salts. The presence of these salts in adequate amounts depends on natural presence, decomposition products of dead plant and animal tissues and excreta of animals, and synthesis by nitrogen-fixing bacteria present in the soil and in the roots of leguminous plants. Small amounts are derived from rain water if the nitrogen in the air has been oxidized at the time of lightning. The addition of fertilizers and organic manures serve to restore nitrogen and other nutrients removed from the soil by plants.

Manures increase soil fertility either directly, by supplying nutrients required, or indirectly by their action on other substances that might be present already in the soil but not in a suitable state for being absorbed. Manures may be composed of degradation products or biological material or chemical fertilizers prepared on a commercial scale.

Inorganic or artificial or chemical manures or fertilizers, as they are variously called, are either specially manufactured or are found in nature as such. They are phosphates, potash salts, salts containing nitrogen, and those containing other elements. Just as the administration of nutritional supplements such as vitamins and minerals to man must be decided in terms of his present nutritional status and need, the addition of inorganic manure must be in relation to the composition of the soil and the age and species of the plant. Inorganic manures should be used in addition to, and not instead of, organic manures, because if used without enough humus in the soil they may prove harmful. It should also be remembered that artificial fertilizers have to be added every year.

The indiscriminate addition of fertilizers also disturbs microorganisms present in soil. These microorganisms play an important part in maintaining the texture of the soil in a state fit for cultivation. They also help in nitrogen fixation. Their destruction will result in poor texture of soil, disturb the nitrogen cycle and decrease the resistance of the crops to pests so that the use of insecticides becomes necessary. Enough emphasis should be laid on the fact that chemical fertilizers must be used in combination with organic manure.

The presence of earthworms in the soil enables the aeration of the soil which is necessary for a good texture of the soil and for the survival of beneficial microorganisms. They are destroyed by the indiscriminate use of fertilizers.

Allowing cattle to graze in the fields after harvest will help to remove residual fodder and loosen and enrich the soil.

As mentioned earlier, legumes can help improve the quality and quantity of protein in our diets. Their cultivation also enriches soil nitrogen as their root nodules contain bacteria which can convert atmospheric nitrogen into nitrates and nitrites (one of the organisms involved is *Rhizobium leguminosae* and sometimes the soil is inoculated with the same before the cultivation of legumes). Legumes can, therefore, be grown as a second crop after the cereal is harvested. Even if there is not enough water for the maturation of legume crops, they can be allowed to grow to the extent permitted by the water supply and the greens ploughed back into the soil. If it is not possible to raise a second crop, crop rotation can be practiced so that all parts of the land are used for legume cultivation at least once in two or three years. For instance, the farmer may allot 1/3-1/5 of the land for legume cultivation and shift the region used for cultivation from year to year. Incidentally, in studies carried out in the author's laboratory, the cultivation of cowpeas is found to enrich soil nitrogen to a greater extent than other legumes.

In some countries, the seeds are inoculated with nitrogen-fixing bacteria such as *Rhizobium* to ensure or speed up nitrogen-fixation.

Household food security

The supply and demand position of food grains gives a satisfactory picture as shown in projected figures in Table 72. The data is based on agriculture productivity and population growth. However, the actual household level availability is limited on account of various factors. One of the factors that limits the availability is post-harvest losses at farm level, transportation and storage. The tropical climate of the country is conducive for growth of fungus and the consequent deterioration of quality which renders the grains unsuitable for consumption. The second factor is storage losses on account of rodents attack and infestation by insects. A third factor is accessibility of food grains in sections of the population whose income levels are low and hence unable to buy the food at prevailing market rate. The National Food Security Mission mentioned earlier envisages to ensure food security at household level. However, in order to sustain the objectives of the mission the post-harvest conservation of food gains needs to be strengthened with inputs of appropriate technology.

Rodent spoilage of the harvested grain can be prevented by having godowns with well-plastered walls which do not permit the entry and survival of rats. For small scale storage, closed metal containers can be used.

Attempts have been made at the Central Food Technological Research Institute to develop techniques for the prevention of food losses. They include fumigation of the storage rooms or godowns (Durofume-process), pest-proofing of gunny bags used for storing grains and the use of 'non-toxic grain protectants' or chemicals toxic for insects but not for man. Fumigant tablets (Minifume) are available for use by housewife. A low dosage, low cost compound based on indigenous fumigants has been formulated to disinfest rat burrows and termite colonies. Incidentally, many field snakes are not poisonous and are effective in keeping the rodent population down. Unfortunately, they are killed indiscriminately.

Methods have also been developed for the better preservation of fruits, vegetables, eggs, milk etc. They include identification of the optimum temperature for the storage of different commodities, application of plant growth regulators before or after harvest, simple hot water-dip treatment to minimize microbial spoilage during ripening for certain commercial varieties of mangoes, skin coating of fruits by a wax emulsion, etc. Irradiation of onions, potatoes, etc. has also been found to reduce spoilage but the effects are controversial. Household methods for the storage of these commodities need to be developed and evaluated. Some methods used have been described earlier.

Table 73. Status of land usage for cultivation of crops vis-à-vis requirements in India.*

Foodstuff	Amount suggested per capita		Yield (kg/acre)	Land required per capita (acre)	Cultivated land per capita (acre)	Additional land required per capita (acre)
	g/day	kg/year				
Cereals	375	140	800	0.175	0.180	-
Pulses	70	26	224	0.120	0.060	0.06
Roots & Other Vegetables	150	50	5000-10000	0.008	0.006	0.002
Leafy vegetables	100	40	5000-10000	0.003	0.002	0.001
Fruits	50	18	6000	0.009	0.008	0.001

Sources: *figures compounded from data obtained from India Horticulture data base 2011 National Horticulture Board.

Agriculture Statistics Division, Dept.Agriculture & Coperation

Govt. of India. Planning Commission Govt.of India.

Dairy farming

We have the largest cattle population in the world both in terms of absolute numbers and the number of cattle per capita, the same accounting for about 1/5 of the world's cattle population.

For a flourishing dairy farming we need to breed our stocks selectively and care for them well. Although we have some of the finest cattle in the world, most of our cattle are of poor stock in addition to which they do not receive good food and care. Our well-nourished cows from good stock yield about 1500 kg (5 kg per day) with individual animals giving 300–500 kg. Yet most animals yield less than 1 kg per day. The buffaloes which are good producers yield about 10–15 kg per day but the yield is less than 2kg in most cases.

We have one lactating animal for every 8 persons. Even if these cattle yield 4 kg of milk per day, which is quite a moderate yield for a well-nourished animal, the availability of milk should be of the order of 250 g per capita per day, not taking into account the fact that buffaloes which account for about one-third of our cattle population are expected to give higher yields. Yet it was estimated to be less than 140 g per day in 1961 and is believed to have come down to 100 g per day at present. Consequent to the Dairy development in India the per capita availability of milk has gone up substantially. National Dairy Development Board, Anand has come out with statistics giving per capita milk availability in India from the year 1991-92 to 2010-11. All India milk availability has gone up from 178 g per day in 1991-92 to 281 g per day in 2010-11. The States vary considerably in the per capita availability of milk. The figures are as low as 31 in Mizoram and Tripura and as high as 586 in Haryana. Where dairy development has not taken place due to several reasons milk supplies have to be made good by importing from neighbouring states.

Contrary to popular belief, our problem is not unproductive animals which account for about 1.5% but underproductive animals. The poor productivity of our cows and buffaloes is due to several factors. In our agricultural economy, draft animals are considered more important than milch animals. We have three categories of breeds. In draft breeds, the bulls are good for the plough but the cows are poor milk producers. Dairy breeds produce good milkers but poor draft animals. Dual purpose breeds produce moderately good draft and milk animals. In the case of draft breeds, the cow is considered more or less as an incidental by-product and not given much attention.

The productivity of a cow depends not only on breed but on nutrition in early life as well as during their productive years. Poor nutrition during early life results in delayed maturity. Well-nourished animals mature about half to one year earlier and the undernourished animals later than the average age of about 3 years. During pregnancy and lactation, the cow has to be fed well as only the surplus nutrients left over and above the amounts needed for its own metabolism can be used for the production of milk. Poor nutrition results in poor milk production and this results in poor nutrition of the progeny as well. In draft breeds, the male calf is fed better than the female. So we end up with successive generations of poor milk producers. The average lactation period is about 300 days but poorly nourished animals dry much earlier.

It is also necessary to ensure that the cow gets good rest and nutrition at the end of a lactation period before it is bred again. During this period it must be fed well so that it can recuperate from weight and tissue losses suffered during the milking period. In this country, once the animal is dry, it is allowed to fend for itself so that it begins each subsequent pregnancy in a poorer nutritional state.

We also need to improve our breeds. Some of our breeds have cherished qualities such as their ability to use coarse fodder and withstand the heat of a tropical climate. They are docile and have good endurance. They have been used for cross-breeding with animals in North and South America with good results. Similarly, cross-breeding of our better producers with good milkers such as the Jersey, the Holstein-Friesians has resulted in increasing yields by 50–100%.

Also, it is our better milkers which are removed to the cities and slaughtered for meat. This results in bringing down average yields. In this country cow slaughter has acquired religious overtones. Even in Pakistan, which is not guided in this regard by religious scruples, steps are being taken to prevent the indiscriminate slaughter of cows.

Apart from selective breeding, even with existing stocks we should be able to more than double the average yield with better feeds.

Like any other animal the cow requires adequate energy, protein and minerals. Although many of the 'B' vitamins are synthesized in the rumen of cattle, a supply of vitamins is also needed, particularly carotene.

Our cattle are fed mainly cereal straw and hay which have less than 1% protein and are deficient in lysine. Legume hay and legume grass are far better. Lucerne grass and agathi leaves also constitute good fodder. Concentrated sources of protein such as oil cakes and cotton seeds are also valuable.

The position can be expected to improve with increase in agricultural yields. There is also another possibility worth exploration, namely, the planting of agathi trees around agricultural land at, say, 10 feet intervals. These trees grow tall and do not spread out their branches wide and will therefore, neither shade the fields nor impose an extra requirement of land.

Each tree can be expected to yield per year at least 100 kg of green fodder and agathi fodder is of proven value as cattle feed. Twenty to forty trees can be planted around the outer edges of an acre of land and will provide 2000–4000 kg of fodder, a quantity enough to increase the availability of fodder to the required level. The trees will not require extra care once they are firmly established.

Varieties of grass such as lucerne are found to give high yields per acre.

The fodder of certain pulses and legumes can be used along with that of cereals. For instance, the fodder of cowpeas is quite rich in carotene. Cowpeas and cowpea hay have been found valuable as cattle feed. Groundnut cake, guar, etc. also form valuable supplements. Fenugreek (methi) is believed to be a valuable supplement as it is believed to have a lactogenic factor and the oil of fenugreek is found to promote lactation in guinea pigs. Dehusked guar seed, which is now available as a by-product of the plastic industry, is a valuable source of protein and minerals and can be used in cattle feeds. Fermented feeds which are byproducts of the malting and brewing industry as well as the antibiotic industry are considered good cattle feed.

At present, whole cotton seed is given as cattle feed. This is found to be poorly digested because of its high fat content. The defatted meal is much more suitable and the fat extracted can be used for edible purposes. In any case coarsely ground seeds are better than the whole seeds. Attempts are also being made to introduce breeds which give high yields and to control the breeding of cattle by artificial insemination. By and large, the cow or buffalo can live on the incidental by-products of agriculture such as hay, bran, rice and pulse washings (in south India it used to be a standard practice to collect these washings from households for supply to cattle) and foliage for which man has no use. In return it contributes a most valuable item in the diet of normal people as well as those in need of 'special' nutrition. Milk compares favourably with other foods of animal origin in terms of cost and nutritive value. Its dung and urine constitute most valuable manure for the soil. Its leather and horns are also valuable to man.

A feed concentrate supplying vital nutrients needed by cattle is currently manufactured at the animal feed centre at Anand and has found popularity with dairy farmers in surrounding areas. This has resulted in increased yield and record yields of more than 16 litres per day have been obtained. Similar measures in other parts of the country should help increase the per capita availability of milk. It is also necessary to ensure an adequate supply of carotene through green fodder. Yellow maize is a better source than other grains. In this connection, some studies have shown that if the grain is harvested a week earlier than is done normally, the fodder contains nearly twice as much carotene as when the plant has completely dried up.

It also contains somewhat greater amounts of protein and fat. On the other hand, delaying the harvest beyond the normal time is found to result in further losses of these nutrients.

The cultivation of vegetables such as cabbage, cauliflower, turnips, etc. can give valuable fodder as a by-product. The net profit from both fodder and vegetable in these cases can be as high as that from tobacco cultivation.

If the feed is mainly based on fodder, it is also likely to be deficient in minerals. The addition of salt and limestone is necessary. In some areas bone-meal and fish-meal are also used.

The provision of adequate drinking water is also necessary and poses a problem in the summer months in drought areas. Apart from nutritional care, the animals must be housed comfortably in clean surroundings and protected from disease and pests.

Poultry-farming

Although the consumption of eggs is becoming popular, the management of poultry farming is far from efficient. People such as the Bhils in Gujarat have at least one hen and cock per family but they get only about 40 eggs per year, a third of which are lost because of damage by crows as well as the mother hen. Eggs with thin shells which break easily are generally due to a deficiency of calcium in the diet. This can be provided in the form of oyster shells, limestone or powdered and steamed bone-meal. Powdered egg shells may also be given, but they must be washed well in hot water, dried and powdered. Otherwise, the birds fed eggshells may start destroying their own eggs. Some of the chickens hatched do not survive till they are ready for sale. About 200–250 eggs per year are obtained in western countries. In India egg productivity is much less.

Several factors contribute to the poor productivity of hens. They are often kept in damp crowded conditions and do not have enough fresh air. The surroundings are unhygienic so that they are more prone to disease and infestation with lice. The cages are infested with mosquitoes, flies, etc. The poultry houses should be constructed on a raised floor in such a way that they are easy to clean and do not become damp. Provision of nesting space which is secluded and dark is necessary. The eggs laid may be fertilized or unfertilized (without an embryo). Infertile eggs have a better keeping quality and are more suitable for marketing as such. For the production of the same, the laying birds are separated from the males.

Poor breeds are partly responsible for the poor yield. At present high-yielding strains such as the white leghorn and the Rhode Island Red, which are good laying birds, are being imported. Other varieties such as White Cornish from England are used for raising chicks. Some strains such as New

Hampshire are suitable for both purposes. Birds obtained by cross-breeding these strains are found suitable for Indian conditions.

Poultry kept in homes are mostly allowed to fend for themselves and to subsist on worms, etc. They are given some substandard grains. But this does not give a balanced diet. The feed must provide enough protein, minerals and vitamins apart from being adequate in quantity. In addition, except when the feed is made into a fine mash, the feed must contain 'hard grits' which settle in the gizzard and help to grind the food consumed.

Feed concentrates to be mixed with grains and bran used for feeding poultry are available. Maize and jowar are found to be suitable. Yellow maize may be better because of its carotene content. It may be worthwhile trying ragi and kodri in poultry feeds as they contain more methionine. Broken dals obtained as a by-product in the pulse mills are also used. The poultry farmer can prepare his own concentrate according to the following composition:

Groundnut cake	10 kg
Fish-meal	2.5 kg
Hay of lucerne or clover grass (dried and ground)	2.5 kg
Bone-meal	1.0 kg
Fine gravel or sharp sand or metal grits	0.5 kg
Manganese sulphate	30 g

Twenty kilos of the above concentrate can be mixed with 30 kilos each of crushed grain and bran for young chicks and with 60 kilos of the latter for older chicks. If fish-meal does not contain enough salt, 1/4 to 1/2 lb salt must be added. Limestone, oyster shells or dicalcium phosphate may be used in place of bone-meal. Green leaves can be substituted for ground hay. Manganese sulphate may be omitted if rich bran is used. For laying birds, about 5 lb of ground limestone should be added to the concentrate. A vitamin supplement may also be added.

Alternatively, the birds can be given a mixture of grains and bran supplemented with equal quantities of mixture of groundnut cake, bone-meal and fish-meal (given in the form of a mash) and chopped greens.

Poultry farming can be taken up as a subsidiary occupation by the farmer. It has the advantage that the capital required is not large and returns can be expected within six months. Further, poultry can be looked after by women, children and the elderly specially, those who are not engaged in agriculture.

Poultry manure is very good and has a high content of nitrogen, phosphorus and potassium. It is better to use it when fresh. Dry manure has to be mixed with it and used as otherwise it might burn the plants. At present, grading and marketing facilities are to be found only near urban areas. Poultry farming would, therefore, be particularly profitable in villages near big cities or towns.

Fisheries

Fishing has the advantage that it can be carried out in rivers and seas and does not involve additional pressure on land. The annual production of fish in this country is about 1.2 million tons. More than half of this is exported. The amount available per capita for internal consumption is about 4 g per day. Much greater quantities can be obtained with improved techniques.

Vegetables and fruits

As stated earlier, vegetables and fruits give high yields per acre and form a welcome and valuable addition to our meals. At least 2-3% of cultivated land must be allotted for cultivation of the same.

In South India, the distribution of leafy green vegetables to the poor was considered a meritorious act (Tamil proverb—"Pachai koduththal pavam theerum" meaning "If you give Greens your sins will be forgiven"). The author wishes we could take this seriously.

Kitchen gardens can go a long way to help increase the supplies of vegetables and fruits. Even a peasant living in a hut can grow a few trees (say, agathi, drumstick and papaya) and a patch of greens such as spinach, amaranth or fenugreek. Creepers such as pumpkin, which can be trained over the walls or roof, do not require much land. Even in urban areas it is possible to grow greens such as coriander and fenugreek in flower pots, discarded tins, cases, etc. Vegetables and fruits can also be cultivated by the hydro-ponic method. A bed of gravel enriched with a solution containing all the nutrients needed by the plant is used. The plants are grown indoors in verandas near window sills where they can get exposure to sunlight at least for a few hours. Cultivation in pots over the house terrace has now become a common practice. This method has found popularity with housewives in Bombay.

If land is available for cultivation of a kitchen garden perennial trees such as drumstick, mango, agathi, lemon, wood apple, jamun, curry leaves, etc. can be planted on one side and seasonal vegetables on the other. These trees yield year after year without much additional care beyond the first few months. Colocasia, yam, mint, etc. which do not require much sunlight can be planted between perennial trees. Agathi trees, redgram, etc. can be grown near the fence. Creepers such as pumpkin, bitter gourd and field beans give generous yields without much care and can be run on corners of the plot over pandals or the fence.

Details regarding vegetable cultivation in kitchen gardens are available from Krishi Vigyan Kendras of various states.

The consumption of fruits and vegetables is of the order of 30–40 kg per capita per year in this country, whereas in Israel, where there is water scarcity, it is of the order of 240 kg per year. Israel also exports a large quantity of vegetables and fruits to Europe. The phenomenal success of Israel is due to its intensive and painstaking efforts. Wine barrels and cane baskets are used for cultivation of flowers, vegetables and fruits. The barrel is drilled with holes on the sides and different plants are allowed to grow butting out of different holes. It is filled to the brim with rich soil and the plants are watered by water oozing out of a pipe which runs through the centre of the barrel. Beans, brinjals and fruits such as strawberries are cultivated by this method which reduces dependence on the availability of land.

Our immediate problem

At the prevailing level of agricultural yields, to produce the diets recommended we would require at least about 0.6 acre of land per capita according to computations made in **Table 73** (p. 388). This figure does not take into consideration land used for rearing animals for milk and poultry for eggs. When all these factors are taken into consideration, the requirement may be of the order of 0.50-1.00 acre per capita at present levels of productivity. In contrast less than 0.7 acre is cultivated per capita. This has resulted in an appreciable gap between amounts recommended and consumed as can be seen from Table 73 which also suggests that additional land is required at existing levels of production. The gap can be met by either bringing more land under cultivation or using some of the land for as second crop or by increasing agricultural yields. However, unless the increase in agricultural productivity is more than that of population, the gap cannot be bridged. This has already been achieved in the case of cereals although the benefits of increased production have not reached the poorest segments of the population.

The gravity of problem of food spoilage by rodents and insects in the case of grains and decay of fruits and vegetables cannot be overemphasized. Adequate measures to reduce the spoilage of food raw materials and improvement in the supply chain to the people are matters of great urgency in terms of food and nutritional security in the country.

Future prospects of agricultural production

The computations in the preceding section have been made on the basis of recent figures available for population as well as agricultural productivity. On the one hand, land required per capita will be less with improved productivity. On the other hand, the land available per capita will also be less with increase in population. The two have, therefore, to be considered in relation to one another.

As stated earlier, increases in agricultural productivity are offset by increases in population. However, increasing agricultural yields at the rate of about 5% per annum seems possible, given the necessary inputs. If this can be achieved and the increase in population growth brought down to 1.5% we may be able to strike a balance between production and need at least within the next one or two decades.

Incidentally, the rate of population growth can be expected to come down with improved standards of living, literacy rate and increasing urbanization. It has been the experience everywhere that with an improved standard of living and urbanization, rate of population growth decreases. In this country, people in urban areas are having much smaller families than their parents did.

Conclusion

Thus, with the current levels of productivity and population growth, we are far from becoming a land flowing with milk and honey. But with the knowledge provided by the progress of nutrition as a science there is no reason why we should not at least take immediate steps to eradicate nutritional deficiency diseases from our midst and make them a bad dream of the past.

Thus, with relatively minor changes in the diet, namely, the greater consumption of pulses and leafy vegetables, the diet consumed by the adult in this country can be made nutritionally adequate. The adult diet can be made suitable for children by simple processing and with increased and diversified agricultural production, it should be possible to meet the gap between production and need. Education is necessary for the better use of available resources.

The role of human effort in agricultural productivity and material prosperity has been beautifully expressed by Tiruvalluvar (1st century A.D.) in his book Tirukkural: "When a man remains idle and complains of want, the good mother earth smiles to herself."

The author would like to end this chapter with the hope that the advances in science and technology achieved by man can be used for his own benefit. She shares the ancient hope expressed in the following verses for the prosperity, well-being and continued survival of mankind and the realization of freedom from hunger and fear.

"Glory to the people;
May the rulers of the world rule with justice;
May cows* and Brahmins prosper;
May all the peoples of the world be happy!" "May it rain in time;
May the earth bear plenty;
May this land be free from want;
May the good be free from fear !"
"May those without sons get Sons; May those with sons get grandsons;
May those who are poor become wealthy;
May all live to a hundred years !"
*Cows and brahmins were considered symbolic of material and spiritual progress.

Appendices

Preservation of Foods

Sterilization

It is very important to ensure that the food to be preserved and the container to be used are both in a sterile condition at the time of 'packing' and that the entry of microorganisms is prevented by rapid sealing. Otherwise, the foods may become subject to spoilage by molds or bacteria.

Examine bottles and lids carefully for cracks, nicks or sharp edges. Do not use imperfect ones. Bottles with screw-type lids, preferably of hard plastic, are to be preferred. Wash jars and covers thoroughly in hot water and soap.

Method I

Sterilize jars and lids by boiling in water for 15 minutes. Leave submerged in the simmering water until ready to fill.

When the food to be packed is ready, take out the jar, one at a time, with tongs (Use the tongs with a light touch. If too much pressure is used, the bottle will break).

Place the bottle on a clean wooden board. If one is not available use several layers of paper or cloth or wooden surface. Immediately pack with food to the brim and close with lid. Do not tighten the lids till the bottles are cold. Screw the lids completely and then turn back by about half an inch.

Allow a space of 2 to 3 inches between jars to allow for circulation of air.

To test for seal, tap the lid gently with a spoon after the jar is completely cool. If the sound is. clear and ringing the seal is good; if it is dull and low the jar is not properly sealed. It is a good plan to examine the seal a second time 4 or 5 days after processing.

Store the bottles in a cool, dry and dark place, away from the stove and other sources of heat.

Method II

If the bottles are to be sterilized after packing in jars, rinse the washed jars and lids with hot water and let them stand in hot water until ready to use.

Fill the bottles and close with lids (turn back by half an inch after complete sealing). Lower carefully into water so that the lids are at least an inch below the surface. Make sure that the temperature of the water is not appreciably different from that of the bottle. (If the bottles are hot, lower into simmering waters.) Alternatively, place the bottles in the pan and add water at the right temperature till the bottles are covered.

Bring the water to a boil and close the pan. Let simmer for about 30 minutes.

Equipment for sterilizing bottles

Use a large aluminium pan with a flat bottom and a lid that fits well. Invert a perforated lid over the bottom of the pan and place the bottles on the same. Alternatively, use a wire-mesh rack made so as to fit the pan. If the rack is equipped with handles the bottles can be placed in and removed from the pan easily. A large colander with a flat bottom and somewhat straight edges or a sieve with a thick wire-mesh (the type used for grains) can also be used.

Canning of fruits and vegetables

Fruits and vegetables selected for canning must be of good quality. Fruits are best for canning when mature, and vegetables, when young and tender. The flavour and texture of fresh vegetables change more rapidly than fresh fruits so that vegetables should be processed as quickly as possible after they are harvested.

For a quality canned food, fruits should be sorted for size, colour and ripeness. Over-ripe and blemished (spotted) fruits should be discarded. First, they should be thoroughly scrubbed and washed, preferably under running water. If necessary they should be peeled.

Preservation with sugar

Fruit preserves: Preserves are fruits or pieces of fruit cooked in sugar syrup until tender and plump. The fruit remains whole and the syrup becomes transparent and thick.

Preserving soft fruits such as mango: Wash the fruits and drain thoroughly. Remove skin and stone and cut into pieces. Weigh the fruit and the sugar. For each pound of fruit take 3/4 to 1 pound of sugar. Add ½ to 1 cup of water for each pound of sugar.

Bring the sugar and water to the boiling point, stirring until sugar is dissolved. Add the fruit. Cook on slow heat until the fruit is clear and tender, stirring frequently and carefully. Pack the fruit into hot sterilized jars; boil the syrup if necessary to thicken it; pour over the fruit in the jars. Wipe the edges of jars and seal at once. Cool and store.

Preserving firm fruits such as pineapple: Wash the fruit, drain thoroughly, peel, cut and remove cores. Weigh the fruit. Allow 3/4 pound of sugar for each pound of fruit. Combine the sugar with water, allowing ¾-1cup of water for each pound of sugar. Bring to a boil, stirring until the sugar is dissolved. Add the fruit, bring to a boil, and cook on slow heat for 1 to 1 ½ hours or until the fruit is tender. Pack the fruit in hot sterilized jars. If the remaining syrup is thin, boil until thickened, then pour over fruit in jars. Wipe the edges of the jars and seal at once. Cool and store.

Squashes: May be prepared from berries such as chani bor and from the juice of oranges and lemons.

Chani bor squash: Wash and boil the fruit with equal volumes of water. Crush and boil again. Churn and strain through a double layer of cheese cloth. Allow the sediment to settle down. Mix the clear juice with 1-1 ½ volumes of sugar and lemon juice. Bring to a boil and let simmer for 30 minutes.

A suitable quantity of edible colour may be added to bring out the desired colour in the finished product. Pack into hot sterilized bottles and seal.

Lime squash: Select fresh, fully ripe limes which are free from blemishes. Wash fruit thoroughly in cold water. Soak in warm water for some time and then cut the fruits with a stainless steel knife. Extract juice and strain using a metal strainer. For one cup of juice, take 1-2 cups sugar and 3-4 cups water for medium sugar squash and 2 cups sugar and 3 cups water for high sugar squash. Boil till all the sugar dissolves and strain through muslin cloth. Boil again, let simmer for a few minutes, add the lemon juice, bring to a boil and pack in hot sterilized bottles or jars. If bottles with corks are used leave a head space 1-1½ inches. Seal the cork with paraffin wax by covering the cork and the adjacent area with molten paraffin wax.

Alternatively, boil the sugar and water together, add the juice, bring to a boil and pack in hot sterilized jars. Cardamom and saffron may be added.

Jams and conserves: They are made by cooking crushed fruit with sugar. Select fresh, fully ripe whole fruits with sweet taste. Wash, peel, remove seed and cut into small pieces. Mash the pieces thoroughly to obtain a uniform mass.

Depending on the acidity of the fruit, add one cup or more of sugar per cup of fruit. Add lemon juice, cook in a greased pan on medium fire with frequent stirring and crushing, till a sufficiently thick paste, which does not stick to the spoon, is obtained. Pack into hot sterilized screw-type jars and seal them immediately. A thin layer of molten paraffin wax may be poured on top before sealing (1 teaspoon per bottle) to prevent recontamination.

Jam may be prepared from fruits such as papaya and fleshy mangoes by the above method.

Jam from fruit juices: Jams may be prepared from the juice of mangoes, chani bor, etc., by the following procedure: Ingredients:

fruit juice	...	1 cup
sugar	...	1 cup
lemon juice	...	8 teaspoons

Mix the ingredients and boil down to jam consistency.

Ripe tomato jam : Select ripe firm tomatoes. Blanch, peel and crush. Allow 3/4 to 1 lb of sugar per pound of fruit. Add lemon juice, thinly sliced lemon peel and a few whole cloves, a few sticks of cinnamon and small pieces of ginger if desired. Proceed as for jam from mango juice.

Raw mango preserve:
Ingredients:

raw mangoes (skinned and grated) ...	1 cup
powdered jaggery	...	1 cup
salt	...	a pinch.

Prepare a thick syrup with jaggery and add the grated mangoes to the same. Cook to jam consistency. Pack in sterilized jars. Lemon juice, salt and spices may be added.

Jellies: They are prepared from the clear juices of fruits rich in pectin.

A good jelly is clear, sparkling and transparent and retains its shape when unmoulded, but is tender.

To make jelly the fruit juice must contain proper proportions of pectin, the jellying substance, and acid, which gives the jelly its firmness and tenderness. Some fruits contain in themselves sufficient pectin and acid to make jelly when properly concentrated. Other fruits lack pectin or acid or both, A fruit naturally low in pectin content may be combined with another fruit rich in pectin or be concentrated in an open vessel until the volume is reduced by a third to half. Commercial pectin in liquid or powder form may be added. If a fruit is low in acid content, lemon juice or another fruit juice may be added.

Test for pectin: To determine the pectin content of fruit juice, stir gently together one tablespoon of the juice and one tablespoon of alcohol. If one large firm mass of jelly is formed, the juice is rich in pectin; if several less firm pieces of jelly are formed or none at all, it is poor in pectin. Do not taste the jelly unless grain alcohol is used.

Guava jelly: Select sound, firm fruits free from blemishes. Soft fruit does not possess good setting quality and hence should be avoided as far as possible.

Wash, cut into small pieces and cover with water. Boil the mass for about an hour till the extract shows good stickiness. Churn and strain through cheese cloth. Add to the residue one-fourth its weight of water and take another extraction. Get a similar extraction once again.

To every cup of the clear extract add about 3/4 cup of sugar according to pectin content. Concentrate the extract if necessary before adding sugar. Add lemon juice or citric acid and cook on slow heat till it forms a sheet when dropped from the spoon. Pack in sterilized bottles.

Woodapple jelly: Scoop out the pulp from just ripe fruit and proceed as in the case of guava jelly.

Common defects in jelly in jelly-making and their causes

- *Tough jelly:* Too little sugar for the amount of pectin; also over-cooking.
- *Syrup jelly:* Too much sugar for the amount of pectin ; juice too low in pectin or acid content or both.
- *Cloudy jelly:* Juice not properly strained; slightly over-cooked; cooled before pouring; fruits too underripe so that starch is present.

Formation of sugar crystals in jelly: Too much sugar; sugar added too near the finishing point of the jelly.

Use of earthenware jars

Earthenware jars (mutka) are much less expensive than glass-bottles and can be used for preserving jams and jellies. Wash the earthenware jar and heat over an open flame, both inside and outside, till it is quite dry. Pack with the material and pour molten paraffin wax over the top. Coat the neck and the sides with a thin layer of molten wax so that the pores on the jar are sealed.

Canning of fresh fruit juices

Fruits suitable for this method: tomatoes, juicy mangoes. Extract the juice from clean sound fruit after blanching. Strain through several thicknesses of cheese-cloth. Warm the juice to about 45°C; pour at once into clean hot jars; partly seal. Heat the jars for 30 minutes in a simmering water-bath. Remove from the bath and seal completely at once.

Tomato paste

Tomatoes are plentifully available for only two months in the year. They are very 'handy' to use in soups and curries and made into a paste and preserved by the following procedure:

Blanch and crush the tomatoes, churn well in a mixer or mash or grind to a smooth paste. Add salt, boil down to 1/4 by volume. Pack into hot sterilized bottles.

Bottling of vegetables

Select firm, sound and tender vegetables. Avoid those with decayed or bruised spots. Grade according to size and maturity. Wash thoroughly, peel, cut and cook. Non-acid vegetables should be cooked-under pressure.

Pack the cooked vegetables loosely in clean hot jars to allow for proper heat circulation and for the vegetable to retain its shape. Pour the boiling water in which the vegetable was cooked to within half an inch of the top of the jar except when canning tender corn or peas. For these vegetables, fill the jar to within an inch of the top. Add boiling water if there is not enough vegetable water. Run a thin spatula down along the sides of the jar to permit the release of air pockets. Seal the jars.

Sterilize the jars under simmering water as in the case of fruit. Cans can also be used in place of bottles if equipment for sealing is available.

Lemon juice, vinegar, tamarind juice or citric acid may be added to ensure an acid medium.

Dehydration

Mango: Select fresh raw green mangoes, wash, peel and add enough salt to coat the slices and dry in the home drier or in the sun.

Bittergourd: Cut into small pieces and dry in the sun.

Cluster beans: Cut into small pieces. Cook in boiling water (containing salt) for 5–10 minutes. Take out and dry in the sun.

An alternate procedure for the above and for other vegetables such as green chillies, field beans, pink beans, manathakkali fruits, neem flowers, etc. is as follows. Steam over a colander for 10–15 minutes, soak in curd or buttermilk with salt added for 12–24 hours and then dry in the sun. Vegetables dried by this method may be deep-fried and used.

Dried potato wafers

Wash, peel and slice into boiling or simmering water and let simmer for 2–5 minutes till it appears cooked. Place on greased aluminium plates and let dry in the sun. Add lime juice, green chilli extract and hing to the boiling water to improve colour and flavour. Wafers can be prepared from sweet potatoes similarly.

Sago papadi

Wash and keep sago ready. For one cup sago, take 3–5 cups water depending on the texture desired and boil. Add lemon juice, salt and an extract prepared from green chillies. Put in the sago, bring to a boil, let simmer until transparent (10–15 minutes) and let rest for 10–15 minutes. Drop by the spoon over greased aluminium plates or cheese cloth and dry in the sun. If cheese cloth is used, water has to be sprinkled from the reverse side after drying to peel off the papadi. Large aluminium plates about 30" diameter are much more convenient. They can be transported easily and shifted readily to different areas with the movement of the sun. As they retain the heat of the sun, the drying is also much quicker. The papadi can be easily turned over when one side is dried.

Rice flour papadi

For 1 cup rice flour take 1 cups water and boil adding lemon juice, salt and chilli extract. Put in the flour gradually, mix well and let cook in simmering heat for 10–15 minutes. Knead well and roll into balls, put in a 'sev' press and press out on a greased aluminium plate to get a macaroni or spaghetti type product. Dry and store. To get a fool-proof product, steam the balls for 5 minutes in an idli vessel or colander and then process as described.

Flours of maize, kodri and jowar can be substituted in the above recipe.

Appendix IA. Common adulterants in foods and methods of detection

Food Commodity	Adulterant	Method of detection
Rice	Stone chips	Place the grains on palms of hand and gradually immerse hand in Water. The stone chips will sink
Pulses	Metanil yellow	Put 5g of pulse in 5ml water. Add a few drops of HCl. Pink colour shows metanil.
Dhals	Kesari Dhal	Visual method. Kesari dhal is Wedge shaped.
Bajra seeds	Ergot	Put some grains in a glass containing 20% salt solution. Ergot will float while bajra seeds will sink.
Rawa (Sooji)	Iron filings	Pass a magnet through the rawa. Iron filings will cling to it.
Milk	Water	Measure sp. gravity with Lactometer. Normal value is 1.03–1.034

contd. ...

contd. ...

Ghee	Vanaspati	Take 1 teaspoonful of ghee and mix with equal quantity of con.HCl in a test tube. Add 2-3 drops furfural solution. Appearance of pink colour in the lower layer means presence of vanaspati.
Ice cream	starch	Perform iodine test for starch
Mustard oil	Argimone oil	Heat the oil with little amount of Nitric acid. Heat for 3 min. Red Colour shows argemone oil.
Coffee powder	Tamarind seed powder	Sprinkle a little coffee powder on a piece of blotting paper. Spread a few drops of KOH solution over the paper. Brown colour develops around particle of coffee powder.
Sugar	Chalk and dust	Dissolve sugar in water. Impurities will settle down at bottom.
Bura sugar	washing soda	Gives effervescence with HCl.
Turmeric, chilly Powder	colouring matter	Sprinkle power on surface of water. Extraneous colouring matter will dissolve.

Heavy Metal Contaminants in Foods

Contaminant	source
Lead	Lead contaminated water from industrial effluent. Improperly tinned copper vessels.
Cadmium	Cadmium plated vessels for processing of foods.
Copper	Water from industrial discharge
Zinc	do
Mercury	do

(Safe limits have been fixed for heavy metals)

Natural Contaminants and Toxicants in Foods.

Contaminant	Source
Fluorine	Drinking water
Gossypol	Cotton seed powder
Cyanogenetic glycosides	Bitter almond, apple seeds, cassava
Polcyclic Aromatic Hydrocarbons (PAH)	Smoked fish, meat, mineral oil contaminated water, oils and fats
Phalloidine (alkaloid)	Toxic mushrooms
Nitrates and Nitrites	Drinking water, processed meat products
Asbestos	Environment
Pesticide residues	Excessive use of pesticides
Antibiotics	Meat from antibiotic fed animals
Steroid hormones	Meat from hormone fed animals

Some Foods Suitable for Young Children and Others

A. Foods already described in the text

- Conjee
- Fruit juices
- Soups
- Salads
- Mashed vegetables
- Mashed bananas
- Softly cooked rice
- Khichri
- Savoury and sweet pongal
- Idli
- Dhokla
- Khaman
- Chapatis soaked in dal, milk or curd
- Biscuits
- Bread.

B. Other foods

Rava idli (savoury)

Roast 1 cup rava and prepare a batter with salt and 1.5 cups or more of curd or buttermilk. Add suitable seasoning and a pinch of baking powder or baking soda. Steam in an idli steamer. Coconut, groundnut, cashewnut, crushed black pepper, ginger, curry leaves, etc. may be added as seasoning.

Rava idli (sweet)

Prepare a batter as described above substituting milk for curd and 1/2 cup jaggery. Add raisins and coconut and steam.

Suji porridge

Roast 1/2 cup suji, add 1/2 cup water and cook on slow heat. When all the water is absorbed, add 1 cup of milk and raisins and cook on simmering heat for 15-20 minutes. Add sugar or jaggery and seasoning such as nutmeg, saffron or cardamom.

Sweet poha

Wash 1 cup poha and add to medium syrup prepared from 1/2 cup jaggery. Continue cooking on slow heat till done to the consistency of cooked rice. Add cardamom, coconut, raisins, roasted til and roasted and crushed groundnut. Roasted and cooked greengram dal (2 tablespoons) can also be added.

Tomato poha

Blanch ripe tomatoes and crush into a pulp. Fry chopped onions in a little fat, add the tomato pulp (1 cup), washed poha (1 cup), salt and seasoning and cook on slow heat till done. Cooked rice or macaroni may be substituted for poha. Grated cheese or the cheesy residue may be added.

Lemon poha

Make a vaghar of mustard seed, add Bengal gram dal and groundnut and roast to a brown colour. Add a pinch of turmeric powder and washed poha. Add salt and cook on slow heat. Add lemon juice. Garnish with curry leaves. The same seasoning (i.e. vaghar, salt, turmeric powder, lemon juice, curry leaves and hing) can be added to cooked rice or macaroni.

Poha kheer

Roast 1/2 cup poha in a little fat. Soften by cooking with 1/2 cup water. Churn, add two cups of milk and churn again. Bring to a boil and add sugar, raisins, nuts and spices. Rose-water of a tea prepared, from rose-petals may be added.

Steamed bread

To one cup wheat flour add 1/2 cup each of mashed banana and jaggery, 1/2 cup groundnut paste, 1/2 cup curd and one tablespoon fat. Prepare a thick batter from the same adding more water or curd if necessary. Add baking soda and steam in a greased and closed container. Groundnut paste can be prepared from roasted and skinned groundnuts.

Biscuits

Prepare a biscuit dough with wheat flour 1 cup, bengalgram flour 1/4 cup, crushed groundnut 1/4 cup, til 1 teaspoon, fat 1 tablespoons, and salt. Shape into biscuits and roast in an oven or a tava. Flours prepared from other cereals and millets can be substituted for wheat flour.

Buttermilk-khaman

Prepare a thick batter with 1 cup Bengal gram flour and 1 cup curd or buttermilk. Add salt, seasoning and baking soda. Steam in a greased and closed container, cool, cut into pieces and serve.

Puttu

Roast rice, maize or jowar flour and make a loose dough with warm water and salt. Let keep for half an hour, steam in an idli-steamer or over a colander, cool and crumble the steamed 'puttu' to grains, add to syrup prepared from jaggery and cook on slow heat. Add suitable seasoning and ghee. Alternatively, roast puffed rice, grind into a coarse meal and treat similarly. For each cup flour use 1/2 cup jaggery.

For savoury puttu, add salt, lemon juice and other seasoning to the steamed puttu.

Proforma for use in Diet Surveys*

Interviewer ...   Family No.

Date   Address

General Information

1. Head of the family   ——————————
2. Composition of family——————————

No.	Name	Sex	Age	Education	Occupation**	Income	Relation to head
1							
2							
3							
4							
5							
6							
7							
8							
9							
10							

* The form given is a comprehensive one which seeks to collect information on socio-economic aspects. A shorter form with selected items may be used according to the information desired.

** Include subsidiary occupations.

1. (a) Information on married women
      Number of children born
      Number of children living
      Miscarriages
      Still births

   (b)

	Present Family	Father's Family	Mother's Family
Number of children born			
Number of children surviving			

(a) Record of deceased family members

No.	Name	When occurred	Relation to head	Age at death	Cause of death
1					
2					
3					
4					
5					
6					
7					
8					
9					
10					

4. Approximate monthly expenditure on :
   a) Milk and milk products
   b) Vegetable and fruits
   c) Groceries,
   d) Fuel
   e) Rent.

5. Surroundings :
   a) Water supply
   b) Ventilation
   c) Lighting

    d)   Sanitary facilities

    e)   Garbage disposal

    f)   Cleanliness of surroundings

6. (a) Kitchen garden:
      For rural areas
      Vegetables and fruits cultivated

  (b) Poultry
      Hens
      Cocks
      Number of eggs got per year
      Number of eggs consumed by family
      Number of eggs marketed
      Chicken consumed by family
      Feed given

  (c) Farm animals
      Milch animals

Number	Condition*	Yield per day	Use of milk**
Cows			
Buffaloes			
Goats			

  * Specify whether resting, pregnant, lactating or sterile. "Specify whether
  ** consumed, sold or used for buttermilk.

Other farm animals

Number	Condition	Use
Bullocks Calves Male buffaloes		
Use of cowdung: as manure	as fuel	not used
Feed used for: milch animals working bullocks resting animals		

  (d) Storage of foodgrains
        Estimate of food losses

II. Dietary Survey

1. Food habits :

   Vegetarian/non-vegetarian/non-vegetarian but usually takes vegetarian food

   Common dietary pattern

   Morning

   Mid-day

   Afternoon

   Evening

   Others

(c) During different seasons

Season	Foods recommended	Foods avoided
Summer		
Winter		
Monsoon		

(b) For religious or other reasons (include data on 'fasts' undertaken by family members and foods taken during 'fasting')

Occasion	Foods permitted	Foods avoided

2. Special foods:

(a) For different groups

Groups	Foods recommended	Foods avoided
Adults		
Infants		
Pregnant women		
Lactating women		
Invalids		

(b) During illness	Foods recommended	Foods avoided
Cold		
Fever		
Diarrhoea		
Dysentery		
Other conditions		

a) For religious or other reasons (include data on 'fasts' undertaken by family members and foods taken during 'fasting'

Occasion	Foods permitted	Foods avoided

(d)   (i) Foods consumed by previous generation and not consumed now
      (ii) Foods consumed now and not consumed by previous generation
      3. Methods of

3. Methods of cooking cooking :
   a)   Roti
   b)   Rice
   c)   Dal
   d)   Vegetables

4. Food sharing practices :
   Members eating out and guests or servants eating with family

6. Foods consumed at home :

	Foodstuff	Amount consumed (g) @	Source from which obtained
1.	Cereals and millets*		
	Rice		
	Wheat		
	Other Grains		
	Other cereal or starch foods		
	Processed cereal foods		
2.	Dals		
	Whole legumes		
	Groundnut, til, etc.		
	Other nuts		
	Parched legumes		
3.	Vegetables (see sepa		
	rate check list)		
	Leafy vegetables		
	Roots and tubers		
	Others		
4.	Animal foods		
	Fish, meat and chicken		
	Egg		

5.	Milk and milk products		
	Whole milk		
	Toned milk		
	Milk powder		
	Curd		
	Baby food		
	@ Specify per day, week or month.		

* Specify the type of rice used, parboiled, milled or handpounded; for (c) specify grain used; for (d) include macaroni, sago, suji, poha, refined flour, tapioca, etc; for (e) include bread, biscuit, cakes, cornflakes, parched grains, etc.

Foodstuff	Amount (g) consumed	Source from which obtained
Cheese		
Mava		
Milk sweets		
Ice-cream		
Other milk products		

6 Fats and oils
   Butter
   Dalda
   Groundnut oil
   Ghee
   Refined oil
   Other oils (specify)

7 Sugar
   Refined sugar
   Jaggery
   Others (honey, molasses, etc.)

8 Condiments
   Tamarind
   Cocum
   Chillies
   Mango slices (e).
   Other spices

9   Preserved and processed foods
     Pickles
     Papadi
     Jams and jellies
     Other canned or bottled foods

10   Beverages
     Tea
     Coffee
     Cocoa
     Malted foods
     Carbonated drinks
     Alcoholic drinks

11   Miscellaneous
     Betel nut
     Betel leaves
     Chewing tobacco
     Smoking tobacco

Vegetable and fruit check list

To get an idea of the pattern of vegetable consumption throughout the year, make a list of the vegetables or fruits available in the area and in the case of seasonal vegetables indicate the months in which they are available. Find out how the family consumes the vegetables when in season and how much each time. Then make an estimate of total consumption. Reliable information on this is necessary for arriving at valid estimates of the availability of nutrients such as carotene, vitamin C and iron.

Where possible, get actual records of vegetables consumed by a few families in different groups for a period of time so as to get some idea of the proportions in which different vegetables are consumed. The vegetable sellers in the market may also be able to give this information.

Foodstuff	Amount consumed (g) per day*		
	per family	per capita consumption	per Unit**
Cereals (rice + other grains)			
Pulses			

Leafy vegetables			
Root vegetables			
Other vegetables			
Flesh foods			
Fats and oils			
Milk			
Sugar and jaggery Nutrients:			
Calories			
Protein (g)			
Fat (g)			
Carbohydrate (g)			
Calcium (mg)			
Phosphorus (mg)			
Iron (mg)			
Vitamin A as :			
carotene (i.u.)			
pre-formed vitamin (i.u.)			
Thiamine (mg)			
Riboflavin (mg)			
Niacin (mg)			
Vitamin C (mg)			

* Unless otherwise specified.
** Consumption units:

Consumption*	Coefficient	Approximate Range@ of Intakes	
		Poor	Upper Class
Adult male	0.8–1.0	2000–3000	2000–2400
Adult female and adolescent girls	0.6–0.8	1500–2000	1800–2000
Adolescent boys (16–19 yrs)	0.8–1.0	1800–2400	2000–3000
Adolescent boys (13–15 yrs)	0.8-0.8	1500–1700	2000–2500

Children (9–12 yrs)	0.6-0.7	1200–1500	1800–2000
Children (5–7 yrs)	0.5-0.6	1000–1200	1500–1800
Children (3–5 yrs)	0.4-0.5	700–900	1100–1500
Children (1–3 yrs)	0.4	900–1100	

Add up the appropriate coefficients to obtain total consumption units for the family surveyed.

* According to ICMR energy allowance assuming 3000 calories for one unit. @ Use the lower limit to check for underestimation and the upper limit to check for overestimation.

A. Volume-Weight Equivalents of Selected Food-stuffs (Approximate values)

	Foodstuff	Weight (g) of one cup (225ml)	Weight (g)as fraction of volume (ml)	Volume (ml) of 100 g
1	Rice	185	5/6	120
2	Flaked rice (poha)	75	1/3	300
3	Puffed rice	18	1/12	1200
4	Parched rice	55	¼	420
5	Wheat(whole)	200	5/6	115
6	Wheat flour	115	½	200
7	Suji	150	2/3	150
8	Jowar flour	120	½	185
9	Bajra flour	120	½	185
10	Parched jowar	30	1/8	750
11	Corn flakes	25	1/9	900
12	Dals	190	5/6	120
13	Bengalgram flour	100	½	225
14	Greengram (whole)	175	¾	130
15	Groundnuts	150	2/3	150
16	Til	150	2/3	150
17	Copra(grated)	75	1/3	300

contd. ...

contd. ...

	Foodstuff	Weight (g) of one cup (225ml)	Weight (g)as fraction of volume (ml)	Volume (ml) of 100 g
18	Cashewnuts(whole)	150	2/3	150
19	Sugar	205	9/10	110
20	Groundnut oil	205	9/10	110
21	Raisins	150	2/3	150
22	Greens (chopped)	90	2/5	250
23	Carrots (grated)	100	4/9	225
24	Fruit juices	225	1	100
25	Milk	225	1	100

B. Approximate Composition of Cooked Foods

Foodstuff	Quantity	Weight (g)	Raw ingredients* (g)		Calories	Protein (g)
Rice	1 cup	200–240	Rice	50–60	175–210	3-4
Pongal (savoury)	1 cup	200–240	Rice	40		
			Greengram dal	15–20		
			Fat	5–10	270–330	8-9
			nuts	5		
Pongal (sweet)	1 cup	200–240	Rice	40		
			Greengram dal	15–20		
			Fat	5–10	450–550	8-9
			Jaggery	40–50		
			Nuts and raisins	5–10		
khichri	1 cup	200–240	rice	35–40	180–210	6-8
			Tur dal	15–20		
Lemon rice	1 cup	200–240	Rice	50–60	220–255	3-4
			Fat	5		

Foodstuff	Quantity	Weight (g)	Raw ingredients* (g)		Calories	Protein (g)
Coconut rice	1 cup	200–240	Rice	40		
			Coconut	25	300	4
			Fat	5		
Curd rice	1 cup	200–240	Rice	40–50		
			Curd	100–150		
			Fat	2-3	270–350	
			nuts	5		
Idli	I serving (2 idlis)	80–100	Rice (par boiled)	40–45	190–230	7-8
			Black gram dal	15–20		
dosa	1 serving (2-3 dosas)	80–100	Rice (par boiled)	40–45		
			Black gram dal	15-20	240–270	7-8
			Fat	5		
Sweet poha	½ cup	100	Poha	30		
			Jaggery	20–25		
			Fat	5–10	250–320	2-3
			Nuts and raisins	5		
Chevda	1 serving	50–60	Poha	25		
			Ground nut	10		
			Chana dal	10	270	7
			fat	10		
Chapati	1 medium size	40	Wheat flour	25	100	3
"	I thick size	55	Wheat flour	35	140–150	4
"	1 very thick size	75–80	Wheat flour	50	190–200	6
Parathas	1 medium size	55–60	Wheat flour	35	150–170	4
			Fat	3–5		
Poories	1	15–25	Wheat flour	10-15	50–80	1-2
			Fat	2-3		
Upma	1 cup	180–200	Rava	50	220–265	6
			Fat	5–10		

contd. ...

contd. ...

Foodstuff	Quantity	Weight (g)	Raw ingredients* (g)		Calories	Protein (g)
Nimki	1 serving	80–100	Wheat flour	50	265	6
			Fat	10		
Suji halwa	1 serving (½ cup)	100–120	Rava	25		
			Sugar	15–20		
			Fat	5–10	210–270	3-4
			Nuts and raisins	5		
Bread	1 slice	20–30	Wheat flour	15	50	2
Samosa	1 serving (2-3)		Wheat flour	20–25		
			potatoes	25		
			Onions	25	200–260	3-4
			Fat	10–15		
Vada (crisp type)	1 serving (2-3)	60–70	dal	25		
			fat	10–45	185	6
			Vegetables	20–30		
Bhajya	1 serving	80	Chana flour	20		
			vegetables	40	175	6
			Fat	10		
Khaman	1 serving	7–80	Chana dal	25–30	105–130	6-7
			Fat	2-3		
Whole legume Or dal –moist Without surplus Liquid (sundal type)	1 cup	200–240	Whole legume Or dal	50–60	200–255	12–14
			Fat	3–5		
Liquid dal	1 cup	200–240	Dal	20–30	90–130	5–7
			Fat	2-3		
Dals cooked with vegetables	1 cup	200–240	dal	20–25		
			Vegetables	40–50	105–135	5–7
			Fat	2-3		
Sambar	1 cup	200–240	Tur dal	25		
			Vegetables	25	115–125	6

Foodstuff	Quantity	Weight (g)	Raw ingredients* (g)		Calories	Protein (g)
			Fat	2-3		
Vegetables (pan cooked without surplus moisture)	1 serving	80–100	Vegetables	100	70–90	3
			Fat	3–5		
Vegetables (gravy type)	1 serving	100	Vegetables	50–75	50–80	1-2
			Fat	3–5		
Tea	1 cup	225	Milk	50	80	2
			Sugar	10		
Coffee	1 cup	225	Milk	100	120	3
			Sugar	10		

* only those contributing significantly to calories listed.

Appendix V

Nutrition Education— Specimen Lessons

A. Primary school level: Papaya

You have just planted papaya trees in your garden. I am now going to talk to you about how good this fruit is from the point of view of health.

Papaya is a delicious fruit which can be easily grown and is very good for health. Its rich yellow colour is due to the presence of a substance called 'carotene'. This substance is also present in other yellow fruits and vegetables such as yellow pumpkin, carrot, sakarteti (rock melon with a rich yellow colour) and mango. Carotene is also present in dark green leafy vegetables such as amaranth, fenugreek (methi), spinach and some red vegetables as tomatoes.

What is the importance of carotene?

The carotene present in food can be converted to a substance called vitamin A in our body. Vitamin A is present in milk, butter, eggs' and fish, which most of us are not able to afford. As carotene can be converted to vitamin A in the body, a person, who cannot afford milk, egg, etc, can remain healthy by. taking foods rich in carotene.

What does vitamin A do in our body?

It protects against infection and helps growth. It is also necessary for the functioning of the eyes. When a person does not eat foods which are rich in either carotene or vitamin A, he may develop night blindness and also total blindness.

Use of papaya

Besides carotene, papaya also contains another vitamin called vitamin C. This vitamin is also present in orange juice, so that it has the same value as orange juice from the point of view of health. Vitamin C is necessary for several body functions. Fruits such as papaya also help to maintain proper intestinal functions.

We can eat papaya as such after removing the skin and seeds. Its taste is improved if we cut it into pieces and add some lemon juice and sugar. This will also help to prevent the destruction of vitamin C. We should not keep papaya long after cutting as the fruit may get spoiled! If we have to keep it, it must be kept covered and no flies should be allowed to sit on it. Keeping the papaya exposed to air after cutting results in two bad effects:

Some of the vitamins get destroyed

The fruit may get contaminated with germs derived from the air and from physical contact with flies and mosquitoes. We must wash the fruit well with clean water before cutting. These precautions are particularly important during the summer and rainy seasons as there are plenty of flies and mosquitoes around during this season with the result that diseases such as cholera, dysentery, etc., spread more easily in this season. Freshly cut papaya can be mashed well and given to very young children.

We can also make jam with papaya. For making jam from fruit, the fruit is cut, mashed and cooked with sugar and lemon juice. The consistency of the cooked jam is like that of halwa. It contains very little water so that it can keep longer. For instance, ordinary milk will not keep for more than a few hours but the same milk, boiled down with sugar so that most of the water is removed, can keep for a few days.

It is necessary to put the papaya jam in clean bottles or mud-pots and keep them covered airtight so that they "do not spoil. The air contains very small organisms which we can see only through microscope. The fermentation of khaman and dhokla batter or the fermentation of curd is due to such microorganisms. Other microrganisms cause the bread dough raise. There are other varieties of microorganisms which can cause food to spoil and others which cause disease to men. So, if we want to keep foods in a good condition it is necessary to prevent harmful microorganisms from entering the foods. This is achieved by packing the jam into a cleaned jar or mudpot when it is hot and by sealing it with wax. If we do not do this, the jam may get spoilt. By boiling the jam to right consistency, packing in clean jars and sealing with wax, we can preserve it for a long time.

Table 1. Protein content of common foods.

Food	Calories/100 g	% protein	% calories from proteins
Sago	350	0,2	0.2
Tapioca	160	0.7	2
Potatoes	100	1.6	6
Rice	345	7	8
Maize, jowar	340–360	10	12-13
Wheat	345	12	14
Buffalo milk	120	4.3	14
Cow milk	70	3.2	19
Groundnut	550	27	20
Pulses and dals	330–370	18–24	23–29
Eggs	170	13.3	31
methi leaves	50	4.4	36
Soyabean	430	43	40
Meat	200	20	40
Fish and chicken	100–150	20-25	70–95

How can we grow papaya?

Papaya plants should be planted during the rainy season, either from June to October or from February to March. First the seeds are sown in pots, boxes or beds. They germinate in 10–12 days. The beds should be raised and pots and boxes well drained to avoid water stagnation. Usually, out of 500 seeds, 125 do not germinate. Out of those which germinate about 200 are fruit bearing (called MADl Plants) and the rest would only give flowers (called NAR plants).

The plants start bearing fruit in one year and last for 7-8 years, but the best fruits are obtained during the first three years.

Care of the plant

Like any other plant, the papaya plant needs three things: water, manure and sun-shine, for its growth. Lack of anyone of these necessities causes the leaves to become pale and yellow.

The plant needs to be protected from diseases, pest and birds. Due to a contagious disease that affects the plant, the foliage, gets curled. The affected plants should be removed and burnt so that the infection does not spread to the other plants.

Sometimes a kind of insect penetrates the stem: and eats the flesh causing the plant to weaken and die. The insects should be picked out, if possible and the holes should be plugged with wax after putting crude kerosene oil into these holes,

Birds should be prevented from doing any harm to the fruits by wrapping jute cloth around the fruit. If not, newspaper can be used.

Exercise

1. What is carotene?
2. What nutrients do we get from papaya?
3. What happens when the diet is lacking in carotene and vitamin A?
4. Which are the foodstuffs that prevent the deficiency of vitamin A?
5. How do we grow papaya?
6. At what age does the papaya start giving fruit?
7. For how long does a papaya tree last?
8. What do the papaya plants need in order to grow?
9. How can we prevent the birds from doing any harm to the fruit?

B. High school level: Protein

All living things have the capacity to assimilate substances from their environments and convert them to their own cells and tissues. For instance, plants convert water, salts and carbon dioxide to protein, carbohydrates, fats, vitamins, etc. We eat rice and dal and take milk and our body converts them to blood, muscle, brain, bone, etc. As a poet says, "It is a very odd thing, As odd as can be, That whatever Miss T eats, Turns into Miss T." Living tissues are made of cells. All cells, whether of plants, microorganisms or animals, share some characteristics. One of these is that they all contain protein which indicates their vital nature. The body of an adult man contains about 16% protein which is, quantitatively, the major constituent next to water.

Proteins are compounds made of carbon, hydrogen, oxygen, nitrogen and usually sulphur. They are composed; of units called amino acids.

As mentioned earlier, the body has the capacity to convert food materials to body tissues. How does the body have this capacity? The foods we eat are digested to simple substances, which can be absorbed by the action of digestive enzymes. Similarly, the absorbed materials are synthesized to body substances by other enzymes. All these enzymes are proteins.

Proteins form major building material of the body and are also needed for making good the wear and tear of the body. Barring water, they are also the chief constituents of vital body fluids such as blood.

The protein content of some common foods is shown in Table 1. It can be seen from the same, that foods such as mutton, fish, chicken, egg, dals, etc., contain more protein than cereals. Roots and tubers contain even less. However, the percentage of protein is not always a reliable guide in the case of foods such as milk or leafy vegetables. Both these foods contain a lot of moisture, but in terms of dry matter, they are quite rich in protein. That is why the percentage of kcals, provided by protein, is a better index.

One gram of protein yields 4 Calories on oxidation in the body.

Most proteins are made of some 18 amino acids. The number of proteins that can be formed from these amino acids is practically unlimited as they can be combined in different proportions and in different orders. For instance, although all the ragas are composed of only a few notes, each raga has a certain unique combination and arrangement of notes.

Plants can synthesize all the amino acids needed for protein synthesis from nitrogenous compounds and carbohydrates. The animal body can synthesize only some of these amino acids and the rest have to be provided in the diet. The former are called 'non-essential', meaning that the body can do without them in the diet, and the latter, 'essential', meaning that they have to be provided in the diet. However, both essential and non-essential amino acids are necessary for protein synthesis and for the many metabolic reactions carried out by the body.

The proteins we eat are broken down to amino acids during digestion and absorbed as amino acids. This was recognized from early experiments in which pieces of meat were packed in metal capsules and given to birds. The meat was found to disappear because the protein in meat is broken down to amino acids by the action of digestive enzymes, and the amino acids, being soluble in water, dissolve in the digestive juices. The amino acids absorbed are synthesized to proteins and other nitrogenous substances in the body.

The amino acid composition of different proteins varies considerably depending on the structure and function of the tissue in which they are present. For instance, even a grain of rice or wheat contains four different kinds of proteins. The proteins in different tissues are also very different. For instance, gelatin, a protein present in the bone contains no sulphur whereas, keratin, a protein present in hair contains more sulphur than other proteins. For the synthesis of the different proteins, the body needs the amino acids of which they are composed in the right proportion. To give an example, if I knit a sweater with a particular pattern in red, white and black, needing the three colours of wool in the proportions 4:2:1, unless I get the three colours in these proportions, I cannot use all the wool. Suppose I get them in the

Table 2. Dietary protein requirements.

Age (yrs)		Height (cm)	Weight (kg)	Desirable amount of dietary proteins (g per day)
1		74–84	9–11	20–25
2–4		84–102	13-14	25–30
5-6		107–111	17–19	30–35
7–10		116–135	22–24	30–40
11-12		135–140	29–32	35–45
13–15	males	144–160	38–42	45–55
	Females	144–155	39–43	40–55
16–19	males	160–165	46–50	45–60
	Females	155–158	43–47	40–50
20–40	males	165–170	55–60	45–60
	Females	155–158	45–50	40–50

proportions 1:1:1, I shall be able to use them only in the proportion 1:1/2:1/4 and 1:1/4 out of 3, or 42% of the wool will not be utilized. In the case of knitting, I can unwind the whole thing and change the pattern according to the proportions in which the three colours are available, but the pattern of body proteins is fixed by the genes and cannot be changed. Further, I can put away the unused wool for future use, but the body cannot hold on to unutilized amino acids for more than a short interval and if they are not used within this interval they are partly converted to urea and excreted in the urine. It is, therefore, clear that our diet must not only provide enough protein, but the amino acid composition of the protein must resemble the overall composition of the proteins in the body. If not, some of the amino acids in the diet will not be used for protein synthesis and more protein will be needed in the diet to cover the wastage.

Milk is the food provided by nature for the growth of the young and can, therefore, be expected to contain all the essential amino acids in the right proportions. The amino acid composition of human milk has, therefore, been used as a standard for evaluating the quality of different proteins. Other standards, such as egg protein and a special pattern formulated by the FAO, have also been used.

The major sources of protein in our diet are cereals, pulses, milk, eggs, fish, mutton, etc. In poor diets, cereals provide most of the protein consumed. Cereal proteins are deficient in the essential amino acid, lysine. Consequently, diets based mostly on cereals are likely to be deficient in lysine. However, the other foods mentioned above are rich in lysine, so that as long as we take a mixed diet consisting of cereals, pulses, greens, milk, etc., we are likely to get proteins of satisfactory amino acid composition.

If a protein is deficient in one amino acid and another rich in the same, the two together can make a good mixture. For instance, wheat is deficient in lysine and bengalgram is rich in the same and a mixture of the two is superior in nutritive value than either alone. Such proteins are called 'complementary' proteins or proteins which enhance the value of one another. The protein value of cereals can be greatly improved by adding pulse to the same. For instance, rats fed only wheat were found to gain only 6 g per week as compared to 12 g by those fed on a mixture of wheat and bengalgram dal. Our ancestors seem to have realised the soundness of this combination of cereal and pulse as preparations such as khichri, pongal, debra, idli, dhokla, dal-roti, sambhar rice, are all based on the same. Two proteins which are of complementary amino acid composition must be taken at about the same time in order to derive the maximum benefit from the combination. For instance, if dal is taken in the morning and wheat at night, the surplus lysine from the former cannot be stored in the body till the amino acids from wheat become available.

Most cereals and legumes have less methionine than other sources such as millets (ragi, kodri, bajra, etc.), sesame and animal foods. Similarly maize, jowar, kodri and most pulses contain less tryptophan as"compared to milk, sesame and bajra. Because the proteins in animal foods resemble body proteins more closely than those in vegetable foods, it used to be fashionable to advocate animal proteins. However, there is no special virtue in taking animal proteins as all proteins are degraded to amino acids during digestion and it does not matter to the body from which source the amino acids are derived. Animal proteins are not only unnecessary, but also impracticable for the majority of mankind. Plant proteins are easier to produce, as land can be used directly for the cultivation of cereals, pulses, oilseeds, nuts, etc. For the production of animal protein (e.g. pork or chicken) we have to first produce plant foods and feed these plant foods to animals. Part of the protein we feed to the animals is needed for their survival and only a part is used for growth. It is estimated that we have to feed 5–10 kg of plant proteins to an animal before we can get back one kilogram of meat protein. This means that we need more land for the production of animal protein. The land available in this country is only of the order of 0.7 acre per capita and it is hardly sufficient to produce even enough plant foods for everyone.

Among animal proteins milk is more economical to produce as the dairy animal needs about 3 kg of protein to produce 1 kg of milk protein and also manages to live largely on foods not consumed by man.

How much protein do we need? As tissues are constantly being renovated in the body, protein is needed for this renewal. In the case of children, additional protein is needed for growth. Detailed estimates of requirements have been made, but generally it is quite sufficient if our diet contains 8–10% of protein or protein calories, provided it is a mixed diet containing cereals, pulses, milk, leafy vegetables, etc. People consuming the amounts of protein suggested in Table 2 are found to be quite well-nourished.

What happens when our diet does not contain enough protein ? If the diet does not contain any protein for a long period, the animal will die, as Magendie discovered in his experiments with dogs some 200 years ago, When the diet is poor in protein, -the amount of protein in the blood and tissues decreases. In the case of young children, growth slows down. If the diet is severely deficient, oedema or retention of water in the tissues results. In the case of the young, bone development is affected. The muscles lose their tone and the child is unable to stand or walk because of oedema and weak muscles. Digestion and absorption are also affected. This means that other nutrients such as vitamin A and iron are also not properly utilized by the body. The child has swollen extremities, is pot-bellied and moon-faced, and is very apathetic and not interested in his surroundings. The hair becomes coarse brittle and discoloured and acquires a reddish tinge. The eyes look muddy and brown instead of being clear and glistening. Patches of the skin become inflammed (dermatitis). The psychological development of the child is also affected. Often the child dies if his diet is not improved in time.

Are our diets adequate in protein? The middle class diet 250–300 g of cereals, 50 g pulse, 300 g of milk are generally adequate with regard to protein. But many people are not able to afford these quantities of milk or pulse or other foods such as meat and their diets may not be adequate specially in the case of children.

To what extent is protein deficiency prevalent in this country: In rural areas and among the very poor sections in urban areas about one-third of the population is found to show mild symptoms of protein deficiency. In health, the plasma of blood contains about 6.6–7.5% of proteins. With mild deficiency, this may be only 5-6%.

Severe deficiency is seldom found in adults except in famine conditions when enough foodgrains are not available and people start eating starchy root and tubers. As the growing child needs more protein (and other nutrients) in relation to body weight than the adult, children are more affected by deficiency. In regions such as Kerala, Tamil Nadu, Orissa, etc. rice is the staple and it contains less protein than other grains. The adult in these regions takes rice with fish or legume or mutton. The child is not given these side dishes or given the same only in small quantities because of the belief that they are not suitable for the child. This makes the child deficient in protein. The child often gets diarrhoea as a result of undernutrition, protein deficiency and intestinal infection and this makes the mother restrict the diet of the child still further and the child is given rice conjee (liquid from cooked rice), sago conjee or tapioca instead of rice. This makes the child worse and he soon develops severe protein deficiency. About 1-2% of the children in such regions are affected by severe deficiency.

In other regions, the young child just weaned from the breast may not get enough to eat because of the unsuitable nature of the foods offered (e.g. hard roti and highly spiced dal) and this may also result in deficiency of not only protein but other nutrients as well.

How can we prevent protein deficiency, particularly in children; The main problem is that when a child is weaned from the breast and the mother is unable to buy enough of cow or buffalo milk, the child is given a little of coffee or tea and the foods mentioned earlier. It would be far better to give children a conjee made of wheat and bengalgram or ground rice and greengram or some such combination. Wheat and dals can be roasted, ground coarse and made into a porridge and given along with jaggery and milk. This would make a nourishing drink for the child. Groundnut can be roasted, ground and used in this preparation.

It is important to recognize that foods such as eggs, meat, dal and fish are more necessary for the child than for the adult. A portion of the same should be removed for the child before spices are added, and the foods should be seasoned mildly for the child. Fermented foods such as idli and dhokla and cereal-legume combinations such as khichri should be popularised.

It is also important to realise that diarrhoea is not always the result of indigestion and if the diet is restricted for a long period, the child will develop malnutrition. If the diarrhoea continues, it is necessary to give easily digestible foods in sufficient quantities.

Malnutrition in children is also sought to be prevented by organizing school lunch and balwadi lunch programmes, where the children are given a meal satisfactory with regard to protein and other critical nutrients such as calcium, iron and vitamin A. Organizations such as the FAO, UNICEF, CARE and the state and central governments have taken steps to organize such feeding programmes in selected areas.

Now there is popular recognition of the fact that severe protein deficiency may affect normal intellectual development. All this talk of protein and lysine deficiency has resulted in advertisements advocating the use of lysine-rich and protein-rich foods, beverages and tonics. Parents persuade children to take these in the hope of making them brighter. If the child is given a well-balanced diet consisting of whole-grain cereals, dals, leafy vegetables, milk or milk products, etc. his diet would be quite adequate with regard to protein and there is no point in giving these special foods unless of course the child likes them and prefers them to other foods and the family can afford them. Otherwise it is much more sensible to spend the money on more milk, curd, etc.

Exercise

What are proteins?

Rank order the following with regard to protein content: tapioca, rice, bengalgram, potatoes, mutton, wheat, egg, soyabean, bajra, jaggery and groundnut.

Would you consider the following combinations to be favourable or unfavourable:

- (i) rice and wheat
- (ii) wheat and bengalgram
- (iii) Wheat and groundnut
- (iv) groundnut and sesame
- (v) milk and mutton
- (vi) wheat and milk?

Gita prefers chapatis and milk to chapatis and dal. Is it necessary to force her to eat some dal so that she may get enough lysine?

Mr. Ram, on learning that cereals and pulses are of complementary amino acid composition decided that the children in his family should get daily either mumra or parched chana with lemon juice for afternoon snack. Do you think this is a sound practice?

Mohan excels in sports but lags behind in his studies. His parents think that perhaps he needs protein-rich and lysine-rich beverages and tonics. Do you agree?

Sudha likes rice, dal and curd but no meat. Her mother is worried about her not eating enough animal foods. Do you think her worry is justified.

A certain tonic is reported to contain lysine and, therefore, promote growth. Bhaskar is rather short for his age, but is very active, playful and cheerful and takes plenty of milk Do you think he should take this tonic?

The following are the diets of two children A and B aged 5 years. Find out whether the diets are adequate with regard to protein:

	A	B
Wheat	100	100
Rice	100	50
Cow milk	500	200
Dal	20	10
Egg	30	0
Sugar	30	10
Ghee+oil	15	10
Vegetable +fruits	100	50

Points for emphasis

Proteins are present in all living tissues and are indispensable for life. Proteins are made of amino acids some of which have to be provided in the diet. Different proteins vary with regard to amino acid composition. For the synthesis of body proteins, the essential amino acids of which they are made must be provided in the diet. Utilization of dietary proteins is more efficient when their amino acid composition resembles that of body proteins. Proteins differing in amino acid composition from body protein can be combined so that the mixture resembles body proteins.

The major amino acid deficiencies in cereals and some other foods are lysine, methionine and tryptophan. These can be made good by including in our diet other foods which are rich in the same. When the diet is lacking in protein, growth and body functions are affected. Children are affected more than adults. When enough milk is not available, the diet of children can be made adequate with regard to protein by giving them generous amounts of cereal, pulse, groundnut, etc. in suitable form. People consuming mixed diets consisting of cereals, pulses, milk, leafy vegetables, etc. do not need special protein foods.

Suggestions for the preparation of audiovisual aids

Chart showing the composition of the human body. Charts comparing the amino acid composition of common foods with standard proteins. (This can be done by a bar diagram.)

- Charts showing the amino acid composition of complementary proteins and their mixtures (for instance, wheat, bengalgram and wheat + bengalgram).
- Chart showing the size of rats reared on different diets. (Area depicting body surface can be made proportional to body weight.)
- Recipes—can be given and demonstrated in class.
- Photographs of children suffering from severe protein deficiency.
- Chart or photographs showing the appearance of a well-nourished and poorly nourished child.
- Chart suggesting some do's and don'ts for mothers.

The story in cartoon strip of the progressive deterioration of a child due to malnutrition and its recovery with a good diet.

Selected References

Albanese, A.A. (1963-1972). Newer Methods of Nutritional Biochemistry Vols.I-V. Academic Press, New York.

Alikunhi (1957). Fish Culture in India. Farm Bulletin No. 20. CIFRS, Cuttack.

Altschul, A.M. (1965). Proteins, their Chemistry and Politics. Chapman and Hall, London.

Aykroyd, W.R. and Doughty, J. (1964). Legumes in Human Nutrition. FAO Nutritional Studies No. 19. Food and Agricultural Organization of the United Nations, Rome.

Beaton, G.H. and McHenry, E.W. (1964/1966). Nutrition, Vols. I-III. Academic Press, New York.

Best, C.H. and Taylor, N.B. (1958). The living Body, 4th edition. Chapman and Hall Ltd., London.

Best, C.H. and Taylor, N.B. (1967). The Physiological Basis of Medical Practice, 8th edition. Scientific Book Agency, Calcutta.

Chatfield, C.C. (1964). Food Composition Tables. Food and Agricultural Organization of the United Nations, Rome.

Davidson, S., Passmore, R. and Brock, J.F. (1973). Human Nutrition and Dietetics, 5th edition. The English Language Book Society and Churchill Livingstone, Edinburgh.

Directorate of Economics and Statistics, Ministry of Food and Agriculture, Community Development and Cooperation (1973). Indian Agriculture in Brief, 12th edition. Government of India Press, New Delhi.

Directorate of Economics and Statistics, Ministry of Agriculture, Government of India (1972). Bulletin on Food Statistics, 22nd edition. Government of India Press, New Delhi.

FAO (1957). Calorie Requirements. FAO Nutr. Studies No. 15. Food and Agricultural Organization of the United Nations, Rome.

FAO (1962). Calcium Requirements. FAO Nutr. Meet. Report Ser. No. 30. Food and Agricultural Organization of the United Nations, Rome.

FAO (1965). Protein Requirements. FAO Nutr. Meet. Report Ser. No. 37. Food and Agricultural Organization of the United Nations, Rome.

FAO (1967). Requirements of Vitamin A, Thiamine, Riboflavin and Niacin. FAO Nutr. Meet. Report Ser. No. 41. Food and Agricultural Organization of the United Nations, Rome

FAO (1970). Amino Acid Content of Food and Biological Data on Proteins. FAO Nutritional Studies No.24.Foods and Agricultural Organization of the United Nations, Rome

FAO (1973). Energy and Protein Requirements. FAO Nutr. Meet. Report Ser. No. 52. Food and Agricultural Organisation of the United Nations, Rome.

Girdhari Lai, Siddappa, G.S. and Tandon, G.L. (1960). Preservation of Fruits and Vegetables. Indian Council of Agricultural' . Research, New Delhi. Gopalan, C. and Vijaya Raghavan, K. (1969). Nutrition Atlas of India. National Institute of Nutrition, I.C.M.R., Hyderabad.

Gopalan, C. and Narasingrao, B,S.(1971). Dietary Allowances for, Indians. I.C.M.R. Sp. Rep. Ser. No. 6. Nutrition Research Laboratories, I.C.M.R., Hyderabad.

Gopalan, C, Rama Sastri, B. and Balasubramanian, S.C. (1971). Nutritive value of Indian Foods. National Institute of Nutrition, I.C.M.R., Hyderabad. Jelliffe, D.B. (1955). Infant Nutrition in the Subtropics and Tropics. WHO Monograph Series No. 29. WHO, Geneva.

Jelliffe, D.B. (1966). The Assessment of the Nutritional Status of the Community. WHO Monograph Series No. 33. WHO, Geneva.

Jolliffe, N (1962). Clinical Nutrition, 2nd edition. Harper and Harper, New York.

Kon, S.K. (1959). Milk and Milk Products in Human Nutrition. FAO Nutritional Studies No. 17. Food and Agricultural Organization of the United Nations, Rome.

Krishnamurthi, S.(1967). Home Vegetable Gardens for Health. In the Vegetarian Way. Special Number XIX. World Vegetarian Congress. The Indian Vegetarian Congress, Madras.

Kuppuswamy, S., Srinivasan, M. and Subramanyan, V. {1958). Proteins in Foods. I.C.M.R. Sp. Report Ser. No. 33. Indian Council of Medical Research, New Delhi.

Leverton, R.M. (1960). Food Becomes You. Iowa State University Press, Ames, Iowa.

Mahtab S. Bamji, Kamala Krishnaswamy, Brahmana, G.N.V. (2009). Textbook of Human Nutrition. Oxford & IBH Publishing Co. Pvt. Ltd., New Delhi.

McArdle, A.A. (1963). A Simple Approach to Low Cost Feeding and Housing of Poultry in India. Literacy House Publication, Lucknow.

McArdle, A.A. and Panda, J.N. (1964). A Poultry Guide for the Villager. Literacy House Publication, Lucknow.

McCollum, E.V. (1957). A History of Nutrition. Houghton Miffin Company, Boston.

Mitchell, H.H.(1962, 1964). Comparative Nutrition of Man and Domestic Animals. Vols. I and II. Academic Press, New York.

Moore, T. (1957). Vitamin A. Elsevier Publishing Co., Amsterdam.

Munro, H.N. and Allison, J.B. (1964-1970). Mammalian Protein Metabolism. Vols. I-IV. Academic Press, New York.

Patwardhan, V.N. (1961). Nutrition in India. Indian Journal of Medical Sciences, Bombay-4.

Rajalakshmi, R.(1972). Perspectives in Nutrition. Published by Department of Biochemistry, University of Baroda, Baroda, India.

Sebrell, W.H.Jr.and Harris,R.S.(1954). The Vitamins. Vols.I-11I. Academic Press, New York.

Shils, M.E., Moshe Shike, Catherine Ross, A. Benjamin Caballero, Robert Cousins (Eds.) (2005) . Modern Nutrition in Health and Disease. Lippincott Williams and Wilkins.

Sukhatme, P.V. (1965). Feeding India's Growing Millions. Asia Publishing House, Bombay.

Swaminathan, M. (1977). Essentials of Food and Nutrition Ganesh Publications Pvt. Ltd., Bangalore.

Underwood, E.J.(1971). Trace Elements in Human and Animal Nutrition. Academic Press, New York.

Watt, B.K. and Merril, A.L.(1963). Composition of Foods. United States Department of Agriculture, Washington, D.C.

West, E.S., Todd, W.R., Mason,H.S. and Van Bruggen,J.T.(1966). Textbook of Biochemistry, 4th edition. The Macmillan Company, New York.

WHO (1960). Endemic Goiter. World Health Organization, Monograph Series No. 44. WHO, Geneva.

Williams, R.J. (1962). Nutrition in a Nut-Shell. Dolphin Books, U.S.A.

Wohl, M.G. and Goodhart, R.S. (1964). Modern Nutrition in Health and Disease, 3rd edition. Lea and Febiger, Philadelphia.

Books and Reports on Foods, Nutrition, Agriculture, Fisheries, Horticulture, Poultry, Dairy, Farming, etc. are published periodically by the following organizations :

1. Food and Agriculture Organization, New Delhi.
2. UNICEF, New Delhi.
3. World Health Organization, New Delhi.
4. Central Food Technological Research Institute, Mysore-2.
5. Indian Council of Agricultural Research, New Delhi.
6. Indian Council of Medical Research, New Delhi.
7. Ministry of Information and Broadcasting, New Delhi.

Scientific Names of the Foodstuffs with their Hindi Versions

Name of food stuffs	Scientific name	Hindi name	Other names
Agathi	Sesbania grandiflora	Agasti	-
Ajma	Trachy spermum ammi	Ajwan	Omum
Allspice	Pimento amygdalus	-	Pimento
Almond	Prunus amygdalus	Badham	-
Amaranth	Amarantus gangeticus	Chaulai sag	Lal sag, mulaikeerai
Amla	Emblica officinalis	Amla	Nellikai

		Seb	Safarjan
Apple	*Malus sylvestris*		
Apricots	*Prunus armeniaca*	Khubani	Khurmani
Arecanut	*Areca catecgu*	Supari	Betelnut
Argemone	*Argemone Mexicana*	-	Darudi
Arrowroot	*Maranta arundinacea*	Araroot	Kuvamavu
Asafetida	*Ferula foetida*	Hing	Hingra, perungayam
Ash gourd	*Benicasa hispida*	Petha	Pushinikai
Asparagus	*Asparagus officinalis.*	-	Satavari
Bajra	*Pennisetum typhoideum*	Bajra	cambu
Banana	*Musa paradisiacal*	Kela	Vazhapazham plantain
Barley	*Hordeum vulgare*	Jau	Juv
Basil leaves	*Ocimum busilicum*	-	Dumbro,ramtulsi
Beet root	*Beta vulgaris*	Chukandar	Beet
Bengalgram	*Cicer aretinum*	Chana	Chickpea
Betel leaves	*Piper betle*	Pankapata	Vethilai
Betelnut	*See arecanut*	-	-
Bitter gourd	*Memordica charantia*	Karela	Pavakkai
Black gram	*Phaseolus mungo*	Urd	Adad
Black pepper	*See pepper*	-	-
Bor	*Zizyphus jujube*	Ber	Elanthapazham, oblong berry

contd. ....

Name of food stuffs	Scientific name	Hindi name	Other names
Bottle gourd	*Lagenaria siceraria*	Lowki	Dudhi, calabash cucumber, suraikkai
Brinjal	*Solanum melongena*	Baigan	Egg plant, ringna
Broad bean	*Vicia faba*	Bakla	Fafda papdi,
Cabbage	*Brassica oleraceavar, capitata*	Band gobhi	Kobi, muttgose
Calabash cucumber	*See bottle gourd*	-	-
Cane sugar	*Saccharum officinarum*	Chini	Sakkar.
Capsicum	*Capsicum annum var grossa*	Papkria	Karamila milagai,giant chillies
Caraway	*Carum nigrum*	Kalajira	Cumin
Cardamom	*Elettaria cardamomum*	elaychi	elakkai
Carrot	*Daucus carota*	Gajar	Manjal mullangi
Cashew fruit	*Anacardium occidentale*	Kajuka phal	Kaji badam mundiripazham, kashuandi
Cashew nut	*Anacardium occidentale*	Kaju	mundiriparuppu
Cauliflower	*Barassica oleracea var botrytis*	Phool gobhi	phulevar
Celery	*Apium graveolens var dulce*	Ajmud, Chana	Randhuni, shalri
Chandal (bengalgram dal)	*See bengalgram*	-	-
Chain bor	*Zizyphus nummularia*	-	Beri, kokamber
Charoli	*Buchanania latifolia var chironji*	Chiraunji	saraiparuppu

contd. ...

Chekkur manis	*Sauropus androgynuns*	-	-
Chicory	*Cichorium intibus*	-	-
Chiku	*Achras sapota*	Chiku	Sapota
Chillies	*Capsicum frutescens*	Mirch	Milagai, marcha
Chowli	*See cowpeas*	-	-
Cinnamon	*Cinnamonum zeylanicum*	Dal-chini	taj
Cloves	*Syzyium aromaticum*	laung	lavang
Cluster beans	*Cyamposis tetragonola*	Guar kiphali	Govar
Cocoa	*Theobroma cacao*	Koko	Coco
Coconut	*Cocosnucifera*	Nariyal	Nariel,thengai
Cocum	*See garcinia*	-	-
Coffee	*Coffea Arabica*	-	-
Colocasia	*Colocasia esculenta*	Arvi	Seppan
Corpa or korpa(dry coconut)	*See coconut*	-	-
Coridander	*Coriandrum sativum*	Dhania	Kottimir
Corn	*Zea mays*	Makkai	Maize, bhutta
Cotton seed	*Gossypium sativum*	Kapas ka beej	-
Cowpea	*Vigna catajang*	Lobia bada	Chavli, cowgram, karamani
Cucumber	*Cucumis sativus*	Khira	Vellarikai, kakri

contd. ....

Name of food stuffs	Scientific name	Hindi name	Other names
Cumin seeds	*Cuminum cyminum*	Zira	Jira, jeeragam
Curry leaves	*Murraya koenigii*	Gandhela	Karuveppilai, mithalimdo
Date palm	*See dates*	-	-
Dates	*Phoenix dactylifera*	Khajur	Perichampazham
Dhaniya dal	*See coriander*	-	-
Double beans	*Faba vulgaris*	Chastang	Papdi
Drumstick	*Moringa oleifera*	Saijan	Sragavo, murungaikai
Dudhi	*See bottle gourd*	-	-
Egg plant	*See brinjal*	-	-
Elephant yam	*Amorphophallus Campanulatus*	Zaminkand	Suran, senaikizhangu,
Fenugreek	*Trigonella foenum graceum*	Methi	Venthayam
Field bean	*Dolichos lablab*	Val	Mochai, walspapdi
Figs	*Ficus caria*	Anjeer	Anjur, athipazham
French beans	*Phaseolus vulga*	bakla	Fansi, French avarai, kidney bean
Galka	*Luffa cylindrical roem*	taroi	Smooth gourd,Ghiya turai
Garcinia	*Garcinia xanthochymus*	-	-
Garlic	*Allium sativum*	-lehsan	Lusoon, lassan
Gingelly seeds	*Sesame indicum*	til	Ellu, sesame

Ginger	Zingiber officinale	Adrak	Adu, inji
Grape fruit	Citrus paradisi	Chakotra	-
Greengram	Phaseolus aureus	Mung	Mug
Groundnut	Arachis hypogeal	Moongphali	Singdhana, peanut, nilakkadalai
Guar	See cluster beans	-	-
Guava	Psidium guayava	Amrud	Jam phal, peru
Hing	See asafetida	-	-
Horsegram	Dolichos biflours	Kulthi	Kollu
Jack fruit	Artocarpus heterophyllus	Kathal	Palapazham, phanas
Jaggery	Saccharum officinarum	Gur	Gud
Jambu	Syzygium cumin	Jamun	Jambu, nagapazham
Jowar	Sorghum vulgare	Juar	Cholam
Kankoda	Momordica dioica	Golkandra	Paluppakkai
Kesari dal	Lathyrus sativus	Langdhal	Khesari
Knoll-khol	Brassica oleracea var caulorapa	Kohl rabi	Nolkol
Kodri	Paspalum scorbiculatum	Kodo	Varagu
Kovau fruit Kuppakeerai	Coccinia cordifolia Amaranthus virdis	Kundree-	Kavakai-
Ladies fingers	Ambelmoschus esclentus	bhindi	Bhendi, vendaikai
Lathyrus sativus	See kesari dal	-	-

contd....

contd. ....

Name of food stuffs	Scientific name	Hindi name	Other names
Leeks	*Allium porrum*	Vilayaiti lasson	-
Lemon	*Citrus limon*	Bara nimbu	Elumichai
Lemon (sour)	*Citrus acida*	-	Neebu
Lemon grass	*Cymbopogon citrates*	-	
Lentil	*Lens esculanta*	Masur dhal	Mysore paruppu
Lettuce	*Lactuca sativa*	Salad	Salad pata
Lichis	*Nephelium litchi*	-	Litchi
Lima beans	*Phaselous lunalatus*	-	Lobia
Lime	*Citrus aurantifolia*	Neembu	Nimbha
Lucerne	*Medicago sativa*	Lasun ghas	Gadhab, vilayughas
Mahuva flower	*Bassia latifolia*	Kaccha mahua	Iluppampoo
Maize	*See corn*	-	
Manathakkali or manathakkalikkai	*Solanum nigrum*	Makoy	Piludi
Mango	*Mangifera indica*	Aam	Mampazham
Maple sugar	*Acer sp*	-	-
Marjoram	*Organum marjorana*	Sathra	-
Methi	*See fenugreek*	-	-

	Menthe spicata	Pudina	Pudhina
Mint	*Menthe spicata*	Pudina	Pudhina
Moth bean	*Phaseolus aconitifolius*	Moth	Matki, mutt
Musammi	*Citrus sinensis*	-	Musambi
Mushroom	*Entoloma marcocarpum*	Tila chhattoo	Koon
Musk melon	*Cucumis melo*	kharbuza	Sweet melon, sakkarteti, rock melon
Mustard green	*Brassica campestris var sarson*	Sarson ka sag	Kadugu ilai
Mustard seeds	*Brassica nigra*	Rai	Sarisha, kaduku
Neem	*Azadirachta indica*	Neem	Nim, limdo
Nutmeg	*Myristica fragrans*	Jaiphal	Jathikai
Olive	*Olea europea*	-	-
Omum	See *ajma*	-	-
Onion	*Allium cepa*	Pyaz	Piaja, kanda, vengayam
Orange	*Citrus aurantium*	Narangi	Santra
Palmgur	*Borassus flabellifer*	Tar gur	Tad gud
Palm oil(red)	*Elaesis guinensis*	Surkh khajur katel	Khajuri tela
Palmyra	*Borassus fabellifer*	Tar	Panam nugu
Papaya or papaya	*Carcia papaya*	Papita	Papaiya
Parsely	*Petroselium crispum*	-	Kothambalari
Paruppukeerai	*Portulaca oleracea*	Chiura sag	Kurfah

contd. ...

contd. ...

Name of food stuffs	Scientific name	Hindi name	Other names
Parwar	*Trichosanthes dioica*	Parwal	Padwal. Potala
Peeches	*Amygdalis persica*	Aadoo	Satalu
Pears	*Prunus persica*	Naspati	Berikkai, goshbub
Peas	*Pisum sativum*	Mattar	Field pea, watana, pattani
Pepper (black)	*Piper nigrum*	Kalimircha	Gole mirch, milagu
Phalsa	*Grewia asiatica*	Falsa	-
Pine apple	*Ananas comosus*	Annanas	-
Pink beans	*Phaseolus vulgaris*	Babril	Avarakkai
Pistachio	*Pistacia vera*	Pista	-
Plantain	*See banana*	-	-
Plums	*Prums domestica*	Alubukhara	Aladu
Pomegranate	*Punica granatum*	Anar	Dalim, madalampazham
Ponnangani	*Alternanthera sessilis*	Saranti sag	Ponnanganni keerai
Poppy seeds	*Papaver somniferum*	postdana	Khaskhas
Potato	*Solanum tuberosum*	Alu	Batata
Prunes	*Prunus salicina*	Jardalu	-
Pumpkin (yellow)	*Cucurbita maxima*	Kaddu	Kohlu, lalbhopia
Radish	*Raphanus sativus*	Muli	Mula

Ragi	*Eleusine coracana*	Mundal	Finger millet
Raisins(dried grapes)	*Vitis vinifera*	Kishmish	Khismis
Rayan	*Mimusops hexandra roxb*	Khirni	Khukhajur
Redgram	*Cajanus cajan*	Tur	Pigeon pea
Rice	*Oryza sativa*	Chawal	Arisi, tandool
Ridge gourd	*Luffa acutangula*	Torai	Juria, peerkangai
Rock melon	*See musk melon*	-	-
Rose	*Rosa sp*	Gulab	
Safflower	*Carthamus tinctorius*	Kardi	Kusumb, sendurkam
Saffron or saffiran	*Crocus sativus*	Kesar	-
Sakkarteti	*See musk melon*	-	-
Sago	*Metroxylon sago*	Sago	Sabudana , javvarisi
Sesame	*See gingelly seeds*	-	-
Sitaphal	*Annona squamosa*	-	Custard apple
Snake gourd	*Trichosanthes anguina*	Chahchinda p a n d o l a , podalangi	-
Sowa sag	*Peucedanum sowa*	-	-
Soya bean	*Glycine max merr*	Bhat	Bhetmas
Spinach	*Spinacea oleracea*	Palak	Pasalai keerai

contd. ...

contd. ....

Name of food stuffs	Scientific name	Hindi name	Other names
Strawberry	*Fragaria vesca*	Straberry	-
String beans	*see cow peas*	-	-
Sundaikkai	*Solanum tiroum*	-	-
Sweet lemon	*Citrus limetta*	Meetanimbu	Limbu, malta
Sweet potato	*Ipomea butatas*	Shakarkuand	Sakkaria
Tamarind	*Tamarindus indica*	Imli	Amii, puli
Tomato	*Lycopersicum esculentum*	Tamatar	Tamata, thakali
Tapioca	*Manihot esculenta*	Maravalli	Cassava, kappa
Tea	*Cameilla thea*	Chaie	Chah
Thyme	*Thymus serpyllum*	Bonajown	-
Til	*See gingelly seeds*	-	-
Tindola	*Coccina cordifolia cogn*	Tinda	Gilodia, little gourd
Tulsi leaves	*Ocimum sanctum*	Tulsi	-
Turmeric	*Curcuma longa*	Haldi	Manjal
Turdal (redgram dal)	*See redgram*	-	-
Turnip	*Brassica rapa*	Shalgam	-
Valore	*See pink beans*	-	-
Variyali	*Foeniculum vulgare miller*	Sonf	Variali, fennel

Walnut	Juglans regia	Akhrot	Akrot
Water melon	Citrullus vulgaris	Tarbuz	Tarbuja
Wheat	Triticum estivum	Gehum	Ghau
White melon	See musk melon	-	-
Wild yam	Dioscorea versicolour	Suar alu	Kodikizhangu
Wood apple	Limonia acidissima	Kaitha	Elephat apple, kothu
yam	Typhonium trilobatum	ratalu	Goradu, karunai, kizhangu

Glossary

A. Food terms

Atta — whole wheat flour.

Aviyal — a mixture of vegetables is cooked together and coconut paste and other seasoning are added towards the end of cooking.

Basundhi — a sweet dish resembling kheer prepared from milk by prolonged boiling so that it acquires a granular structure.

Bhajya — 1. vegetable fritters : vegetables are cut into slices or pieces, covered or mixed with a fritter cover batter made of chana flour and deep-fried; called bhajji in south India. 2. steamed product shaped like roly-pollies prepared from colocasia leaves and chana flour.

Brew — infusion prepared by boiling and/or fermentation.

Bulgar wheat — parboiled wheat.

Chakli — deep-fried product prepared from chana or rice flour. A dough is made from the flour which is pressed through a press into hot fat so as to come out as thick noodles with a smooth or corrugated surface.

Channa — curdled cheese obtained from milk

Chana flour — flour prepared from dehusked bengalgram dal

Chapati — the Indian equivalent of unleavened bread; whole wheat flour is kneaded into a firm pliable dough,

	shaped into balls, rolled out, partially cooked on a tava
Chevda	(also called chooda): 1. savoury mixture made of deep-fried poha, groundnut, chana dal, kopra, etc. 2.an upma type product prepared from tender corn.
Chutney	a relish usually containing spices.
Conjee	gruel or porridge
Cordials	fruit juices preserved with sugar syrup
Cottage cheese	cheese obtained by curdling sour milk. This is pressed and further fermented to make mature cheese,
Cracked wheat	coarsely ground whole wheat
Cream of wheat	rava, suji or semolina; coarse meal prepared from wheat flour of low extraction.
Curd	yogurt; fermented milk.
Curry	spiced vegetables, dals or meat. A tamil term which originally meant meat and was later stretched to include vegetables.
Curry powder	a mixture of spices used in making curries; a spice powder made of coriander, fenugreek, chillies, black pepper, cumin seed, turmeric, hing, roasted dals and other ingredients.
Dahi-vadas	vadas soaked in curd to which suitable seasoning has been added.
Dals	dehusked and split legumes.
Debra	pan-cooked roti prepared from dough to which chopped greens, other vegetables, seasoning etc. are added.
Dhokla	a steamed product prepared from fermented batters usually made of cereals and dals.
Dosa	pan-fried product resembling pancake, usually prepared from a fermented batter made of rice and blackgram dal. Other batters are also used.
Doughnut	deep-fried product, usually prepared from fermented doughs and coated with powdered sugar.
Dumplings	balls used in sauces or gravies; steamed balls prepared from dals, vegetables, cheese or meat.
Ghee	butter from which the moisture is removed by heating; the resulting clear liquid acquires a granulated structure on cooling.

Grams	a term used collectively for black gram, bengalgram, greengram and redgram. Also used synonymously with bengalgram.
Gulabjamun	sweet prepared from khova which is mixed with a little flour and curd, kneaded into a dough, rolled into balls, deep-fried and put in sugar syrup.
Halwa	a pasty sweet, prepared from ghee, sugar and starchy material such as flour, fruit (e.g. chikku) or vegetable (e.g. carrots)
Kabab	fried meat balls; they are used as dumplings in curries
Khadi	soup or broth prepared from buttermilk.
Khaman	steamed product prepared from fermented batter of made of bengalgram dal.
gur	a solid brown mass obtained by boiling down sugarcane juice. Also prepared from the sap of palmyra tree.
Kheer	(also called payas or payasam): a semifluid dessert prepared from milk, sugar and starchy material such as rice, poha, vermicelli, sago, etc.
Khichri(or khichedi)	rice cooked with dal with the addition of salt, turmeric powder and sometimes fat.
Kopra (copra)	dehydrated coconut.
Khova	the solid mass obtained by evaporating milk till almost all the moisture is removed.
Laddu	1. a sweet made of chana flour. A batter prepared from chana flour is dropped in the form of globules into hot fat by passing the batter through a colander or perforated ladles; the deep-fried product is mixed with sugar syrup, spices and seasoning and shaped into balls called laddus. 2. other similar products such as mumra laddu, prepared from jaggery or sugar syrup.
Ladu	more commonly a product resembling laddu, prepared from roasted flour of dals (chana dal, moong dal, etc.), ghee and powdered sugar. Also used synonymously with laddu.
Magaj	sweet prepared from roasted chana flour, sugar and ghee.
Maida	refined wheat flour

Malai	top scum formed when milk is boiled and cooled.
Malt	processed food prepared from cereals by partial germination followed by fermentation.
Masala	seasoning; dry masala-spices; green masala herbs such as coriander and curry leaves, green chillies, fresh garlic and ginger etc.
Mawa	khova.
Mocha	a drink prepared by mixing coffee and cocoa.
MPF	multipurpose food; a processed food mixture made of groundnut cake and bengalgram and enriched with vitamins and minerals
Mumra	puffed rice, parched product prepared from dehusked paddy
Mysore pak	sweet prepared from chana flour, ghee and sugar which are blended together to form an emulsified product.
Natto	a fermented product prepared from soya bean
Neera	the fermented sap obtained from coconut and palmyra trees.
Nimki	a deep fried product prepared from flour. Chapati-type dough prepared from plain flour, seasoned suitably, rolled out thin, cut into squares or diamonds and deep-fried to give a crisp savoury product.
Pakora	a crisp deep-fried product prepared from a dough made of chana flour, onions, fat and seasoning.
Pancakes	product resembling dosa or poora
Papad	dehydrated product prepared from dals or rice. A firm but pliable dough is made from the flour of dals or rice with addition of suitable seasoning. It is shaped into balls, rolled out thin, dried and stored. It is toasted over open fire or deep-fried in hot fat so as to give a light, crisp product. Also called appalam or papadam.
Papdi	dehydrated product prepared from cooked sago or rice flour and deep-fried like papads before consumption. Also called vadam, vadi, phool-papdi, etc
Parathas	pan-fried chapatis. Chapati dough is rolled out and the top coated with fat and folded over to form a semi-circular shape; the process is repeated once more and

	the folded chapati, now a quadrant in shape, is rolled out and cooked on both sides in a greased pan.
Pastries	baked products prepared from doughs made of flour.
Peda	milk sweet. Milk boiled down to a solid with a low moisture content and combined with sugar and spices. This is rolled into balls and flattened to form small thick circular sweets
Pies	usually, pastries baked with a filling inside
Poha	flaked rice; paddy is soaked in water, roasted and pounded to yield a flaked product resembling flaked oats.
Pongal	prepared from rice and roasted greengram dal or other dals with suitable seasoning.
Poora	product resembling dosa or pancakes.
Poories	dough prepared from whole wheat flour, shaped into small balls, rolled out and deep-fried.
Pork	meat of pigs.
Potato	wafers dehydrated potato slices. Potato slices are semi-cooked, dried and stored. They are deep-fried as needed
Pudding	usually, a steamed or baked dessert of a soft texture
Puffed	rice see mumra
Pulav	a special variety of cooked rice. Rice is roasted before cooking and spices and dressings such as peas, onions and other vegetables and meat are added.
Puran polis	a pan-fried pastry containing a sweet filling
Puttu	a steamed product prepared from flour. In Madras, a steamed sweet dish with a granular texture prepared from rice flour and jaggery. In Kerala, a main dish prepared from tapioca flour, salt and seasoning.
Rabdi	1. a pasty sweet prepared from milk and sugar. The milk is boiled down so as to remove most of the moisture. 2. a steamed product prepared from a batter made of flour and butter milk.
Rasam soup	type liquid prepared from red gram dal, salt, spices and some acid source such as tamarind, lemon or tomatoes; incidentally mulligatawny soup (a distortion of milaguthanni, meaning pepper-water) is a misnomer for pepper rasam.

Rasgollas	a milk sweet; cheese obtained by curdling milk kneaded into a dough, rolled into balls and put in sugar syrup.
Rava	see cream of wheat
Roti	chapatis or chapati-type product prepared from cereal or millet flour; also called rotla. The term is also sometimes used for yeast breads which are more commonly called pav-roti.
Rusk	bread slices baked so as to give a crisp biscuit-like product
Sakkarpara	see nimki. Sugar may sometimes replace salt in this preparation
Sambhar	broth prepared from redgram dal, vegetables, tamarind juice, salt and spices; coconut paste and herbs are also added.
Samosa	deep-fried pastries with a vegetable filling usually made of peas, potatoes and other vegetables.
Sandesh	a sweet resembling pedas prepared from curdled cheese and sugar.
Scotchbread	short-bread; a rich biscuit prepared from flour, sugar and butter with or without the addition of rice flour.
Seasoning	spices etc. added to foods to improve their flavour and taste.
Semolina	rava, suji, cream of wheat
Sev	1. deep-fried noodles prepared from chana dough which is pressed through a press into hot fat to form noodles. 2. steamed noodles; cooked doughs prepared from flour, rolled into balls, steamed and pressed into noodles. 3. products resembling vermicelli, macaroai spaghetti etc., also called sevaiya or semiya.
Sirrah	halwa-type product prepared from suji.
Spaghetti	macaroni or sev-type product prepared from plain flour
Stuffed paratha	parathas containing a filling.
Suji	see cream of wheat
Tandoori chicken	chicken stuffed with rice and roasted in a special charcoal oven
Tempeh	fermented soya bean preparation

Toddy	alcoholic drink prepared from the sap of coconut or palmyra tree
Upma (or upuma)	a product prepared from rava or ground rice with addition of salt, seasoning as well as onions, peas, etc., and having a granular structure
Usal	steamed product prepared from dal paste. Dals steeped in water, coarsely ground and steamed With or without the addition of vegetables and seasoned suitably to yield 'usal' which resembles upma in texture.
Vadas	deep-fried product prepared from dal paste. Dals steeped in water, wetground and the dough deep-fried after appropriate additions to yield vadas; the soft vada are shaped like doughnuts.
Vaghar	special types of seasoning; mustard seeds are put in hot fat and allowed to crackle to make vaghar. Cumin seed, ajman, black pepper, fenugreek seeds, etc. may be treated similarly. Red chillies and dals are fried in oil and added.
Vinegar	acetic acid obtained by fermentation from sugar

B. Other terms

Achlorhydria	a condition in which hydrochloric acid is absent in the gastric secretion
Acid-alkali balance	or more commonly acid-base balance; the balance maintained between acids and bases in blood so that normal blood is slightly alkaline with a pH of 7.4
Acidosis	a term commonly used to describe acidaemia or a condition in which the pH of the blood is lowered.
ATP	adenosine triphosphate
Adipose tissue	fatty tissue or tissue in which excess fat is stored
Adrenals	glands situated at the upper end of each kidney which secrete the adrenal hormones
Aetiology	of factors causing disease; their study disease
Afforestation	planting of forests.
Agglutination	aggregation of cells in small masses so that they lose their power of movement

Albumin	a water soluble protein present in blood whose synthesis is influenced by several factors including protein nutritional status
Alcoholic	a person addicted to excessive consumption of alcoholic drinks
Alkaloids	organic substances of a basic nature found generally in plants
Alkalosis	a term commonly used to describe alkalaemia or a condition in which the pH of the blood is increased.
Allergy	an abnormally high sensitivity to specific factors including heat, cold, drugs, foods, etc; allergy to specific foods is common
Alloxan	a substance which produces diabetes by destroying the cells of the pancreas which synthesize insulin.
Amoebic	dysentery dysentery caused by the parasitic presence in the intestine of one-celled organisms called amoeba such as Endamoeba coli, Endamoeba histolytica and Endamoeba nana.
Amines	organic compounds containing nitrogen. They are formed from ammonia (NH) by the replacement of one or more hydrogen atoms by organic radicals
Amino acids	substances forming the chief structure of proteins; they contain an amino group (—NH2) and a carboxyl group (-COOH).
Amino sugar	sugar containing an amino group.
Anaemia	a condition in which the blood is deficient in either the number of red blood cells or their hemoglobin content.
Anti-allergic	drugs which counter act the effects of abnormal amounts of histamine produced in allergic conditions.
Antibiotics	chemical compounds used to prevent the growth and survival of harmful organisms. They are usually produced by microorganisms.
Antidiuretic Hormone	hormone secreted by the pituitary which regulates the secretion of urine and prevents excessive urination. A deficiency of this hormone results in diabetes insipidus.
Antioxidants	substances which prevent oxidation.

Antitoxins	substances present in blood which can neutralise the effects of specific toxins.
Anti-vitamin	a substance which inactivates a vitamin
Aplastic anaemia	deficiency in the formation of new red blood cells generally associated with defective functioning of the bone marrow
Arteriosclerosis	a condition marked by loss of elasticity and the thickening and hardening of arteries.
Atherosclerosis	arteriosclerosis with the formation of masses containing small drops of fat
Artificial Insemination	breeding of animals by injecting the semen of the male into the female of the species.
Bacillary	dysentery caused by bacilli
Basal metabolism	oxygen consumption of the body at rest. Energy production at basal condition.
Blanch	plunge or steep in boiling water.
Bone marrow	soft fatty substance found in the bone and concerned with the formation of red blood cells.
Cardiac muscle	heart muscle
Cardio-vascular	disease affecting the heart, blood vessels and disease circulation.
CARE	Cooperative for American Relief Everywhere
Catalyst	a substance which speeds up a chemical reaction but appears to remain unchanged at the end of the reaction
Cheese-cloth	coarse cloth used for straining liquids
CFTRI	Central Food Technological Research Institute, Mysore
Collagen	1. connective tissue; 2. a protein with a high content of amino acids hydroxyproline
Coma	a state of deep unconsciousness; may be caused by several conditions including uraemia and diabetes.
Compost	manure made from cow-dung, dry leaves and other organic matter.
Conjunctiva	the mucous membrane covering the anterior surface of the eye-ball and lining of lids.
Conjunctivitis	inflammation of conjunctiva.
Convalescence	period between end of a disease and the restoration of normal health.

Convulsions	violent and involuntary muscular contractions; in popular language fits.
Coronary thrombosis	formation of a clot in the arteries which supply blood to the heart.
Cretinism	a condition caused by thyroid deficiency at the time of birth and marked by arrested physical and mental development and lowered basal metabolism.
Deaf mutism	condition of being both deaf and dumb.
Defecation	the evacuation of faecal matter from the bowels.
Dehydration	removal or loss of water.
Dementia	impaired mental function.
Demineralisation	excessive loss or removal of minerals.
Dental caries	decay of tooth, dissolution and disintegration of enamel and dentin in tooth.
Dermatitis	inflammation of the skin.
Detergent	cleansing agent.
Detoxification	counteracting the toxic effects of substances. This is achieved by their conversion to harmless substances.
Diabetes insipidus	a condition caused by a deficiency of antidiuretic hormone in which there is excessive loss of urine but the urine is free from sugar.
Diabetes mellitus	a metabolic disorder in which impaired utilization of glucose results in its excretion in urine
Diphtheria	infectious disease of bacterial origin marked by inflammation of the throat, nose, trachea and bronchi and by toxaemia
Diuretics	substances which increase the flow of urine
Dropsy	excessive accumulation of clear watery fluid in any of the tissues and organs of the body.
Electro-encephalo-gram (EEG)	record of the electrical activity of the brain obtained by attaching electrodes to the brain.
Enteritis	inflammation of the intestine
Epidemic	a disease attacking many members of a locality at the same time
Epidemiology	study of the causes of epidemics
Estrogen	female hormone
FAO	Food and Agricultural Organization

Fermentation	chemical decomposition brought about by microorganisms
Femur	thigh bone
Fetus	the unborn offspring of mammals; the term embryo is used in the earlier stages before it has assumed the characteristic form of the species
Fluorescence	the re-emission of light following its absorption. The re-emitted light is visible although that absorbed may not be.
Gall bladder	a pear-shaped structure found under the liver which acts as a reservoir for bile.
Gastritis	inflammation of the stomach
Globin	a protein present in the blood serum
Globule	small spherical mass.
Globulin	the protein present in haemoglobin.
Glomeruli	coils of blood vessels surrounding the tubules in the kidney
Glutathione	a tripeptide composed of glycine, cysteine and glutamic acid. Its synthesis is influenced by protein and methionine status.
Goitre	chronic enlargement of the thyroid gland
Gout	a disease commonly associated with an excess of uric acid in blood
Heme	an iron-protoporphyrin; constituent of haemoglobin
Haemoglobinuria	the presence of haemoglobin or related compounds in urine
Haemosiderin	one of the forms in which surplus iron is stored in the liver.
Haemagglutinin	a substance that causes the agglutination of red blood cells and thus interferes with the circulation of blood.
Haemorrhage	bleeding.
Hepatic coma	coma caused by failure of liver function
Histamine	amine formed from histidine by decarboxylation. It dilates blood vessels and stimulates gastric secretion. Excessive amounts of the same are released in allergic conditions
Hormones	chemical substances secreted into the body fluids by endocrine glands which have specific effects on the activities of other organs

Humus	soil containing decayed vegetable matter
Hybrid	strain (or breed) obtained by cross-fertilization of two different strains (or breeds).
Protein hydrolysate	a mixture of amino acids prepared by hydrolysing a protein; used in special diets when ordinary food proteins are not utilized well.
5-hydroxy-tryptophan	a compound formed from tryptophan.
5-hydroxy-tryptamine	serotonin; a compound formed from 5-hydroxy-tryptophan which elevates blood pressure and has an important role in brain function
Hyperacidity	excessive acidity of the gastric secretion caused by hyperchlorohydria
Hypercalcemia	increased levels of calcium in blood.
Hypercholesterol-aemia	increased levels of cholesterol in blood
Hyperglycemia	increased levels of glucose in blood
Hypertension	increased blood pressure; renal hypertension hypertension caused by kidney disease.
Hypoacidity	decreased acidity of gastric secretion caused by hypochlorhydria
Hypochlorhydria	decreased amounts of hydrochloric acid in the gastric juice.
Hypochromia	anaemic condition in which the haemoglobin content of red blood cells is decreased.
Hypoglycemia	condition in which blood sugar level is decreased
Hypothyroidism	condition in which the functioning of the thyroid gland is affected; e.g., in iodine deficiency
ICMR	Indian Council of Medical Research
ICNND	Interdepartmental Committee on Nutrition for National Defence (U.S.A.).
Inanition	condition resulting from lack of food.
Ingestion	the act of taking food.
iu	international unit.
Jaundice	a disease caused by the accumulation of bile or bile salts in blood; the accumulation of bile pigments results in the yellow colouration of the skin and mucous membranes.

Kadai	frying pan.
Keratin	a protein present in skin, hair, nails and horny tissue.
Keratomalacia	softening of the cornea; dryness with ulceration of the cornea which may result in its perforation.
Keto acids	chemical compounds containing the keto group (> CO) and carboxy group (—COOH) formed in the body during the oxidation of carbohydrate and fat.
Ketones	compounds containing a keto group.
Ketosis	a condition marked by excessive accumulation of ketone bodies in the body.
Lethargy	drowsiness; lack of interest, will-power and energy.
Metabolic	antimetabolite; substance which replaces a antagonist closely similar substance essential for metabolism.
N'-methyl nicotinamide (N'MN)	a substance formed from nicotinic acid. Its excretion in the urine is believed to indicate nicotinic acid status.
Milch animals	animals maintained for milk production.
Miscarriages	abortions.
Molasses	syrup obtained as a by-product during the manufacture of crystalline sugar.
Mottled teeth	discolouration of teeth due to deposits of calculus usually caused by excessive intake of fluorine.
Mucilage	gum; substance resembling gum.
Mucin	the chief constituent of mucus.
Mucopolysaccharide	polysaccharid which contain hexosamine which form mucins when dispersed in water.
Muscle cramps	painful muscular contractions.
Mutka	earthenware/pot.
Mucus	sticky fluid secreted by certain membranes called mucous membranes.
Myelin	the fat-like substance forming a sheath around the nerve fibres.
Nausea	tendency to vomit.
Necrosis	death of cells in contact with living tissue.
Neuritis	inflammation of nerves,
Norepine- phrine	an amine present in the adrenals; also called noradrenalin.

Nucleic acid	substances such as DNA and RNA which are present in the nucleus of the cell.
Nucleoprotein	proteins present in the nucleus of the cell containing nucleic acids.
Obesity	excessive accumulation of fat in the body.
Oedema	abnormal retention of water in the tissue.
Organoleptic trials of foods	evaluation of the taste and flavour of foods.
Osteofluorosis	a condition in which the bones become brittle and chalky because of excessive fluorine intake.
Osteoid tissue	bony tissue.
Osteomalacia	a disease characterised by a gradual softening of the bones which become flexible and resulting sometimes in deformities.
Osteoporosis	rarefaction of bone which becomes excessively porous.
Palpitation	unduly rapid action of the heart which is sensed by the patient.
Pancreas	gland situated behind the stomach near the duodenum which secretes the pancreatic juice as well as insulin.
Pandal	an open or closed shed made of branches of trunks of trees and thatched leaves.
Parching	subjecting grains to intense dry heat in the presence of a little moisture, the rapid expansion of which results in the swelling of the grain and results in a light crisp product resembling pop-corn.
Pathological condition	condition in which structure or function or both are abnormal.
Peripheral Neuritis	inflammation of the nerve endings of terminal nerves; a condition in which the limbs particularly the lower ones are affected.
pH	a measure which varies inversely with hydrogen ion concentration, which determines the acidity of a substance. A pH of 7.0 indicates a balance between acids and bases (or between hydrogen (H+) and hydroxyl (OH-) ions), whereas higher values indicate alkalinity, and lower values, acidity.
Phospholipid	a lipid containing phosphorus and a nitrogenous compound. example: lecithin which is found in nerve tissue.

Phrynoderma	alsocalled toad skin. Dry eruptions in the skin resulting in a horny skin generally associated with a deficiency of vitamin A.
Placenta	an organ of flat circular form through which nutrients in the maternal blood are transferred to fetal blood and waste products in the latter are eliminated
Plasma	the fluid portion of circulating blood from which the blood cells are removed; it differs from serum in that it contains fibrinogen
Polymers	compounds formed by the chemical union of two or more molecules of a substance
Proteolipids	lipid protein compounds in which lipid part is more than protein part
Purines	nitrogenous bases of nucleic acids
Radioactive Substances	substances that emit radiation
Radiology	use of radioactive substances for diagnosis of diseases
Renal blood	concentration of a substance necessary for its threshold elimination through the urine
Resistant rickets	rickets which does not respond to treatment with ordinary doses of calcium and vitamin D.
Rickets	a condition in which normal bone development is disturbed. It is marked by bending and distortion of bones and is generally caused by a deficiency of calcium and vitamin D
Ruminants	cud-chewing animals whose stomachs have four chambers
Sedative	an agent that quietens nervous excitement
Sedentary	inactive
Serum	fluid portion of blood obtained after coagulation and removal of blood cells as well as fibrin.
Simmer	cook at a temperature just below boiling point (at about 97-98°C).
Soil erosion	continuous removal of soil from the sides of a river or other sites.
Sprue	chronic diarrhoea found in the tropics caused by inflammation of the mucous membrane in the alimentary tract; it is sometimes associated with undernutrition and a deficiency of 'B' vitamins.

Staple	cereal, millet or tubers used as the main item in the diet.
Sterols	a group of compounds resembling cholesterol.
Still-birth	birth of a dead child.
Syndrome	a group of symptoms associated with a disease.
Tava	a concave or flat iron griddle used for pan-frying.
Testosterone	male hormone
Tetany	a disorder marked by muscular spasms, usually occurring in the hands, trunk and face.
Thyroid gland	a gland which secretes thyroid hormone
Tibia	the large bone of the leg below the knee.
Toxic	poisonous.
Ulcers	lesions on the surface of the skin or mucous membrane.
UNICEF	United Nations Infant and Children Emergency Fund.
USDA	United States Department of Agriculture
Vegans	persons who do not consume foods of animal origin.
Vegetarians	persons who do not include foods obtained by killing animals such as meat, chicken and fish. Most vegetarians include milk in their diets and some include infertile eggs as well.
WHO	World Health Organization.

Index

A

Acetyl CoA 30
Achlorhydria 456
Acid-alkali balance 456
Acidosis 456
Active transport 118
activity increment 42, 45
adenosine diphosphate 37
adenosine triphosphate 37, 456
adipose tissue 15, 31, 33, 34, 38, 39, 51, 76, 89,
    121, 123, 126, 188, 235, 313, 314, 317, 367
adrenal 100, 106, 340, 456
adrenal cortex 100, 340
Adulteration 265
    definition 265
    of Coffee, tea and cocoa 271
    of Fats and oils 268
    of Milk 268
    of Spices 270
    prevention act 265
    types 266
Aerated drinks 226
afforestation 383
agricultural production 6, 381, 395
albumin 457
alcohol consumption 232
alimentary canal 57, 109–111, 115–118
alkaline phosphatase 57
alkalosis 336, 339
Allergy 457
Alzheimer's Disease 142, 143, 145, 235

Amino acids 18, 27, 124, 126, 457
    Essential 21, 27
    excess in foods 24
    glucogenic 16
    imbalance 96
    in common foodstuffs 21–28
    Keto acids 14, 122, 124, 339
    limiting 21
    non-essential 18
amylase 14, 112, 113, 115, 162, 297
anacidity 112
Anaemia 64, 65
    Aplastic 458
    Classification 66
    haemolytic 89
    macrocytic 97
    megaloblastic 98
    microcytic hypochromic 65, 99
    normocytic normochromic 65
    nutritional 347
    pernicious 97
angular stomatitis 93
Anthropometric measurements 355, 356
antibiotics 64, 66, 75, 87, 246, 247, 275, 276,
    304, 337, 338, 341, 343, 457
antidiuretic hormone 340
antimetabolite 462
antioxidant 88, 127, 191, 232, 261
antivitamin 101
aphonia 92, 323
Apolipoprotein 142
appetite 118
Arachidonic acid 31
Ariboflavinosis 322

Arterial hypertension 340
Ascorbic acid (see vitamin C)   63, 64, 72,
    102–107, 127, 136, 150, 151, 174, 227, 233,
    273, 321, 322
Aspergillus flavus 180
Aspergillus niger 244
Aspergillus oryzae 181
Atherosclerosis 32, 143, 332
ATP 8, 9, 10, 11, 34, 37, 62, 66, 119, 120, 121,
    123, 124, 126, 235, 456
Aub-Dubois 39, 46
    standards 46
Avidin 74, 75, 101, 236
Aykroyd, W.R. 435
Aztecs 225

B

Baby foods 61, 295
Bacillus subtilis 181
Bacteria 244
Bajra
    Chemical composition of hybrid 150
    strains 150
Baking powder 216, 239, 407
Balance studies 131, 132, 133
Balasubramanian, S.C. 436
Basal metabolic requirements 39, 40
Basal metabolism 458
    and Age 41
    BMR 40
    brain 43
    environmental temperature 37, 45, 212
    Hypothyroidism 41
    menstrual cycle 41
    Pregnancy 41
    Sex 41
    sleep 41
Basundhi 217, 450
Beaton, G.H. 12, 70, 435
Belavady, B. 96
Benedict, F.G. 40
Beriberi 89, 92, 322
Beta oxidation 10, 97, 123
Betel leaves and nut 416, 439
Beverages 221
Bile salts 76, 115
Biotin 74, 75, 101
Birth weights 135, 302, 347, 366
Bitot's spots 79, 320
Blood

    calcium 57
    Cholesterol 32, 33, 34, 123, 330, 332
    glucose 16
    haemoglobin content 328
    pressure 52, 328, 329, 330, 340, 341, 461
BMR 38, 40, 41, 42, 44, 45, 46, 47, 313, 316
Bodhidharma 224
Body Composition 12
    Surface area 39, 47
    weights 57, 69, 96, 106, 107, 129, 289, 290,
        294-296, 307, 312–320
Bomb calorimeter 36, 37
Bone
    calcium content 57
    demineralization 70
    development 58, 59, 83, 84, 86, 371,
        431, 464
    diseases 58
    effect of calcium deficiency 58, 59, 61,
        299, 311
    effect of Vitamin D deficiency 86
    Effects of vitamin A deficiency 79
    formation 50
    marrow 458
    mineralization 308
    ossification centres 59, 308
Boston norms 300, 301
Bread 245
Breast feeding 32, 292, 308
Bressani 165
British Medical Council 106, 136
Brock, J.F. 435
Burning feet syndrome 101

C

Calcium 54, 55, 58,
    absorption 55
    calcium phosphorus ratio 56
    content of foods 60
    deficiency 58, 59, 308, 309, 311,
    hypercalcemia 61
    in adult human body 57
    in milk 55
    intakes 58
    recommended dietary intake 58
    requirement 58
    utilization 55, 126-27
    and bone formation 56
Calories 13
    definition 35
    from foods 13
    intake 357

recommended dietary allowance 137, 420

Carbohydrates 11, 12, 16
in foods 13
utilization 141, 126-27

Carnegie Institute, Washington 40

Carotene 76, 77, 206, 242, 304, 424
beta carotene 76
gamma carotene 76
Utilization 126, 27

Catering institutions 249

Cellulose 14, 113, 117, 174, 222, 233, 236, 271, 333

Central Food Technological Research Institute 157, 165, 184, 203, 373, 387, 437, 458

Cereals 154–172, 283

Cheese 217

Cheilosis 93

Chittenden 29, 94

Cholecalciferol 84

Cholesterol
conversion to vitamin D 32-35
Hypercholesterolemia 34, 330
in blood 29, 189, 330, 332, 461

Citric acid 9, 55, 159, 186, 199, 226, 228, 233, 237, 239, 244, 246, 403, 404

Clostridium Botulinum 247

cobalamine (see vitamin B12) 97

Cobalt 67

Cocoa 225, 271

Coconut milk 184

cod-liver oil 295

Coenzyme A 9, 100

Coffee 221, 271

Collagen 105

Community Nutrition
suggestion for improvement 370–80
for neonates 370
for other groups 374
for pre-school children 371
for school children 373

Complementary protein 430

Conjunctivitis 458

Cooking
baking 238
broiling 239
methods 238–243

Copper 65, 273, 406
body requirement 65
deficiency 65

Corneal vascularization 79, 93

Corneal xerosis 79

Coronary thrombosis 332

Cretinism 68

Cryptoxanthine 76, 234

Curcumin 234, 235, 333

Curd 245, 263

Curry powder 229, 451

D

DNA 99, 139, 140, 141, 143–146, 232, 463

DNA methylation 143-146

Douglas Bag 42

Dairy farming 389

Dark adaptation 80, 404

Davidson, S. 12, 435

deaf-mutism 68

Dehydration 257

Dementia 94

Dental caries 69, 70, 71, 197, 300

Dental fluorosis 70

Dermatitis 94

De Sweemer 310

Dextrin 14

DHA 32

Dhokla 60, 171

Diabetes insipidus 340, 457

Diabetes mellitus 315, 329, 459

Diets 138
Bhil 34
diabetes mellitus 329–333
digestive disease 333–337
Eskimos 15
Gluten-free 344
Gujarat poor class 192
Gujarat upper class 192
high protein 344
hypercholesterolemia 330–333
liver disease 337-338
major components 72
modification 328–344
renal disease 339–42

Diet (and Nutrition) surveys 347–360
anthropometric measurement 356–358
clinical symptoms 358-359
diet records 353
family survey 351
food intake 354
institution diet 355-56
oral survey 347–350
proforma 410–418
weighment of foods 350

Dietary allownances 128, 138, 286
    formulation 135–138
    recommended 135–138
Digestion 109
    carbohydrate 119–122
    fat 124, 133
    protein 124
Diseases of the digestive system 333–344
    constipation 335
    diarrhea 334
    faulty diet 5
    gastritis 337
    intestinal inflamation 333
    ulcers 335
Diuretics 342, 459
Dosa 171, 451
Drinking water 250, 404, 406
Dutch oven 238
Dynamic State of protein metabolism 18, 19

E

Eggs 219, 272
Eijkman 89
Electrolyte balance 51, 313
Elephant yam 201, 202, 442
eledona 213
Elvehjem, C.A. 96
Emulsion 184, 190, 194, 213, 269, 388
Energy Metabolism 36, 37, 39, 41, 43, 45, 47
    activity increment 42
    energy balance 44
    energy cost 42
    Specific dynamic effect 43, 45
Entamoeba histolytica 117, 333
Enzymes 126, 234
    amylase 14, 112, 113, 115, 162, 297
    cellulase 113
    chymotrypsin 113, 115
    erepsin 116
    in food spoilage 256
    lactase 113
    lipase 112–115, 123, 124
    pepsin 112
    rennin 112, 217
    sucrase 113, 296
    trypsin 113, 115, 172, 178, 236, 240
Epigenetics 139, 141, 143, 145, 146
Ergocalciferol 84, 85
Escherichia Coli 253
Essential amino acids 18, 20–22, 24, 26, 31,
    122, 126, 182, 428, 429, 434

Essential fatty acids 30–32, 34, 80, 188, 327
Exchange system 283, 285
Extracellular water 51

F

FAO 21–24, 26, 27, 29, 58, 81, 93, 136, 137, 152,
    153, 265, 272, 374, 429, 432, 435, 436, 460
FAO/WHO 21, 27, 58, 137
fate of nutrients 119
    carbohydrates 119
    fat 122
    protein 124
    Vitamins and minerals 124
Fats
    adulteration 190
    characteristics 190
    consumption 189
    content of foodstuffs 13
    linoleic acid content 192
    utilization 126-27
Fatty acids 16, 30, 31, 32
Fenugreek 185
Fermentation 169, 172, 460
    changes in vitamin content 241, 242
Fermented foods 169
    Dosa 171
    Dhokla 171
    Idli 170
    Khaman 170
    Natto 181
    Tempeh 181
Ferritin 124, 126
fibre content of selected foods 334
Fibrin 87, 464
Fibrinogen 87, 464
Fish 219, 220, 393
Fisheries 220
Fissured tongue 93, 300
Flatus 114, 379
Flavism 179
Fleisch
    standard 46
Fluorine 67, 69
    deficiency 69
    toxicity 70
    intake 69
    toxicity 70
    in drinking water 70
Fluorosis 70, 326
Folic acid 66, 74, 99, 144
    deficiency 99

history 72
intake 136
requirement 136
Food
adulteration 274
amino acid composition 20, 24, 434
breakfast foods 168
carbohydrate-protein ratio 330
composition 150
consumption 132
fads 378-380
fortified 376
insect infestation 266, 267
intakes 44, 118, 299, 302, 307, 312, 313, 316, 317, 323, 347, 352, 354
lime incorporation 60
mineral composition 53
microbiology and hygiene 244–54
nutrient content 149
Safety 6, 265, 267, 269, 271, 273, 274, 275, 276, 277
Security 169, 381
oxalic acid content 344
patterns 3, 4
pesticide contamination 267
poisoning 273
preservation 255-64, 399-406
preservatives 261
acids 262
chemicals 231
salt and sugar 270
processed 186, 416
Production 28, 29, 154, 381, 382, 383, 385, 387, 389, 391, 393, 395, 397
scientific names 438-449
sodium content 52
spoilage 396
standards 274–277
sterilization 258
storage 388, 412
tables 149–153
volume-weight equivalents 419–423
wrong beliefs 290, 378–380
Fruits 198–209, 263, 393
Fruit juices 206
Fruit salad 208
Fuels
used by the Body 7, 9
Funk 89

G

Galactomannan 14
galactose 12, 14, 115, 119, 126

gamma amino butyric acid (GABA) 107
Gandhiji 383
Gastritis 337, 460
gastroenteritis 70, 326
Gelatin 20, 21
Germination 102, 166, 256, 453
Ghai, O.P. 293
Globulin 460
Glossitis 93, 99, 107, 300
Glucagon 111, 121, 122
Glucose 8
Glucose metabolism 9, 121, 337
glutamic acid 11, 122, 124
Glutathione 62, 71
Gluten 17, 161, 162, 194, 267, 344
Glycemic index 16, 123
Glycogen 11, 121, 126, 272, 337
Goldberger 94
Goiter 68, 325
Goitrogen 69
Goodhart, R.S. 437
Gopalan, C. 13, 46, 137, 149, 436
Gossypol 406
Gout 343, 460
Grainger, R.M. 70
Groundnut milk 184
gulabjamuns 216
Gumastha, A. 96

H

Haemagglutinins 179
Haemoglobin 63, 64
synthesis 64
factors involved 64
haemorrhages 87, 105, 321, 342
Haemosiderin 64, 124, 126
Harper, A.E. 96
Harris, R.S. 74
Hawkins, W.W. 67, 300, 301
heart disease 2, 89, 123, 197, 224, 225, 332
heights 136, 293, 356, 362, 373
Heights 293
hemicellulose 233
Herbs 227
High altitude 75
Hippocrates 102
Histone modification 143, 144
Honey 196
Hookworm 63, 304, 324

Hormones 67
Human development 32
Hunger 118
Hybrid strains 150, 163, 164, 187, 385
Hydrolytic rancidity 191, 192, 194, 267, 268
Hypercalcemia 61, 461
Hyperchlorhydria 112
hypercholesterolemia 197, 329, 336
Hyperglycemia 461
Hypervitaminosis A 83
Hypervitaminosis D 86
Hypochlorhydria 112
Hypoglycemia 461
Hypothyroidism 41, 461

I

idli 61, 170, 407
Incaparina 186
Indian Agricultural Research Institute, Delhi 183
Indian Council of Agricultural Research 187, 437
Indian Council of Medical Research 26, 106, 136, 149, 436, 437, 461
Infant
    anthropometric measurements 293, 356
    body weights 290
    foods 297-302
    mortality 92
    nutritional care 290
infantile beriberi 92, 322, 323
infantile eczema 34, 310
Infection 5, 80, 94, 248, 249, 251, 252, 298, 304, 321, 324, 335, 337, 339, 341, 370, 424, 426, 431
Insect infestation 266, 267
Insulin 16, 121–123, 197, 316, 329, 330, 457, 463
Intermediates 10, 11, 124, 141, 199
Intestinal atrophy 313
Intestinal parasites 66, 250, 333
Intestine 113
Intracellular water 51
Intrinsic factor 66, 74, 98
Iodine 67
    deficiency 68
    functions 67
    goitrogens 69
    iodized salt 69
    radioactive iodine 69

iodine number 190
iodized salt 69
Iron 63
    absorption 63
    and intestinal parasites 63
    and oxalate 63
    and protein quality 63
    and Vitamin C 105⁻
    content in foods 63
        deficiency 65
        requirement 152
        Utilization 126, 27
irrigation 169, 382, 383
Ischaemic heart disease 332
Isoflavone 146, 182, 234,
Isoleucine 18, 22, 25, 95, 164, 185

J

Jelliffe 295, 436
Joule 36
Jowar 164
        amino acid content 22-23
        in aetiology of pellagra 95

K

Keratin 20, 80, 320, 327, 428
keratomalacia 79, 82, 321
Keratosis 80, 327
ketone bodies 15
Ketosis 15, 35, 320
Khaman 61, 169–171, 176, 181, 237, 246, 298, 409, 425
khichri 165, 176, 285, 298, 330, 371, 420, 430, 432
Khova 216, 270, 452, 453
Kidney stone 107, 343
Kodri 154, 155, 164, 165, 171, 202, 283, 391, 392, 405, 430
Kothari, B.B. 104
Krebs Cycle 9, 10, 15, 35, 120, 123
kwashiorkor 306–308, 340, 344, 374

L

Lactase 113
Lactation 28, 46, 100, 107, 269, 296, 367, 378, 389, 390
Lactic acid 90, 120, 212, 245, 246, 257, 272
Lactobacillus bulgaricus 213

Lactogenic factor 390
Lactose 55, 113, 182, 195, 212, 245, 269
Lard 87, 88, 188, 190
Lathyrism 325
Lathyrus sativus 179, 325, 443, 444
Laubina 162, 186
Leavening agents 194
Legumes 173
    consumption of 179
    dals 176
    origin of 173
    production of 180
    sprouting of 174
    toxic materials in 117
Leucine 18, 22, 25, 95, 96, 164
Leverton, R. 361
Lind 102
linoleic acid 4, 32, 34, 163, 192, 235
linolenic acid 15, 32
Lipoproteins 122, 123, 126, 143, 235
Liver
    damage 70
    diseases 337, 38
Lysine
    content in foodstuffs 22-23
    deficiency in cereals 24
    effect of cooking on 152, 240
    enrichment of flour 162
    in maize 96
Magendie 431
Magnesium 3, 11, 49, 62, 160, 182, 226, 343, 344
Maize 163
    amino acid content 165
    in aetiology of pellagra 164
    linoleic acid content 192
    yields 384
Malnutrition
    Diseases 5
    aetiological factors 304
    Anaemia 64
    beriberi 5, 322
    fluorosis 326
    goiter 325
    kwashiorkor 306
    lathyrism 325
    marasmus 307
    obesity 314
    osteomalocia 311
    osteoporosis 311
    pellagra 323
    protein deficiency in adults 314

    retarded skeletal development 308
    rickets 309
    scurvy 321
    skin disease 327
    tetany 310
    vitamin A deficiency 320
    among rich 368
    and mortality 366
    productivity 367
    psychological status 365
Maltose 109, 112, 113, 115, 166, 246
Manage L. 196
Manganese 71, 385
Manures 385, 386
Marasmus 5, 117, 291, 307, 308
Margarine 189
Mayas 225
McCollum, E.V. 436
McHenry, E.W. 12, 435
Meal-Planning 281, 283, 285, 287
Meat 217, 272
Megaloblasts 64, 66
Merrill, A.L. 13
Metabolic antagonists 75
Metabolism 18, 34, 109
Metanil yellow 271, 405
Methionine 18, 24, 25, 26
Microflora intestinal 247
Microrganisms 425
Milk
    adulteration 269, 349, 268–270
    Composition 294
    microcrganism in 213, 248
    standards 248
    yields 384,
    Milk 21, 22
    Buffalo 22
    composition 24
    in infant feeding 294
    Condensed 215
    Cow 22
    composition 294
    in infant feeding 294
    Dry 215
    Evaporated 215
    formulas 294
    goat 211
    Human 22
    pasteurized 248
    skim 189
    Toned 215

Milk-alkali syndrome 336
Millets 154–172, 380, 381, 385, 409, 414, 430
Minerals 49–71, 124
Mitchell, H.H. 434, 436
Mocha 226, 453
Molybdenum 71
Moore, C.V. 12
Mottled teeth 70
Moulds
    Food poisoning 247
    Food spoilage 244
Mucopolysaccharides 80
Multipurpose Food (MPF) 184
Mushroom 445
myocardial infarction 332
Mysore pak 194, 453

N

Nanavati, K. 96
Narasinghrao, B.S. 137
National Academy of Sciences, U.S.A. 136
Natto 181, 453
Nephritis 70, 326, 339–343
Neuromotor development 308, 358
Nicotinic Acid 91, 94
    content in foods 91,
    deficiency 94, 95
    history 72, 73
    recommended dietary allowances 137
    requirement 96
Night-blindness 76, 81, 83
Nikiforuk, G. 70
N' Methyl Nicotinamide 323
Normoblasts 64, 66
Nucleotide 140, 141, 143
Nutrient
    contributed by 155, 282
    recommended allowances 58
    requirement of different organisms 3
    utilization 136
Nutrition Research Laboratories, Hyderabad
    179
Nutritional
    Care of Particular Groups 289
    education 373
    requirements 289
    status assessment 129
Nuts 3, 32, 35, 88, 96, 101, 108, 138, 176, 177,
    185, 186, 188, 190, 208, 236, 282, 406, 408,
    414, 420, 421, 430

O

Obesity 131, 144, 197, 223, 235, 303, 314–317,
    328, 329, 332, 333, 336, 342, 344, 368
Oedema 50, 51, 92, 306–308, 313, 314, 322, 323,
    340, 341, 358, 431
Oilseeds 29, 35, 88, 89, 183, 204, 206, 330, 430
Oleomargarine 189
1 carbon metabolism 100
Opaque maize 385
Osteofluorosis 70, 326
Osteomalacia 59, 86, 134
Osteoporosis 59, 70, 311, 312, 463
Over nutrition 38, 315, 350
Oxalate 54, 55, 63, 65, 203, 343, 344
Oxalic acid 54, 152, 203, 343, 344

P

Palm-gur 195
Pantothenic acid 74, 100
Papyrus 102
Parathyroid gland 57
Parathyroid hormone 85
Parching 152, 166, 167, 168, 178, 239, 240
Passmore, R. 12
Patel, D.S. 384
Pectin 14, 198, 233, 333, 337, 402, 403
Peda 212, 216
Pellagra 5, 73, 94–96, 160, 164, 165, 323
Pellagra preventing factor 94
Peripheral neuritis 107
Peroxide value 191, 193, 194, 268
Personal hygiene 252
Pesticides 241, 267, 273, 385, 406
Phenylalanine 18, 25
Phosphorus 54
    content in foodstuffs 55
    in human body 54
    utilization 126-27
Photophobia 82
Phrynoderma 80, 310, 327
Physical stature 129, 299, 347, 356, 362, 363,
    370
Phytase 55, 85
Phytate 54, 65, 71, 85
Phytonutrient 233
Plants 3, 4, 18, 69, 75, 385, 425, 426, 428
Pliny 102
Polyneuritis 89

Polyunsaturated fatty acids 31, 88, 186, 304, 330
Pongal 176, 177
Poppy seeds 185, 446
Population 381–396
Potassium 11, 54
Potato starch 246
Poultry-farming 392
Pregnancy 28, 41
Priestley 226
Protein
    complementary proteins 24
    content in foodstuffs 13
    content in human-body 12
    efficiency ratio 21
    endogenous losses 26
        FAO 27
        limiting amino acid 25
        malnutrition 298, 304, 337, 351
        novel sources of proteins 429
        nutritive value of 25
        protein-calorie malnutrition (PCM) 308
        recommended allowances 137
Psychological status 365
PUFA 31, 192
Pulses 263
Punekar, B.D. 96
Pyridoxine 64, 65, 107, 166, 343, 344
Pyruvic acid 9, 122

R

Rabdi 164, 214, 216
Radiation 38, 69, 84, 261, 464
Ragi 165
Rajalakshmi, R. 198, 436
Rama Sastri, B. 436
Rama-swami Aiyar, C.P. 383
Ramakrishnan, C.V. 198
Ramalingaswami 65
Ramayana 167, 173, 218
Rancidity 191, 192, 194, 260, 261, 267, 268
Recipes 202, 434
    based on cereal-legume 202
    Cost and composition 201
    preparation 249
    Chutneys 208
    Fruit salad 208
    Gulabjamun 452
    Juices 206

Khova 452
Rabdi 454
Sandesh 455
    vegetable combination 201
    Vegetables 198–210
Red blood cells (RBC) 64, 65, 88, 98, 99, 324, 457, 458, 461
Reference proteins 24
Refractive index 190
Refrigeration 204
Renal disease 339
Renal hypertension 340, 461
Resistance to infection 5, 321
Resistant rickets 87, 464
Retinal 76, 80
Rhodopsin 80
Riboflavin 92
    content of selected foods 93
    deficiency 322
    history 72
    recommended allowance 137
    requirements 93
Rice 156
    Chemical composition 157
    converted 157
    Fortification 160
    linoleic acid content 192
    losses during cooking 157
    Losses during milling 157
    parboiled 156
    Polished 156
    products 160
    storage 158
    unpolished 156
    yields 157
Rickets 59, 83, 309
Roasting 166
Ruminants 464
Russell, B. 361

S

Sakariah, K.K. 5, 234, 235
Salmonella enteritidis 247
Sambhar 176, 455
sambhar powder 171
Sandesh 212, 216
Sandhu, R.K. 293
Saponification number 268
Scrimshaw 165
Scurvy 74, 102, 321, 322

Sebrell, W.H. Jr 74
Selenium 71
Sesame 126
Shortening agents 194
Single Nucleotide Polymorphism 141, 142
skeletal
      growth 86
      maturation 56
      retardation 134
Skin diseases 327
Sodium 12, 49, 52, 53, 132
Sohonie, K. 178
Soups 205, 207
Soy bean 180
      milk 182
      Nutritive value 181
Speakman 226
Spices 227
      All spice 228
      cinnamon 227
      coriander 228
      cumin 228
      fenugreek 228
      garlic 228
      ginger 229
      mustard 228
      nutmeg 229
      Sweet pepper 230
      Turmeric 229
Specific dynamic effect (SDF) 47
Sprouting 55, 93, 96, 166, 172, 174, 175, 179,
      241, 383, 384
Streptococcus lactis 246
Substrate level phosphorylation 119, 120
Sucrase 113, 296
Sucrose 14, 195
Suet 188
Sugar 188, 195
Sukdi 372
Sulpha drugs 66, 304, 341, 343
Swaminathan, M.S. 169

T

Tartaric acid 193, 199, 228, 233, 239
Tea 224, 225, 271
Tempeh 181, 455
Tetany 62, 85, 310
Thiamine 89
      content in foodstuffs 91
      content in human body 12

deficiency 90
history 72
recommended dietary allowance 137
requirements 90
Threonine 18, 22, 25
Thrombin 87
Thyroglobulin 126
Thyroid 41, 98, 126, 465
Thyroid deficiency 98
Thyroxine 126
Torula yeast 186, 213
Trace elements (see individual elements)
      49, 63, 67
Transamination 107
Trigonelline 96
Trypsin inhibitor 172, 178, 236, 240
Tryptophan 18, 21, 22, 25, 94–97, 163, 165,
      430, 434, 461
Tuberculosis 5, 75, 248, 344
Twain, Mark 379
Tyrosine 18, 22, 25, 67

U

Undernutrition
      in adults 312
      in children 305
      in pregnancy 303
      diarrhoea 431
UNICEF 374, 432, 437, 465
United States Department of Agriculture
      152, 368, 465
Uraemia 342, 458
Urea 11, 18, 20, 25, 37, 50, 124, 339, 340, 341,
      342, 429
Uric acid 50, 267, 340, 343, 344, 460
Urinary calculi 343
Usal 454, 456

V

Vasco de Gama 102
Vegans 99, 211
Vegetables 198–210
      carotene content 273, 392
      Leafy 203
      Recipes 202, 434
      Starchy 199
      vitamin C content 104, 105
Vitamin A 75
      Bone development 80
      content in body 81

content in foods 77
deficiency 79
history 72
Vitamin B1 (see riboflavin) 89, 158, 242
Vitamin B12 97
    absorption 98
    anaemia 97
    deficiency 65
    history 72
    in rain water 99
    intrinsic factor 98
    microbes synthesizing 99
    requirement 99
Vitamin C 102
    anaemia 66, 107
    concentration in different tissues 105
    content in foods 102
    deficiency 102
    history 72
    levels in blood 106
    losses during cooking 104
    Requirement 106
    utilization 126-27
    in adult human body 12
    in breast milk 295
    and common cold 107
Vitamin D 83
    vitamin D2 84
    content in foods 84
    Deficiency 84
    history 72
    Hypervitaminosis D 86
    Requirement 86
    utilization 84, 126-27
    and bone development 84
Vitamin E 87
    Amount in the diets 88

deficiency 88
history 72
utilization 88, 126-27
and anaemia 89
Vitamin K 87
    deficiency 88
    history 72
    microflora 87
    utilization 83, 126, 27

W

Walker 312
Water 49–52, 256
Watt, B.K. 13, 437
Wheat 161
    bulgar 162
    gluten content 161, 194, 267
    linoleic acid content 192
    yield 162
Williams, R.J. 437
Wills, Lucy 99
Wodehouse, P.G. 313
Wohl, M.G. 12, 437

X

Xerophthalmia 320

Y

yeast 244–246, 255, 298, 327, 455
    bread preparation 161
    in food spoilage 255

Z

Zinc 12, 71, 406

About the Authors

Prof. Rajalakshmi did her doctoral studies at McGill University, Canada under the guidance of Prof. D. Hebb, FRS famous for his theory on Brain Function and Behaviour. She was the Professor of Biochemistry and Nutrition in the Biochemistry Department, M.S. University of Baroda. She has played an important role in establishing a strong school in teaching and research in Food and Nutrition at M.S. University which is one of the earliest to start Home Science Faculty in the country. Under her guidance a large number of students completed their Masters and Doctoral studies in the field of Nutrition. She became widely acclaimed for her work in the area of Nutrition and brain function and her work in this area has been supported by UNDP, UNICEF, Ford Foundation, UGC and International Brain Research Organization. She was a member of WHO committee on brain diseases, Indian Dietetics Association and International Neurochemistry Society and International Neuroscience Society. She was a plenary speaker in the International Conference on Nutrition and Brain Development and Function. Prof.Rajalakshmi's autobiography was published in "Women Scientists: The Road to Liberation" edited by Dr. Derek Richter of MRC Laboratories, London and published by Macmillan Press and her biography was published in World Women Scientists.

Dr. K.K. Sakariah completed M.Sc. and Ph.D. degrees at M.S. University of Baroda. He had a stint as Faculty member at Biochemistry Department, M.S. University before joining Central Food Technological Research Institute, Mysore as Scientist. At CFTRI he was associated with International Food Technology Training Centre (IFTTC). IFTTC was originally established at CFTRI under the aegis of Food and Agriculture Organization of the United Nations Organization. Dr. Sakariah has been a core faculty member of this centre in conducting M.Sc. course in Food Technology the participants of which included students from India and South East Asian countries. He has a wealth of experience in teaching varied subjects including Biochemistry, Nutrition, Food Chemistry and Analysis and Food Microbiology. A large number of students have undergone research training under his guidance as part of the course requirement. Areas of his research interest have been phytonutrients and bioactive principles in food ingredients and his research publications have been cited in reputed journals. Author of several patents Dr.Sakariah has been associated with Indian Universities in the capacity of Chairman and member of Board of Studies and Board of Examiners in Food Science and Technology. After retirement as Head, Human Resources Development and Deputy Director, CFTRI Dr. Sakariah is presently associated with food ingredient manufacturing industry in product development, research and development and quality upkeep.